LIVE
BEYOND
ORGANIC

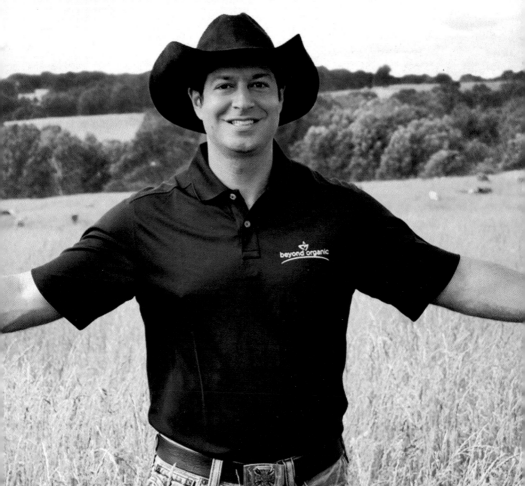

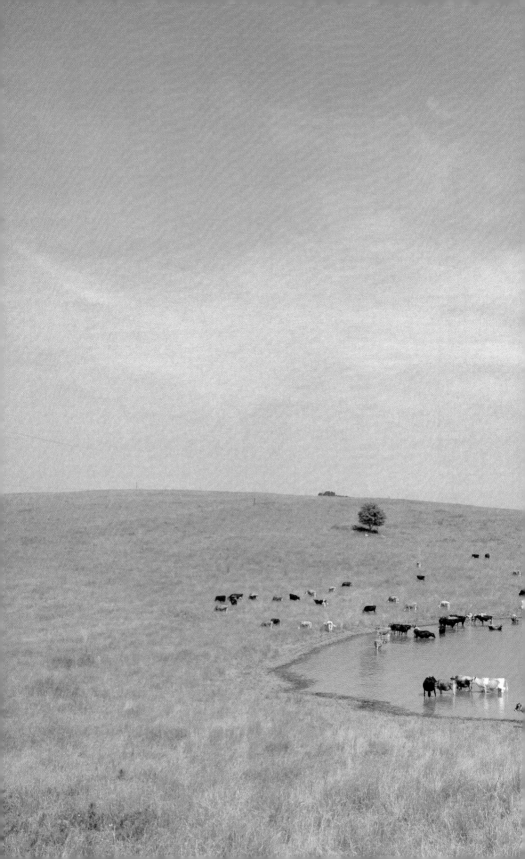

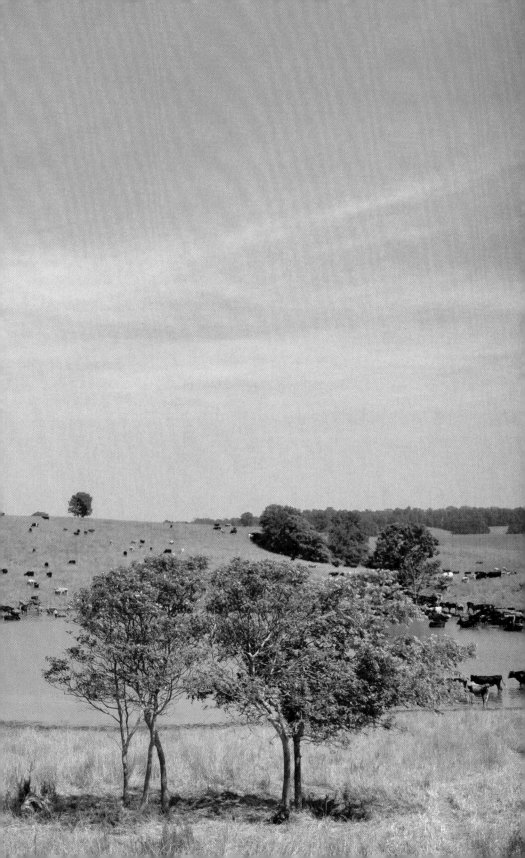

Beyond Organic
1250 Southern Rd
Kansas City, MO 64120
(800) 560-3961
www.LiveBeyondOrganic.com

Printed in the United States of America
ISBN: ISBN-10 0615547796
ISBN-13 9780615547794

TABLE OF CONTENTS

beyond organic

IMPORTANT NOTICE

THIS BOOK IS NOT INTENDED TO PROVIDE MEDICAL ADVICE OR TO TAKE THE PLACE OF MEDICAL ADVICE AND TREATMENT FROM YOUR PERSONAL PHYSICIAN. READERS ARE ADVISED TO CONSULT THEIR OWN DOCTORS OR OTHER QUALIFIED HEALTH PROFESSIONALS REGARDING TREATMENT OF THEIR MEDICAL PROBLEMS. NEITHER THE PUBLISHER NOR THE AUTHOR TAKES ANY RESPONSIBILITY FOR ANY POSSIBLE CONSEQUENCES FROM ANY TREATMENT, ACTION, OR APPLICATION OF MEDICINE, SUPPLEMENT, HERB, OR PREPARATION TO ANY PERSON READING OR FOLLOWING THE INFORMATION IN THIS BOOK. IF READERS ARE TAKING PRESCRIPTION MEDICATIONS, THEY SHOULD CONSULT WITH THEIR PHYSICIANS BEFORE BEGINNING ANY NUTRITION OR SUPPLEMENTATION PROGRAM.

IN ADDITION, BELOW ARE GOVERNMENTAL WARNINGS REGARDING THE CONSUMPTION OF RAW EGGS AND RAW JUICES:

- CONSUMING RAW OR UNDERCOOKED EGGS MAY INCREASE YOUR RISK OF FOOD-BORNE ILLNESS.

- JUICE THAT HAS NOT BEEN PASTEURIZED MAY CONTAIN BACTERIA THAT CAN INCREASE THE RISK OF FOOD-BORNE ILLNESS. PEOPLE MOST AT RISK ARE CHILDREN, THE ELDERLY AND PERSONS WITH A WEAKENED IMMUNE SYSTEM.

RELATED TO THE DIETARY SUPPLEMENTS AND FOODS DISCUSSED IN THIS BOOK:

THESE STATEMENTS HAVE NOT BEEN EVALUATED BY THE FOOD AND DRUG ADMINISTRATION. THIS PRODUCT IS NOT INTENDED TO DIAGNOSE, TREAT, CURE OR PREVENT ANY DISEASE.

From Tragedy To Destiny

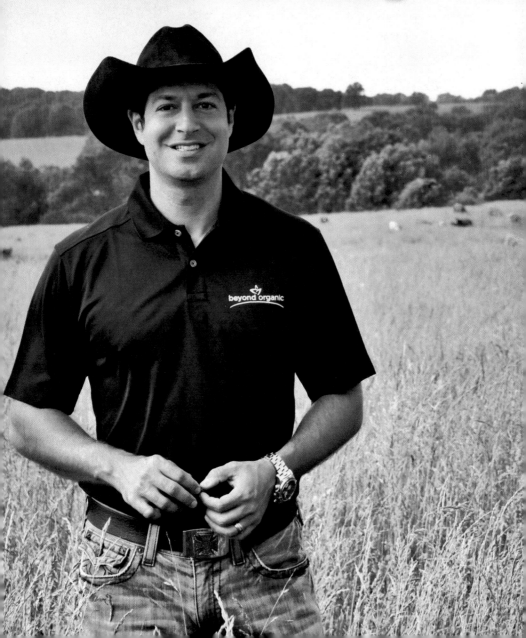

Imaneuvered the '68 Dodge bunkhouse motor home past the manicured lawns and bay windows of the Pacific Beach homes atop Crown Point, a finger of land that overlooked San Diego's Mission Bay, an aquatic recreational playground.

The year was 1996, and I was a few months away from my twenty-first birthday. It was getting late in the day, and I was looking for a place to encamp for the evening and cook dinner. Parking around Mission Bay could be tricky because local authorities didn't want transients—like myself—parking overnight in beach lots or bothering residents in nearby homes. But as long as you were unobtrusive and moved along first thing in the morning, you could usually get away with parking overnight near one of the bay's many inlets.

"How does this place look?" I asked my two passengers, Kenny Duke and Jason Dewberry. Kenny had been my close friend while growing up in Palm Beach Gardens, Florida, and Jason was my college roommate at Florida State University in Tallahassee. Unfortunately, I had to medically withdraw from school during my sophomore year when I became seriously ill with a variety of life-threatening ailments. Now I was living in San Diego, trying to get well.

Kenny shrugged his shoulders. "Fine with me," he said.

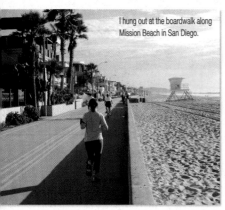

I hung out at the boardwalk along Mission Beach in San Diego.

Kenny and Jason had flown in from the East Coast to check up on how I was doing. They were amazed at my transformation when I picked them up at the airport. I had put on a good thirty pounds since they last saw me—pounds that I desperately needed.

A grin came across Kenny's face. "So is this what you have to do every night, move around like a vagabond?"

"It hasn't been too bad," I replied. "Being near the water is nice."

Actually, looking for a new place to park every night was the least of my worries. Twenty-two months earlier, my good health—something every college student takes for granted—was suddenly ripped away from me. I had been a counselor at a summer church youth camp when I began experiencing nausea, stomach cramps, and horrible digestive problems. I limped home, having lost twenty pounds in less than a week.

As my health continued to deteriorate, my parents took me to doctor after doctor in an attempt to reverse the downward trend, which was threatening to spiral out of control. Over the next few months, I was diagnosed with Crohn's disease and exhibited symptoms of rheumatoid arthritis, chronic fatigue syndrome, fibromyalgia, diabetes, extreme anemia, heart problems, urinary tract and prostate infections, yeast (Candida) overgrowth, parasites, and multiple viral infections.

My body was shutting down. The worst moment happened in the hospital late one night when I overheard a nurse crying in the hallway, telling a fellow nurse, "He's not going to make it through the night."

I did survive my brush with death, but my continuing health problems led to severe depression. I was down and out in every possible way. I looked into the mirror and didn't know who I was seeing in the reflection. Most nights, I slept no more than forty-five minutes at a time. There was no escape. Day after day, night after night, was misery. I felt trapped in a prison that was my own body.

When I wasn't in a hospital room, I visited dozens of doctors and health practitioners and was put on medication after medication. Nothing worked. My parents, feeling the pressure to do *something*, sent me to alternative medicine clinics in Mexico and Germany, but these desperate attempts did not work out as hoped for.

I felt great guilt when my parents mortgaged their future and spent a fortune of money on trying to get me well. My friends didn't come around very much anymore because when you go from being the life of the party to the death of every conversation, people can't really relate to what you are going through.

Except for Kenny and Jason. When they flew out from the East Coast to see me in San Diego, it was great to hang out with them and reminisce about old times.

They knew, when I had landed in San Diego five or six weeks earlier, that I needed wheelchair assistance from the plane to the baggage claim. Waiting for me was a nutritionist named William "Bud" Keith, who my father had reached out to after hearing about him from a friend. Bud told me over the phone that I could become well again by following the health plan in the Bible.

When I spoke with Bud, he offered to introduce me to the Bible's eating plan if I would come to his hometown. "If you come see me, I will teach you how to eat and live, and I promise you in three months, you'll be working out on the beach in San Diego."

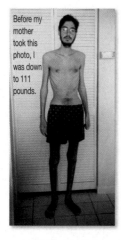

Before my mother took this photo, I was down to 111 pounds.

I don't know why, but I believed him. Hope swelled in my heart. I smiled for the first time in nearly two years and told my mother that I was going to get well.

You see, once my illness set in and I knew the severity, I realized that this wasn't just about me. I suddenly knew how important good health was and that there must be others suffering as I was. I also knew that God doesn't waste our pain. We only go through and overcome painful circumstances in life so we can benefit others who are going through similar experiences. In fact, a year into my illness, there was a moment that would change my life forever when I asked my mother to take a picture of me at the depth of my suffering.

"Jordan, I don't want to take your picture," my mom said. "It breaks my heart just to look at you."

She had a point. I was standing in front of my parents' closet, wearing just boxer shorts, and you could practically count every rib in my emaciated body. I had lost nearly half of my body weight and stood at just 111 pounds. I looked like one of those Holocaust survivors, not much more than skin and bones.

"Mom, you need to take my picture."

"Jordan, I don't want to take your picture. Why do you insist?"

"Because the world is not going to believe what God is about to do in my life." (See my "before" picture with the beard on the top of this page.)

Kenny and Jason couldn't believe how much better I looked when I picked them up at the airport. I had arrived in San Diego weighing an unhealthy 116 pounds, but I had added nearly thirty pounds during my forty-day health experience.

"You guys ready for dinner?" I asked. "The menu is pretty simple. I hope you don't mind."

"Since when did you learn how to cook?" Jason teased.

"I wouldn't really call it cooking, but it's healthy and doesn't taste too bad either," I promised.

I pulled into the bayside parking lot and found an unobtrusive spot. I had purchased the dilapidated motor home in San Diego after spending a few weeks with Bud Keith and his family to get my bearings. He urged me to spend as much time as possible near the beach, breathing in ocean air by the lungful and catching the sun's rays to give my body a vitamin D boost.

Bud also talked nonstop about the importance of eating whole and natural foods as consumed by our biblical ancestors. "I know why none of the other doctors have helped you," he said. "You need to follow a health plan that is based on the Bible, one that's been proven through history and confirmed by science."

Now, I was a young man of deep faith, but during those dark times, I was miserable. Sure, I read the Bible every day, but I never thought of God's Word as anything more than a spiritual book. While the Bible gave me insight into the Creator of the universe and taught me how to act and live, I couldn't recall reading anything about health or nutrition in the Old or New Testament.

But as Bud expounded upon his philosophy, his thinking could be boiled down to two powerful points:

1. EAT WHAT GOD CREATED FOR FOOD.

2. EAT FOODS IN A FORM THAT ARE HEALTHY FOR THE BODY.

Bud gave me an eating plan that outlined what foods he wanted me to eat, and he also gave me plenty of "homework," meaning he handed me several books to read. One of them was called *The Milk Book* by William Campbell Douglass, M.D., which opened my eyes to the virtues of consuming grass-fed cultured dairy products. Bud thought drinking raw unpasteurized milk and cultured dairy such as kefir from grass-fed cows would be greatly beneficial to my digestive tract and help my ailing immune system. He also directed me to eat grass-fed beef, wild-caught fish, as well as drink raw juices made from organic fruits and vegetables.

That made for a limited menu, but for a twenty-year-old nomad with no access to a kitchen, that would have to work.

"Tonight we're having grass-fed beef burgers," I announced to Kenny and Jason.

My well-used RV, which had more than 80,000 miles on the odometer with sleeping accommodations for two above the cab and two bunk beds at the rear, didn't have many of the creature comforts that you'd find in more modern motor

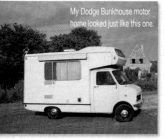
My Dodge Bunkhouse motor home looked just like this one.

homes. I had a two-burner propane stove and a combo toilet/ shower—but no refrigerator. To keep my meat and dairy products properly refrigerated, I filled a cooler with new ice daily and made sure nothing stayed longer than two days.

We're not talking the Four Seasons here.

I had a single stainless steel pan to cook my meat or fish, a cutting board, and a few kitchen utensils. I opened my ice chest and unwrapped the thick butcher paper, which contained a couple of pounds of hamburger. This wasn't your typical ground beef, the most frequently purchased type of meat in supermarkets around America. This hamburger came from cattle that grazed in pastures—in other words from cows that were grass-fed, not given troughs of ground-up corn laced with antibiotics to help these animals overcome digestive issues due to the confined environment in which they were raised.

I reached for a stick of organic butter in the cooler and cut off a half-inch, which I dropped into the saucepan. The guys helped me pat the hamburger into fist-sized patties, and then I set them one-by-one into the pan. The pleasing aroma of sizzling meat filled the tiny motor home.

"What else have you got to eat?" Kenny asked.

"Raw veggie juice and some cottage cheese with fruit and honey. That's pretty much it, although I think I still have some cultured dairy left," I said.

I opened my ice chest and saw that I was down to a quart of cultured dairy. "Sorry, guys. I'm almost out of dairy. There's not enough to share. I hope that's going to be okay." (I'll have a lot more to say about the health benefits of cultured dairy products throughout this book.)

Kenny and Jason looked at each other and grinned. "That's going to be all right," Jason said. "We'll survive."

Okay, maybe my raw kefir didn't look that appetizing to the guys. And maybe my hamburger wasn't the way they were used to eating it since I bought 100 percent whole grain buns—not your typical hamburger buns made with enriched white flour.

I can assure you that my burgers hit the mark for three hungry young men, and the cottage cheese, honey, and pineapple for dessert was a fan favorite as well. Then I reached for my last quart of cultured dairy.

"I hope you don't mind that we have to get going early tomorrow morning," I told the guys. "I need to do a little shopping."

THE PROMISE TO MYSELF

Forgetting to set my alarm was not an issue.

The local water ski club began firing up their outboard engines shortly after 5:30 a.m., no doubt to take advantage of the glassy conditions on Mission Bay. But from our spot near the water, it sounded like a 747 taking off.

I drove us to a nearby health food store—Boney's Market on Garnet Avenue, Pacific Beach's main commercial thoroughfare. (Boney's became Henry's Marketplace before turning into a Sprout's Farmers Market in 2011.) I silently shot up an arrow prayer, asking for the delivery of Steuve's cultured dairy products that morning—kefir, cream, and cottage cheese.

Natural, raw-certified cultured dairy products were hard to come by because so little was produced and local demand was so high. My favorite product was raw kefir, which came in quart-sized cardboard containers. I often consumed two, sometimes three quarts a day because the powerful proteins, important enzymes, and billions of live, friendly bacteria in the raw kefir colonized my gut with good germs and crowded out the bad bacteria that had been making my life miserable for nearly two years.

One of the main reasons why Bud Keith wanted me to come to San Diego was because the state of California was one of only a handful of states that had legalized the retail sale of raw cultured dairy products. In my home state of Florida, for instance, unpasteurized dairy products were not legal to sell.

Not so in California, for which I was grateful. When raw cream was available at Boney's, I liked to mix it with raw carrot juice, a common practice in Europe where they believe the combination improves the absorption and utilization of the fat-soluble vitamins and carotenoids found in carrot juice. But most of the time, I chugged cultured dairy like it was going out of style—more than a half-gallon a day.

My new diet—heavy in cultured dairy, salads made from organic produce, grass-fed beef and wild-caught fish, cultured veggies like raw sauerkraut, raw carrot and vegetable juices, and a powerful probiotic supplement containing beneficial microorganisms from healthy soil and plants—put me on a fast road to recovery.

Within a few weeks, I no longer resembled the proverbial ninety-eight-pound weakling that tough guys kicked sand on over at Mission Beach. As I walked up and down the boardwalk, I performed chin-ups and worked the monkey bars in the beachside parks. I slowly but surely regained my stamina. I was starting to feel like my old self again.

We pulled into the Boney's parking lot at about a quarter to eight that morning— fifteen minutes before opening time. The spacious parking lot was nearly deserted, but I never took anything for granted.

"Follow me, guys."

I led them toward the front door, which was still locked. I leaned against the glass and cupped my hands over my eyes. Then I saw him—Matt!

Matt was the dairy guy at Boney's—and my new best friend. Shortly after I purchased my motor home and began camping out near the Pacific Ocean, I quickly found out that Boney's was my best bet to find cultured dairy and organic meat. Deliveries, however, were sporadic, and it wasn't uncommon for Boney's to sell out of their shipment of cultured dairy products within an hour of opening. Sometimes Matt stashed away a few cartons in the back for me, but I couldn't count on that.

Since I was pounding at least two quarts of cultured dairy every day—and could keep only a two-day supply on hand in my ice chest—this presented a problem. I counted on a regular supply of cultured dairy to provide the proteins, vitamins, minerals, probiotics, and healthy fats that helped me tremendously with my digestion, my immune system, and my weight gain. If Boney's was out of cultured dairy, then I could check two other stores in San Diego, but both were a good half-hour drive from Pacific Beach.

Matt looked up from inside the closed store and noticed me waiting outside. He smiled and waved back, then shot me a thumb's up. The cultured dairy had arrived that morning.

"It's going to be a good day, guys," I said. Then I explained to Kenny and Jason why Matt was smiling.

I purchased eight quarts of cultured dairy that morning, as well as two bags of ice for my cooler, an assortment of fruits and veggies, and dinner that evening—wild sockeye salmon. That would be enough to keep three young guys fed and happy.

We hung out at the beach the rest of the day, and I can remember gazing at the horizon and thinking some deep thoughts. I don't know if my reflections were prompted by having two longtime friends come and show their support by visiting me in San Diego, or whether I was feeling optimistic about the times ahead. Because I *was* going to have a future, thanks to my new biblically based diet and the organic "living" foods I was eating.

But I already knew from personal experience that the foods fueling my recovery weren't always available, and the thought of *not* having access to these healthy organic foods some day gave me pause. That afternoon, something in my heart stirred for the first time. I knew it sounded crazy, but I could not deny the feeling in my gut.

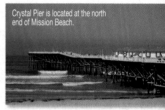
Crystal Pier is located at the north end of Mission Beach.

While gazing out at the blue Pacific, I decided that one day I would have my own ranches and farms where I could grow and raise these powerful foods for myself, my future family, and my friends and loved ones. I can remember that feeling like it was yesterday.

Keep in mind, I was a penniless ex-college student still dependent upon my parents when this thought formed in my mind. I was just twenty years old with no college degree, no opportunities on the horizon, and no job. But the thought was so real that I decided to tell Kenny and Jason what I was thinking— that one day I would raise and grow my own food, go beyond organic with uncompromised quality, and provide people everywhere with foods and beverages of biblical quality.

"Awesome," Kenny said. "If anyone can do it, you can."

Jason thought it was great, too. "You be sure to remember me when you start this ranch and produce these products because I want to be there with you when it happens."

We serve an amazing God whose nature is to give us immeasurably more than we can ever ask or imagine. Today, sixteen years later, Kenny and Jason are both key members of the Beyond Organic team, but I'm getting ahead of my story.

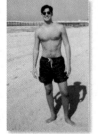
The fact is, even though I had this desire to raise and grow my own food that day in San Diego, my imagination wasn't nearly big enough to envision what God had lying ahead for me.

But the first thing God did was to complete His healing of my body during my forty days in San Diego. I was physically reborn and gained twenty-nine pounds during that time. In fact, you can see the results in the photo of me at Crystal Pier pictured on the previous page.

Considering my diseases were considered medically "incurable," and with what I'd been through for nearly two years, this was an absolute miracle.

NEXT STEP

There is something powerful about having the faith to take action. My action first required an eight-step walk from my bedroom to my parent's closet to ask my mom to take my picture. Eight steps might not seem like much, but many times during my illness I would attempt to walk those eight steps only to wake up hours later with my face planted in the tile, glasses broken having blacked out due to my extreme anemia. Another step of faith I ventured on required a 2,300-mile trip to learn from a man I'd never met and follow principles that I had never heard of.

If you had asked me at any time during my illness—"Jordan, what can I pray for?"—I would have responded, *I want my health back. I want my old life again.*

I got my health back, all right, but I didn't get my old life back. Instead, I received a *new* life and a vision, a passion, and a mission to see the health of this nation—and world—transformed one life at a time.

When I returned to South Florida, I was eager to share my testimony with anyone and everyone who would listen. Those who had seen me at my lowest were amazed to see me in good health.

You know how it goes: people tell other people and word of mouth gets around. One of those persons who heard about me was Dr. Morton Walker, a medical researcher and columnist for the *Townsend Letter for Doctors & Patients*, a newsletter that publishes information about the latest news in alternative medicine written by researchers, health practitioners, and patients. Dr. Walker was keenly interested in talking to me after hearing how I had overcome Crohn's disease and other ailments by following a biblically based health plan and supplementing my diet with probiotics.

Dr. Walker called me in the spring of 1997, and we had a friendly interview. Then he wrote a lengthy article about my battle back from "death's door." The story entitled "One Man's Journey from Sickness to Health" was a detailed account of my two-year battle against incurable diseases and the health program that brought me life again.

I don't know how many people read the *Townsend Letter*, but I'm not exaggerating when I say that several thousand people contacted me asking about the diet and the probiotics that helped me. Many of these letters and phone calls were from hurting folks with inflammatory bowel disease and other health challenges. They were desperate to know where and how they could eat the foods and acquire the probiotics that helped nourish me back to health.

I really believed I could help these people, and Lord knows I was touched by their stories of how illness had brought ruin on their lives. It was then, out of my parents' friends' garage, with my dad's credit card and a dream, and based on my belief that food is the best medicine, that I began to formulate whole food nutritional supplements and started a company called Garden of Life®.

At the time of my interview with Dr. Walker, I was working in a health food store in Palm Beach Gardens, stocking shelves and earning a whopping $4.25 per hour. I didn't really like what I was doing since stacking cans of organic black beans wasn't exactly my passion. But each and every day, people would walk into the health food store, and I would hear and see them out of the corner of my eye, asking an associate for help with their child with autism, their sister with breast cancer, their mom with osteoporosis, or their dad with arthritis.

My colleagues didn't always have an answer, but I—never being short on words—enjoyed offering my opinion whenever those questions came my way. Though I did not know all the answers, I remember striking up a conversation one time with a woman suffering from psoriasis, a skin disease marked by red, itchy, and scaly patches.

"Ma'am, I don't know a whole lot about psoriasis," I began, and then I reached into my back pocket and showed her a copy of my "before" picture. "What I do know is this: once I was dead and now I am alive. Would you like to know how?"

She nodded her head with a grateful look on her face, and then I told her my story. Often times, I was asked to describe what foods I ate or nutritional supplements I took. On other occasions when I struck up conversations within the store, I would recommend avoiding an entire food group or suggest an important book to read.

Amazing things happened in that health food store. I'd be stocking shelves when customers would walk down the aisle a couple of weeks later with big smiles on their faces. They would seek me out. Some would even be jumping up and down, but nearly all of them would hug me and say:

"Jordan, remember me? I'm the woman with the skin condition. Look at me now."

"Jordan, remember me? I'm the one who had a child who couldn't focus and couldn't behave in school. Now he's doing great in the classroom and is behaving well."

"Jordan, remember me? I had terrible digestive problems, but now I'm symptom-free."

Frequently people would walk in and comment about how my recommendations—from a stock boy, mind you—had helped them. What an opportunity to live my purpose by sharing my struggles and how I became victorious!

While working at the health food store, I also began an exhaustive study on nutrition and natural health. Due to my passion for digestive health, I focused a great deal on probiotics like the *Lactobacilli, Bacilli*, and *Saccharomyces* species. After meeting with hundreds of people in the health food store—and hearing from hurting folks following the publication of my story in the *Townsend Letter*—I knew there was a real need to take the very nutrients and compounds that improved my health and formulate them into whole food nutritional supplements. I named my first formula Primal Defense®.

While I was in no position to start an organic, sustainable ranch and farming operation at this point, I could do the next best thing: put whole food nutrients and compounds into nutritional supplements that would empower extraordinary health. Thus, Garden of Life was born.

Since I also had a deep desire to transform people's health one life at a time, I decided to share my healing story with the world. In 2002, I wrote my first book *Patient, Heal Thyself*, sharing the message of health and hope with more than 1.1 million copies in print. I can't tell you the number of people who contacted me to say, "Jordan, reading your story was like looking in a mirror. You went through exactly what I'm going through now. Our stories are so similar. Your journey from sickness to health made me believe I could get well and by following your suggestions, I am so much better."

Since then, I've authored twenty books and shared this message live in front of hundreds of thousands of people on five continents and forty-four states throughout this great country. I've hosted a pair of TV programs—*Extraordinary Health* and *Perfect Weight America*—that have aired on several cable networks. I've been interviewed and featured in the *New York Times, Washington Post, USA Today* and on TV programs such as *Good Morning America*, *Fox & Friends*, and *Inside Edition*. I've appeared on dozens of faith-based TV programs sharing the message of health and hope.

In the meantime, Garden of Life grew beyond my wildest dreams. By the mid-2000s, our products were being sold in sixty-seven countries and in more than 10,000 health food stores and thousands of doctors' offices.

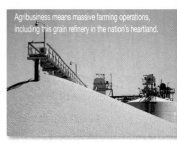
Agribusiness means massive farming operations, including this grain refinery in the nation's heartland.

During my various speaking tours, I would drive by and sometimes visit ranches and farms while I was on the road. Nearly every time I stepped on a working farm or ranch, I was disappointed in what I saw. American agriculture had become "agribusiness," which is a commonly used term that reflects the big corporate nature of many farm enterprises throughout the fruited plain. Huge machinery, chemical fertilizers, and automation had taken over, and the business model could be summed up in a simple sentence: produce the biggest yields possible for the lowest possible cost. If this means dousing your crops with pesticides and herbicides, feeding your livestock genetically modified cornmeal, or picking your fruits and vegetables before they ripen and then gassing them before going to market, then so be it.

Plain and simple, food has become a manufactured commodity these days; all one has to do is watch a few episodes of *Unwrapped* on the Food Network to see firsthand how America's "favorite" foods are processed and packaged. But even before our food is mass-produced in some industrial bakery or far-off factory, the ingredients have been sprayed with pesticides, pumped up with additives and preservatives, and stripped of vital nutrients.

More often than not, I would visit local and organic farms, not conventional farms, in search of healthy dairy and meat products. And while these producers were always much more conscientious than those at the large farms, a lack of resources usually kept these small farmers from producing foods and beverages of the highest quality and safety.

My travels across the U.S. continent added more fuel to the fire burning deep in my gut to one day produce the world's healthiest foods and beverages, without chemicals and preservatives, and as God intended. Food whose quality would go beyond organic.

And then the Lord spoke to me with words I'll never forget.

Jordan, you need to be a Joseph.

LOOKING OUT FOR OTHERS

I'm Jewish, and one of my favorite stories in the Tenach, or Old Testament as we call it today, is about Joseph. It's one of the great stories in history.

Joseph was born in Canaan many centuries ago—long before Moses or Jesus came to this earth. He was the eleventh of twelve sons born to Jacob and the son of the love of Jacob's life, Rachel.

Joseph must have been something special because his father clearly favored him over his older brothers and showed everyone how he felt by giving Joseph an elegant robe "of many colors."

Jacob's favoritism of Joseph caused jealousy in the family, and his older brothers didn't react well. They barely spoke to Joseph and let it be known that they hated him with a passion. They grumbled among themselves and couldn't say a kind word about him.

One day, when Joseph was in his late teens, he told his brothers about a strange dream he had.

"Guess what, guys? Last night I dreamt we were tying up bunches of grain out in the field when suddenly my bunch stood up while all of yours gathered around and bowed to mine."

The brothers looked at each other in disgust, but Joseph continued. "Then I had another dream that the sun, moon, and eleven stars bowed down to me."

"Who do you think you are?" one of his older brothers said. "Do you think that you are better than all of us? Do you think that we would ever bow down to you?"

This made the brothers dislike Joseph even more.

A few days later, Jacob asked Joseph to run an errand for him—check on his brothers out in the fields, which were quite a distance away.

When the brothers saw Joseph approaching, they hatched a plan to kill him. But Reuben, the oldest brother, calmed the hotheads down. "Let's not kill him," he said. "Just throw him in a well out here in the field." Reuben suggested this because he was secretly planning to come back and rescue Joseph when the other brothers had left for the day.

Joseph had a rude reception upon his arrival. His brothers grabbed him, yanked off his beautiful robe, and threw him into the empty well. A little while later, a band of Ishmaelite traders passed through the fields, saying they were on their way to Egypt, where they planned to sell their goods.

"Why don't we sell Joseph to these people?" said one of the brothers. "That way we never have to see him again, but we don't have to kill him."

The other brothers liked the idea, and Reuben wasn't there to stop them. So Joseph was placed on the auction block, and off he went—hands and feet bound—to Egypt. Once there, Joseph found out that he belonged to an important man named Potiphar, an assistant to the Pharaoh of Egypt.

Meanwhile, back at home, the rest of the brothers had to create a storyline about what happened to Joseph since his parents—especially his father, Jacob—would be worried sick about him.

One of the brothers took Joseph's beautiful robe, dipped it in animal blood, and returned to Jacob. When the father saw this, he cried out, "Some animal has killed my son!" Then he fell to his knees in tears, and he was inconsolable for days.

What happened to Joseph? Well, he started out as a slave, but the Lord was with him and no matter where Joseph was placed, he chose to do what was right. So Potiphar made him his helper and put him in charge of everything he owned.

Things were looking better for Joseph, but then he got royally messed with when Potiphar's wife accused him of making unwanted advances towards her. It was her word against his, and she won—despite the horrible lie she told. Joseph was thrown into prison and languished there for years until one day when Pharaoh heard that Joseph had an uncanny ability to interpret dreams. Pharaoh had a crazy dream that he couldn't figure out, and nobody could explain it to him.

Joseph was brought before Pharaoh, who asked him, "Can you understand dreams?"

"I can't, but the God I serve gives me the wisdom," Joseph replied.

So Pharaoh described his troubling dream, which Joseph immediately explained.

"God is warning you," he began. "There will be seven years where nothing will grow and there won't be food for anyone."

This wasn't what Pharaoh wanted to hear. "What can I do?" he asked.

"God has shown you what to do. There will be seven years that will be very good prior to those bad years. So good that there will be extra food for everyone. So you should set aside a portion of each year's harvest. That way you'll have enough to get you through the lean years."

Pharaoh believed everything Joseph said and put him in charge of all the land in Egypt as well as the food storage program.

During the seven years of "plenty," Joseph made sure that enough food was set aside to see Egypt through the coming famine. Sure enough, when the rains didn't fall and crops failed throughout the entire known world, people came from all countries to buy grain from Joseph—including Joseph's brothers.

When the contingent from Canaan arrived, they were led into a palace chamber where Joseph heard requests for food and grain. When his brothers walked in, Joseph recognized them, but they didn't know who he was because it had been more than a decade since they had seen him.

The brothers all bowed to him because he was an important person—just as Joseph had dreamed years earlier.

After a few meetings with his brothers, Joseph couldn't keep it in any longer. "I am Joseph!" he said. "Is my father alive?"

But his brothers couldn't answer him because they were afraid.

"Come here," Joseph said. "I am your brother, the one you sold. Do not worry, and do not be angry at yourselves for selling me because God has put me here to save people from starving." He also said one of my favorite lines in the Bible: "What you meant for bad, to hurt me, God has meant for good!"

How is that for an unbelievable attitude?

So Joseph sent his brothers back with food and provisions, and eventually his father, his brothers, and their families came to live in Egypt with Joseph, where they had all the food that they needed.

Not only did Joseph's provision save the lives in his family, but there is evidence in Scripture that this worldwide famine caused starvation among people everywhere and the only ones who survived were those who obtained food through Joseph by his God-given wisdom.

God used Joseph to save the world. Today, we believe that the story of Joseph was a foreshadowing of the One who was to come that would bring spiritual salvation to the world, Jesus our savior.

Jordan, you need to be a Joseph.

What did that mean?

When I first heard that voice in the stillness of my heart, I went back and reread the story of Joseph in the last thirteen chapters of Genesis. I was struck by the wisdom that God gave Joseph to store up food during seven years of plenty in advance of the seven years of famine that were coming. I'm sure that many people in Pharaoh's court thought Joseph was nuts, but because of his foresight and trust in God that he was given the right interpretation of Pharaoh's dream, there would be enough to eat in the land of Egypt *and in Joseph's own family.* The future nation of Israel would be saved.

So the Lord told me to be a Joseph, a person who could provide food, hydration, shelter, and protection to people in coming years.

I'm thirty-six years old, and those of us in Generation X don't think much about impending doom or the end of the world. We have known only economic prosperity throughout our short lives, although the Great Recession of the last few years have given many of us pause that the U.S. economy will never be as vibrant as the decade from the late-1990s to 2008.

The point is that no one is immune from great hardship and difficulties, and those who ignore history are doomed to repeat it. In fact, those in my own family experienced great tragedy at the hands of outside forces.

My late grandmother, Rose, was born in 1922 in a pastoral Polish village that could have doubled as the set for *Fiddler on the Roof.* She was the youngest of seven children born to Gidalia and Simma Catz.

Her Jewish family faced growing harassment during that uneasy era following World War I, and then Adolf Hitler was elected chancellor of Germany in 1933. He moved quickly to pass repressive anti-Jewish laws—and persecution of Jews intensified elsewhere throughout Europe.

Amid this hostile environment, Rose's family talked about fleeing Poland. Fortunately for them, there was still time to get out. Thirteen-year-old Rose joined her parents and several siblings and immigrated in 1935 to the United States, where the family settled in Queens, New York. They were among the last wave of European Jews to arrive in America prior to World War II.

Two of my great-aunts—my grandmother's oldest sisters, Sonya and Dora— were already married with their own families and felt they didn't need to come to America. They had husbands and jobs, and they believed their government would protect them from the likes of Hitler.

After the war, we learned what happened to Sonya and Dora as well as their families. During the Nazi blitzkrieg that swept Poland in 1939, they were rounded up by the SS and paraded through the streets along with other Jewish families. Then the children—screaming with fright—were separated from their parents and shot before their horrified eyes. Next, the women were ordered to gather, and they were gunned down in front of their husbands.

And then all the men stood shoulder to shoulder in front of the machine guns.

It's hard to believe that such inhumanity could happen, but this massacre—the forerunner of Hitler's "Final Solution" for European Jewry—happened less than seventy-five years ago. In the annals of time, this is a blink of an eye.

I tell this gut-wrenching story because we have no idea what the future will bring. Kingdoms rise, and kingdoms fall. The United States of America has been a great civilization—the shining city upon a hill—since we fought for our independence after our country was formed on July 4, 1776. I realize that I would have never been born if Lady Liberty hadn't opened her arms to my grandmother back at Ellis Island, so I am eternally grateful.

Now I have my own family to look after and care for. I married Nicki in 1999, and we have three children ages seven and under, so following through on the deep desire in my heart to produce my own food and provide places of refuge is very real to me. Whenever Nicki and I talked through my vision, she was on board, especially as we discussed what was happening to our nation in recent years.

We felt as though the scales were coming off our eyes and could clearly see the world around us. We agreed that our economy is based on paper money that is backed by absolutely nothing, and most of us use a piece of plastic to buy things we don't need with money we don't have from someone who doesn't even own them. With federal deficits flying through the roof and state governments straining to balance their budgets, it all seems like a house of cards.

If history is a guide, it reminds us that it wouldn't take much—a run on the banks, a stock market collapse, a cataclysmic event or, God forbid, a major terrorist attack on a U.S. city—to see it all start tumbling to the ground.

WHAT IS WEALTH?

As God spoke to me about Joseph, I was prompted to do a study in Scripture about what He considers wealth. I read that Abraham grew wealthy with cattle, gold, and silver. Isaac planted a field and reaped a hundredfold harvest. Jacob, through his wisdom and discernment, grew his flocks and herds. Job was blessed "twice as much" later in life with sheep, camels, and donkeys.

God describes His own wealth in Psalms by saying, *He owns the cattle on a thousand hills.* After reading that, I realized that it probably would be a good idea to own cattle on a hill or two myself. I also knew I needed to find sustainable sources of water since water is even more important for life than food.

I began a nationwide search to find the right land while crisscrossing the country on a forty-five foot tour bus that was part of a six-month promotional tour for my book, *Perfect Weight America,* during the first half of 2008.

We looked at properties in Idaho, California, and North Carolina but didn't find what we were looking for. In the fall of 2009 after a long search, we found just the right place—seven different pieces of property totaling 8,600 acres in southern Missouri's Ozark mountains and north Georgia's Blue Ridge mountains.

Talk about being "all in."

The best part about my God-given vision is that the dream to produce the world's healthiest foods and beverages, to provide water, food, shelter, clothing and protection to people who need it most, to offer places of refuge and best of all hope to a lost and dying world, isn't mine alone.

This is my invitation for you to join me in my mission to transform the health of this nation and world, one life at a time.

You, too, can live beyond organic.

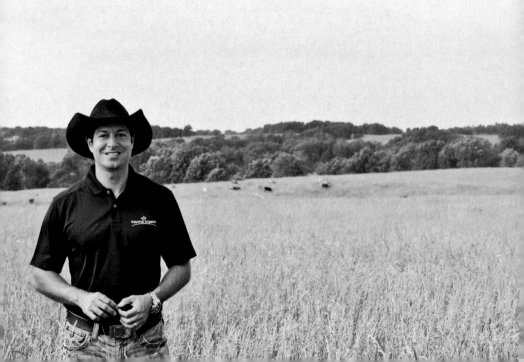

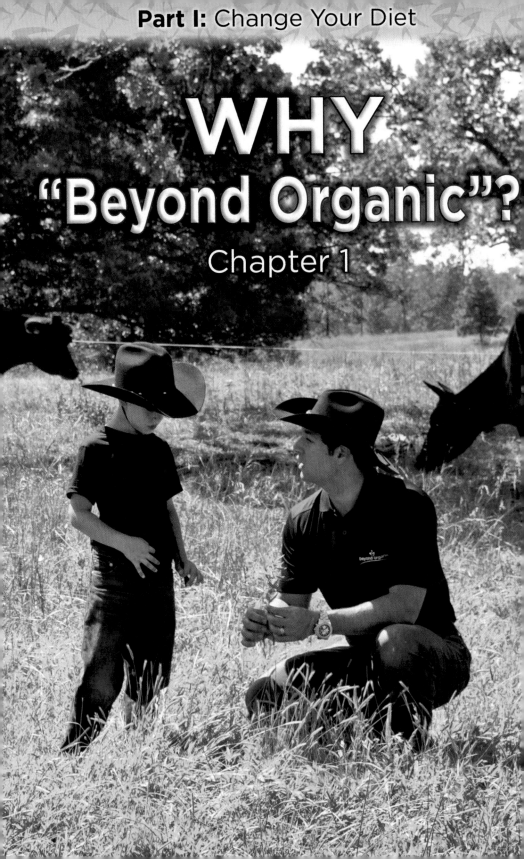

WHY "Beyond Organic"?

Chapter 1

My Baby Boomer parents were part of the counterculture generation that came of age in the late Sixties. Both Mom and Dad were drawn to the hippie lifestyle while growing up in the New York metropolitan area. Then again, just about everyone under the age of twenty back then dressed in tie-dyed T-shirts, hip-hugger jeans, and peasant skirts, wore mood rings and love beads, and spent "lost weekends" at love-ins, from what I've been told.

My parents, Herb and Phyllis Rubin, can say they actually attended Woodstock in midstate New York in the late summer of 1969. They were teenagers and dating each other when they joined 500,000 flower children on Max Yasgur's farm, arriving in time for Joe Cocker's set in the midst of a heavy rainstorm. All they'll tell me is that there were a lot of spaced-out naked men and women sliding around in the mud. I guess what happens in Woodstock stays in Woodstock.

My father went on to become an excellent pre-med student at New York University. He was in the midst of applying to several medical schools when he happened to thumb through a magazine called *Prevention*, a healthy lifestyle periodical founded by J.I. Rodale in 1950. (Don't forget Rodale's name, as you'll see.)

Prevention was hugely popular at the time and still is today with one of the largest readerships in the world and a monthly circulation of nearly three million. Filled with snappy articles about food, fitness, nutrition, beauty, and cooking, the easy-to-read, *Reader's Digest*-sized publication is a staple at supermarket checkout stands around the country.

As Dad paged through his issue of *Prevention* that day, his eyes spotted an advertisement for a school looking to train a "new breed" of doctors. Since he was on the med school track and a bit of a hippie nonconformist, my intrigued father read further. That's when he learned that the National College of Naturopathic Medicine was looking for students interested in treating patients from a whole different perspective than so-called "conventional medicine."

THE PRINCIPLES OF NATUROPATHIC MEDICINE, SAID THE ADVERTISEMENT COPY, COULD BE SUMMED UP WITH THESE BULLET POINTS:

- Nature has tremendous healing power
- Be sure to treat the whole person
- Do no harm
- Identify and treat the cause
- Prevention is the best cure
- The doctor is also a teacher

Dad had always been countercultural, the longhair type who swam against the prevailing tide. Something about pursuing a natural approach to medicine appealed to that sensibility. When he delved further into naturopathy, he learned that the roots of naturopathic healing could be traced back to the teachings of Hippocrates, Galen, and Paracelsus but had died out in the United States in 1954 with the closure of the last naturopathic medical school. The founding of the National College of Naturopathic Medicine two years later in Wichita, Kansas, however, resurrected naturopathic medical education, and the school was looking for interested students just like him.

That single advertisement in *Prevention* magazine changed the direction of my father's career path, as well as his life, when he decided to apply to the National College of Naturopathic Medicine. (The name has since been changed to the National College of Natural Medicine.) After receiving acceptance, he and Mom moved to Kansas in the mid-1970s. A little more than a year later, the school moved just outside of Portland, Oregon, and my parents moved as well. Like any young married couple with their futures ahead of them, they were enjoying every moment of this grand adventure called life.

In the summer of 1975, Dad was taking a course in obstetrics and gynecology while Mom was in her final weeks of pregnancy. The way my father saw things, this was a chance for some hands-on experience.

When Mom's time came due and the contractions intensified, Dad and three other naturopathic students came over to the house to perform the delivery. I don't remember coming into this world, but apparently Dad and his cohorts were effective midwives. Mom, though, likes to joke that she gave the four of them a D- as their practicum grade.

I was born on July 10, 1975, the son of full-fledged, back-to-nature, health-nut parents whose motto in life—"The more natural, the better"—certainly fit with the times. In their spare time, Mom and Dad helped start a food co-op, which is a collectively owned grocery-type store. They filled their pantry with wheat germ, raw honey, and granola and stocked their refrigerator with farm-fresh fruits and veggies. What they didn't put in their refrigerator was meat. After being breastfed, I was raised, a vegan for the first four years of my life until Mom became pregnant with my younger sister, Jenna, and decided we were missing too many body-building nutrients from not eating beef, chicken, fish, eggs, and dairy.

We moved several times following my birth, hopscotching from Portland to New York to Atlanta and then small towns in Georgia and Florida before finally settling in Palm Beach Gardens when I was in elementary school. I quickly learned that I was the odd kid in the neighborhood. None of the youngsters on my block were into wheatgrass smoothies or homemade plain yogurt, so it was hard to invite anyone over to the house when my parents had banned potato chips, store-bought cookies, and ice cream bars.

Whenever my school pals asked why I didn't have a piece of birthday cake at a classroom celebration, I shrugged my shoulders and said, "I eat natural foods."

I don't know if my classmates got it, but adults did. Back then, *natural* was the gold standard. If a jar of peanut butter or box of cereal flakes had a big "Natural!" plastered across the labeling, that meant the food was healthy to eat, at least in the public's mind. We've since learned otherwise, but back in the 1980s, *natural* is where you wanted to be.

If, however, I had said, "I eat organic foods" in the mid-1980s, my statement would have elicited blank stares. The word "organic" wasn't on the lips of many Americans back then. Those who knew about organic foods were usually part of the Birkenstock-wearing, dreadlocked crowd that frequented hippie-esque health food stores.

Interest in organic foods started to swell, though, right around the time I was making my health comeback in San Diego. I believe I know why. As I recall, the mid-1990s was a time when newspapers started publishing stories about the runaway U.S. "obesity epidemic" that was threatening our national health. Newsmagazine shows like *20/20* and *Dateline* followed up with arresting "special reports" that touched the heartstrings—usually weeping mothers describing how their overweight children were teased unmercifully in the schoolyard.

The dramatic TV segments as well as thoughtful op-ed pieces outlined in stark terms that we had a serious obesity problem in this country, one that had been building since the early 1980s. Back in President Reagan's first term, less than half (46 percent) of American adults were considered overweight, but by the mid-1990s, the Centers for Disease Control was saying that more than 60 percent of American adults were considered overweight. That figure has risen to *68 percent* today and shows no signs of receding.

The escalating numbers of obese individuals portends all sorts of public health issues, including the increased health care costs associated with treating those with obesity-related conditions such as type 2 diabetes and cardiovascular diseases. In addition, childhood obesity has *tripled* in the last three decades, which doesn't contribute to good health for our kids *or* our country's future. Some demographers have declared that children born after 2000 could live fewer years than today's current life expectancy, which is 75.6 years for men and 80.8 years for women, according to the National Center for Health Statistics.

Health experts pin the blame on sedentary lifestyles and a permissive society that can't say no to highly processed, low-nutrient, mass-produced foods. The abundance of cheap high-caloric meals and unhealthy sugary snacks, coupled with a lack of fruits and vegetables in the diet, is the reason why so many Americans have bulging waistlines.

As millions of families heard the message ten or fifteen years ago that a steady diet of processed ingredients and fast food meals were causing some serious health issues, attitudes changed. Parents of overweight kids were especially motivated to do something because they knew from personal experience what lay ahead.

Figuring out what to do wasn't so easy, but since we had a "crisis" on our hands, measures needed to be taken. Low-fat eating plans and low-carb Atkins-style diets had their day in the sun, but those regimens were found wanting since the pounds usually came right back once the dieter resumed a "normal" diet.

So what about organic foods? They aren't processed foods, so they have to be healthier for you, right?

They are . . . or at least they were. The message that organic foods gave your body a greater quantity of essential nutrients, were grown or raised without pesticides and synthetic chemicals, and were easy on the calories, seeped slowly but surely into the culture. What's happened over the last twenty years is nothing short of amazing: the market for organic foods has grown dramatically in ways that no one could have predicted. The most telling statistic is that U.S. sales of organic food and beverages grew from $1 billion in 1990 to $26.7 billion in 2010, a nifty 2,600 percent increase.

I'm heartened by the greater availability of organic produce, dairy, and meat products today, but we still have a long way to go. While organic food sales have been showing double-digit increases from year to year, they still account for only about 3 percent of total food sales, and the market for grass-fed beef is less than 3 percent of all U.S. beef sales. That means the other 97 percent is still coming from shopping carts filled with conventionally grown fruits and vegetables, cellophane-wrapped packets of conventionally raised beef, chicken, and farm-raised fish, and assorted boxes and packages of processed foods like breakfast cereals, bakery items, lunchmeats, frozen meals, and sweet treats.

Half of our food dollars—the money budgeted to feed us and our families—are spent inside supermarkets and grocery stores. The other half ends up in restaurants, including the cash registers of fast-food chains that line every busy boulevard in America. From the crack of dawn to late at night, between 20 to 25 percent of the U.S. population zips through a drive-thru lane or lines up at a counter to order burgers, burritos, and bacon-topped sandwiches every day.

America's love affair with fast food and processed treats, however, is sending our country down the road to perdition. As I recently mentioned, obesity rates have continued to rise since the media first sounded the alarm in the mid-1990s. We're ballooning to extremely obese proportions—meaning at least 100 pounds overweight or a Body Mass Index (BMI) of 40 or greater—at an alarming rate; the number of heavyweight travelers who have to buy a second seat on Southwest Airlines is four times more likely than it was twenty years ago. (Have you ever sat next to an obese individual whose excess poundage was spilling into your "space" on a cross-country plane flight? I have, and it was a very unpleasant five hours for me and, I know, very embarrassing for the heavyset person.)

So, even though the evidence demonstrates that organic foods account for around 3 percent of total food sales, and we can't say no to junk food or fast food stops, why does the American public think they eat healthy?

Good question, but we do. When asked if they eat a healthy diet with the recommended servings of fruits and vegetables, a vast majority of Americans answer in the affirmative in poll after poll. One of the most recent surveys, a 2011 poll conducted by *Consumer Reports*, reported that 90 percent of Americans say they eat a "somewhat," "very," or "extremely" healthy diet.

Actually, I'm not surprised that nine out of ten American adults give themselves credit for eating a healthy diet. I've spoken with thousands of people who attend my seminars, and many eagerly tell me the same thing—that they eat "healthy"—

even though I have a sixth sense that it's simply not the case.

Some do eat a clean diet, but I'm afraid that all too many don't because they're confused about what constitutes "healthy food." The reason I can say this is because they describe the sketchy foods they eat—thinking that they're healthy—or they ask me questions about what they should be eating because they really aren't sure what to do.

So, as a public service, as well as to help you comprehend what constitutes healthy food as well as my rationale for creating a new standard I call Beyond Organic, let me begin with a tutorial about the three general categories that foods fall into—conventional, natural, and organic.

After explaining what each of those categories mean, I'll describe why I believe "beyond organic" is the new standard for the healthiest foods that you could ever consume.

THE 800-POUND GORILLA: CONVENTIONAL FOOD

All I can do is shake my head when I see some of the advertisements on TV touting "home cookin'." You know, the ads for TV dinners.

The typical TV dinner ad begins with the image of a homespun meal being served in a warmly lit country home, decorated with oak furniture and a blue-and-white checked tablecloth. The camera lingers with a close-up of an appetizing slice of meat tucked next to a mountainous helping of mashed potatoes and gravy, complemented with fresh-from-the-garden vegetables.

The images say *comfort food.*

But no matter how well the alluring advertisement is shot, the advertisement grossly distorts reality.

The truth is that the dinner meal was thrown together on a conveyor belt by workers in white uniforms and hairnets inside an aseptic factory somewhere in the nation's midsection. Or maybe robots dropped a three-ounce portion of mystery meat on a moving tray, sprayed a brownish sauce loaded with sodium chloride, food coloring, and preservatives on top, plopped five ounces of off-white paste that resembled mashed potatoes into one corner, and released several strands of green beans onto an aluminum tray traveling at lightning speed down an automated assembly line.

TV dinners are downright crummy food. And yet millions of people buy these meals each and every day—and consume them. In our time-starved society, the quicker dinner gets on the table, the better.

TV dinners and other processed meals-on-the-go are sold mainly in brightly lit, gleaming supermarkets—the end product of something I call the food-industrial complex. It's comprised of Big Agriculture, mammoth food production companies, and a sophisticated retail network that works together to grow, harvest, produce, market, and sell conventional foods to 300 million unassuming Americans every day.

These manufactured foods are heavily advertised, widely promoted, and peddled to the masses as cheaply as possible. They must travel well and sit on supermarket shelves or inside refrigerated and frozen food cases for weeks or months at a time—which is possible, thanks to preservatives and food additives. More than 300,000 different processed foods compete for our food dollars—and it seems like every one of them are on display whenever I step into a grocery store.

How these processed foods get shipped to convenience stores and supermarkets begins in farm fields, feedlots, and fisheries. Let's take the farm side first.

The rise of Big Agriculture in the last century means that fewer and fewer farmers are growing more and more food on ever larger plots of land. Taken at first blush, this economy of scale sounds like a good thing: there's plenty to eat (but that's been a problem), the risk of famine is practically nil (something we shouldn't take for granted), and shopping for food is relatively affordable (although food commodity prices have seen a 15 percent leap in 2011).

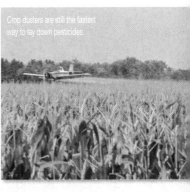
Crop dusters are still the fastest way to lay down pesticides.

To increase crop yields and get the most of their acreage, Big Agriculture plants crops containing genetically modified organisms (GMOs) that are resistant to insect infestation, douses their crops with pesticides and herbicides just to make sure the critters are dead, and relies on mechanized farm operations to harvest their bounty and bring their yields to market.

Sure, chemical pesticides, herbicides, and fertilizers stimulate rapid plant growth and kill or reduce the likelihood of pests devastating the crop, but when crop dusters swoop over fields and lay down a thick spray of pesticides, they're introducing harmful and toxic chemicals to plants, fruits, and vegetables—as well as to our air, soil, and water. Pesticides also kill the *good* microorganisms that are beneficial to plants, our digestive tracts, and our immune systems.

Whenever you consume conventionally grown foods, you receive environmental toxins that leave an unhealthy residue in your body. These chemical compounds find a way to your muscular tissues, circulatory system, and bone marrow. If you had your blood or urine tested for various chemicals and toxins, you'd be in for a big surprise: lab technicians would likely uncover minute traces of PCBs (polychlorinated biphenyls), dioxins, furans, trace metals, phthalates, VOCs (volatile organic compounds), and chlorine. When toxins enter the bloodstream through the foods you eat as well as the air you breath and the water you drink, this residue is referred to as your *body burden,* a chemical legacy that's harmful to your health today and in the future.

Hundreds, if not thousands, of chemical compounds taint your food. First, think of all the pesticides and herbicides used to grow food these days. Then consider all the artificial flavors, colorings, and preservatives *added* to your food in the production process. Although your body was designed by God to eliminate toxins, your immune and eliminative systems can be taxed to the point where they can no longer keep up.

The result is lethargy, allergies, and possible disease. Toxins have been scientifically linked to illnesses like Crohn's disease, irritable bowel syndrome, constipation, Candida, asthma, and even life-threatening diseases like cancer. Toxins can also cause birth defects or abnormal development in children.

Then there's the issue of GMO foods.

Never heard of genetically modified foods? You're not alone. Few Americans are aware of genetically modified crops or how quickly they have made it into the food chain, but their presence is ubiquitous. It's estimated that 60 to 70 percent of processed foods in grocery stores include at least one genetically engineered ingredient. Nearly 90 percent of soybeans and nearly two-thirds of the corn grown in this country come from crops that have been genetically engineered using the latest molecular biological techniques. Since many processed food products contain soybean or corn ingredients—and just think of all the juices and sodas sweetened with high fructose corn syrup—you can figure that genetically engineered foods have successfully penetrated the marketplace.

These plants were modified in the laboratory by taking genes from one organism and inserting them into another to make them grow higher, larger, denser, and more resistant to pests. No wonder my friend Jeffrey Smith, GMO expert and author of *Seeds of Deception*, says that GMO should stand for "God move over" because that's really what we're doing here—playing God by using engineering to force genetic information across the protective species barrier in an unnatural way.

While the idea of creating pest-resistant plant species is laudable, the problem is that scientists have successfully added genes to foods that weren't originally part of that food's creation, which is unnatural and changes the DNA character of the crop. As of this date, these laboratory-created mutations have not been subjected to any sort of rigorous testing. My family and I will not knowingly eat a food made from genetically modified ingredients because we don't know what the short-term or long-term effects will be.

Notice that I used the qualifier *knowingly*. Our family doesn't eat conventional foods very often, but on the rare occasions we do, we would have *no way* of knowing if that product contained genetically modified components because GMO ingredients do not have to be disclosed on food labels. Legislative bills requiring mandatory labeling of genetically engineered foods have been introduced in Congress and the Colorado state legislature, but nothing has been passed.

That breakfast cereal?

Made from genetically modified grain that was sprayed with pesticides.

That artisan bread you buy at a specialty bakery?

Ditto.

That New York steak in your home freezer?

That cut came from cattle fed an abundance of genetically modified corn and soy.

Other processed meats—like turkey lunchmeat, bologna, and chicken nuggets—are no bargain either. This would be a good time to take a closer look at chicken nuggets, a kids' staple everywhere children sit down to eat—at home, in a restaurant, or at a friend's house.

If you've ever wondered how these dinosaur-shaped nuggets are made, it's better that you don't know because the production process is obscenely gross and borderline alien. Even though I'm going to tell you anyway, I'll spare some of the ugly details.

After chicken meat has been removed from the carcasses on the assembly line, there's still a little meat left on the bone, plus some tendons and tissue. Back in the day, millions of these carcasses were buried in a landfill or burned in an incinerator, but machines were invented to mechanically separate those scraps of meat and muscle fiber.

The mechanically separated poultry, or MSP, is run through a grinding machine that turns the meat remnants into a pink goop that resembles strawberry frozen yogurt being dispensed at your local mini-mall. Nobody wants to bite into pink chicken nuggets, so food colorings and artificial flavorings are added to bring back the whitish color and deliver the taste that we've always associated with cooked chicken breast.

As you've probably figured out by now, Nicki and I don't feed our three children chicken nuggets—and wouldn't serve them conventionally grown poultry or corn-fed beef either. Instead, we prepare meals from grass-fed beef, bison, lamb, and venison as well as organic pastured chicken and wild-caught fish.

My biggest problem with conventional meat is that cattle, chicken, and fish are raised and fattened on feed containing hormones, nitrates, and pesticides. Raising livestock on these types of grain is the equivalent of raising children on candy. On top of that, livestock and chickens are penned up on "factory farms" that confine thousands of animals in impossibly cramped conditions with zero access to sunlight, fresh air, or natural movement.

According to the Grace Factory Farm Project, an estimated 70 percent of all antibiotics in the United States are fed to cattle, poultry, and pigs to promote growth and compensate for the unsanitary and deplorable living conditions on factory farms. (To learn more about the untold story of conventional agriculture and factory farming, visit www.themeatrix.com and watch this clever animated feature.)

The situation is no rosier when it comes to the fish sold fresh or frozen these days. The orange flesh of "farm-raised" salmon is one of the most popular items in warehouse clubs and supermarkets—and one of the most affordable—but these "feedlot salmon" pass their days making tight circles in long concrete sloughs gulping oily brown fishmeal pellets containing antibiotics, GMO grains, and even chicken feces. Farm-raised salmon, trout, and tilapia, as you could expect, don't taste as good as wild-caught fish or pack the same nutritional punch as their cold-water cousins that streak through the ocean or fresh-water streams sustaining themselves on small marine life.

The only good news to report on this front is that the U.S. House of

Representatives approved a bill during the summer of 2011 to prohibit the Food and Drug Administration (FDA) from approving genetically engineered fish like salmon.

Let's hope that we never see this sort of Frankenfish in stores, but I'm afraid that the conventional-industrial food matrix—from the huge farming operations to the food manufacturing plants to the supermarket and convenience store—is too entrenched, too powerful, and too ingrained in the American psyche.

I've been doing my best to open eyes and unplug ears regarding the unhealthiness of conventionally raised beef, poultry, and fish, but I've learned that people are creatures of habit. Too many people coast through life without thinking about the significance of what they eat, the quantities they consume, or where the food comes from.

The fact that you're reading my words right now gives me hope, though.

There's still time to change!

NO MEANING ANY MORE: NATURAL FOOD

Remember how I told the kids in my old neighborhood that I ate "natural foods" when I was in elementary school?

Back then, *natural* meant something—a food that didn't contain any artificial ingredients, no chemical preservatives, or, in the case of meat and poultry, was minimally processed. But over the years, conventional food companies and processors chipped away at these standards to the point where "natural" has no meaning these days. In fact, there is no legal U.S. definition for natural foods at the present time, and because of this, the Food and Drug Administration (FDA) discourages companies from labeling their foods "all natural" or "natural."

Since federal authorities have chosen not to define how the word "natural" can be used, we're left with all sorts of shenanigans. You can find the adjective "Natural!" slapped on just about any anything in a supermarket. For instance, food bars give you a "natural energy boost"—whatever that means. You can start your day with "natural fiber" in your breakfast cereal, which may or not be made from genetically modified grains. Potato chips are labeled "natural" because one of the "natural" ingredients is salt. (Most consumers aren't aware that commercial potato chips are fried in cottonseed oil, a partially hydrogenated oil that has been injected with hydrogen gas at high temperatures, which doesn't sound very natural to me.)

The USDA requires natural meat and poultry to be free of artificial colors, flavors, sweeteners, and preservatives, but some poultry producers inject their chickens with saline solution, claiming it adds flavor—after all, salt is "natural"— but that practice conveniently adds 25 percent extra weight to the bird, which is sold by the pound.

Don't trust the popular ice cream cartons boasting "all natural" flavors, either. Those ice creams are produced with factory-made ingredients like fake vanilla, corn syrup, and partially hydrogenated soybean oil as part of the mix.

So, with the meaning of *natural* obliterated, the only good news to report is that natural does *not* mean organic, but there again, the public is confused about what *organic* really means.

GETTING MORE POPULAR BUT NOT PERFECT: ORGANIC FOOD

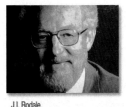

J.I. Rodale, the founder of Prevention magazine

J.I. Rodale, born in 1898 the son of a New York City grocer, started a publishing company in 1930 with an interest in promoting a healthy and active lifestyle. He launched a magazine called *Organic Farming and Gardening* in 1942 that promoted organic horticulture, which was followed by *Prevention*. Until his sudden death in 1971, he pioneered the idea that food grown without harmful chemicals was better for people and the planet.

Rodale, who looked like Leon Trotsky with a little goatee, was not viewed as someone on the fringe. He was well connected in the New York publishing world and best known for producing *The Synonym Finder*, a 1,361-page reference tool that is a thesaurus in dictionary form. In the summer of 1971, he was appearing on the *Dick Cavett Show*, talking up health foods as the publisher of *Prevention*, when he keeled over and died instantaneously of a heart attack—while cameras taped and the audience gasped. (The show never aired.)

Forty years later, Rodale's legacy still lives on because he is credited with popularizing the term *organic*. I also feel a bit of kinship since his magazine was instrumental in my father choosing to go into naturopathic medicine. If Rodale were alive today, I'm sure he'd be smiling at how widespread and how popular organic food has become.

Times have changed.

During my health comeback fifteen years ago, I could count on one hand the number of natural food markets in San Diego. Now there are more than three dozen in the country's seventh largest city—places like Whole Foods, Jimbo's, Sprouts, OB People's Food Store, and Trader Joe's.

I'm sure the shopping scene has changed where you live, too. Perhaps you've seen a Whole Foods or Sprouts open recently in your neighborhood, or your local health food store has expanded to meet the rising demand. Or maybe it's hard to find a parking place at the farmer's market every Saturday morning. The number of farmer's markets in the country have increased 17 percent in the last year, according to the U.S. Department of Agriculture. "There's a yearning for the 99 percent of Americans who are no longer connected to the farm to reconnect," said Kathleen Merrigan, deputy secretary of the USDA.

As more and more people flock to places like farmer's markets and natural food stores to buy their food, traditional grocers like Kroger, Publix, and Safeway—fearful of losing market share—have responded to this shift by stocking organic fruits, vegetables, and dairy products to bring customers back to their stores. According to news reports, Walmart, the world's largest retailer, plans to become the largest provider of organic foods and beverages.

Let's face it: it's cool—and politically correct—to tell others that you eat organic. Our First Lady, Michelle Obama, planted an organic vegetable garden on a patch of the South Lawn at the White House, which was great news because I'm a huge fan of foods grown organically and sustainably. I've been eating organic since I became deathly ill at the age of nineteen; it gives my body the best fuel possible. A hidden camera crew would get bored rather quickly if they tried to find me eating conventionally produced foods.

Organic refers to the way agricultural food products are grown and processed. Organic food production is based on a system of farming that maintains and replenishes soil fertility without the use of toxic and persistent pesticides and fertilizers. Organic foods are minimally processed without artificial ingredients, preservatives, or irradiation—that means zapping them similar to how a microwave oven cooks—to maintain the integrity of the food.

Some people claim that organic food has more flavor than conventionally grown food, but taste is a subjective measure. All I know is that *I* can taste the difference. The aromas are heavenly and the flavors are intense—most likely from the higher average levels of antioxidants and phytochemicals.

Organic agriculture has been around since Adam and Eve were forced from the Garden and had to grow their own food. Farming and raising livestock didn't change much for centuries. As recently as 1900, half of the U.S. labor force were farmers or working a ranch, but as mechanization and technology made huge leaps in the 20th century, that number has shrunk to just 2 percent today—and 60 percent of those hard-working folks are part-time farmers.

I've already described how modern agriculture has morphed into an agribusiness that feeds the world, but the price has been horribly steep. Voices in the wilderness like J.I. Rodale and others like Paul Bragg and Ann Wigmore gave the organic movement a voice in the pivotal 1970s and 1980s, but even then, few knew exactly what "organic" meant as the movement picked up steam.

The U.S. Department of Agriculture stepped in and began working on standards during the 1990s, but I can only imagine the lobbying efforts and political pressures that came to bear on this federal agency. After *years* of bureaucratic infighting, the USDA established guidelines in 2002 that outline what steps farmers, ranchers, dairymen, and other food producers must follow in order to be certified organic by the U.S. government.

THE USDA THEN ESTABLISHED THREE DESCRIPTIONS THAT CAN BE PUT ON FOOD PRODUCTS:

- **100 percent Organic.** This food must be all organic or contain only organically produced ingredients before it can receive this green-and-white USDA seal.

- **Organic.** The food must be at least 95 percent organic before it can receive this blue seal.

- **Made with Organic Ingredients.** The food must contain at least 70 percent organic ingredients. The remaining 30 percent cannot include any genetically modified ingredients.

The USDA regulations on what can and can't be called "organic" is as thick as a Manhattan phone book. (I didn't know that a year ago, but I do now!) The super-digest version is that organic meats must come from animals that eat

100 percent organic feed without any animal byproducts; for dairy cows, the whole herd must have eaten organic feed for the previous twelve months. Organic produce cannot be grown with chemical pesticides or most synthetic fertilizers, and animals cannot be fed or injected with antibiotics and growth hormones. Organic farms undergo a rigorous certification process and are inspected for compliance by an independent agent.

This would be a good place to define the term "sustainably," which is often spoken in the same sentence as "organic practices." Sustainability refers to a system of farming that maintains and replenishes soil fertility without the use of toxic and persistent pesticides and fertilizers. Livestock are pasture-raised, and fish are not pulled from the ocean faster than they can reproduce or caught in ways that destroy other sea life or undersea habitat.

So, are eating foods organically grown and sustainably raised the very best foods you can consume?

The short answer is yes, but let me tell you a dirty little secret: there are loopholes in organic rules that you can drive a Mack truck through. An example would be organic eggs. Do chickens have to spend time outdoors, or can they be kept cooped up in an enclosure? Can they eat a high percentage of their diet as organic grain, or must they hunt and peck for their food in a pasture in order to be called organic?

The guidelines can be murky—and subject to change. Here's a case in point.

IN 2010, THE USDA ANNOUNCED A NEW RULE ON ACCESS TO PASTURE FOR ORGANIC RUMINANT ANIMALS (COWS, SHEEP AND GOATS). CALLED AN "ENHANCEMENT" TO THE NATIONAL ORGANIC STANDARDS, THE NEW RULES LAID OUT THESE ADDITIONAL REQUIREMENTS:

- Animals must graze in pasture during the grazing season, which must be at least 120 days per year.

- Animals must obtain a minimum of 30 percent dry matter intake from grazing pasture during the grazing season.

- Livestock are exempt from the 30 percent dry matter intake requirement during the finish feed period, not to exceed 120 days. Livestock must have access to pasture during the finishing phase.

Notice the workding "access to pasture." Let me translate this last bullet point for you. The rule allows cattle to be taken from a pasture and taken to a livestock yard to "finish"—a euphemism for fattening them up prior to going to the slaughterhouse. During this period, which can be as long as 120 days or four months, the cattle can be fed just about anything—"as long as it's organic"—since they are exempt from the 30 percent "dry matter," which is another way of saying the grasses and forage they find in pasture fields.

When the rule also states that livestock must have access to pasture during the finishing phase, this can be broadly interpreted. Cowpokes could let the cattle out into a fenced-off "pasture" next to the stockyard for ten minutes and still be in compliance with the National Organic Standards.

You can finish your cattle on an almost entirely grain-based ration "as long as the grain is organic," just as the conventional feedlots do, and you can still label your steaks and hamburger meat "organic." But that "organic" cow could be fattened on grains or feasted on corn-based feed just like conventionally raised cows, but only without the hormones and antibiotics, which is certainly an improvement. That's why I tell people, "When it comes to beef, it's not so much how they start, it's how they finish."

In my opinion, the USDA Organic standards can be limiting in scope and potentially misleading to consumers, especially if they think organic is the ultimate standard for what is healthy.

THE NEXT GENERATION OF EATING: BEYOND ORGANIC

Organic standards are not perfect, but choosing to eat organic foods is an excellent and necessary step in the journey of reestablishing health and sustainability. While organic is *far* better than natural and leaps and bounds ahead of conventionally grown foods, I believe we can do better, and that's why I created a new standard called Beyond Organic. I do not seek to tarnish or invalidate the USDA organic standards, but I desire to elevate the level of awareness and knowledge of true health and wellness as it applies to humans and our planet.

My desire, borne out of a vow I made to myself as a twenty-year-old in San Diego, is to produce foods that cut no corners and are completely and totally healthy. To fulfill that desire, we've established higher standards that go beyond the organic guidelines.

OUR TEN-POINT BEYOND ORGANIC LIVESTOCK STANDARDS CAN BE SUMMED UP IN THIS FASHION:

1. **Our animals are GreenFed™ and GreenFinished™.** This means our dairy cattle intensely graze on grasses and a "salad bar" of forbs, herbs, and legumes—with no grains. Our beef cattle partake in our GreenFinishing program, which includes a bovine detoxification program and a diet of fresh organic pasture supplemented in the winter with green foods such as alfalfa and certified organic hay with no grain.

2. **Our grazing lands are free of pesticides, herbicides, fungicides, and chemical fertilizers.** This is a cornerstone of who we are at Beyond Organic.

3. **We do not treat our cattle with antibiotics, hormones, or vaccines.** The conventional cattle-raising business relies on chemical medicines to treat their sickly animals, but on our ranches and farms, we do not.

4. **We do treat our animals with respect and kindness.** God made everything that lives on the earth, including the animals, and He commands us to be respectful and kind to the animals under our care. Proverbs 12:10 reminds us that a righteous man takes care of his animals, yet another reminder that God has called us to be stewards of His creation.

5. **We follow sustainable land and soil management practices.** The earth is God's creation as well, is it not? Then it behooves us to be responsible for the way we treat the land by not polluting it and by managing it well for future years starting with the micro- and macro-organisms that improve the health of our soil.

6. **We never use GMO feed or plants in the field.** Genetically modified organisms are widespread in conventional agriculture, but they have no place at our Beyond Organic ranches and farms.

7. **We use Olde World production methods.** We want to revive the ancient methods of producing foods and beverages that enhance, not destroy, their health benefits.

8. **We use "fair made" ethical business practices.** We treat others as we would want to be treated, guided by principles of financial stewardship, economic self-sufficiency, and environmental integrity. We pay fair wages to our employees and seek higher social standards.

9. **We use biblically based processing methods.** Our beef and poultry animals must be slaughtered in accordance with biblical principles, which are described in Deuteronomy 12. This method of slaughter is widely recognized as the most humane method possible. We do not process animals that have died of natural causes or been killed by other animals, and we make best efforts to thoroughly drain the blood.

10. **We pursue quality and safety for our finished products.** We combine the best of ancient wisdom and modern science to ensure that our foods and beverages deliver maximum health benefits and minimal toxicity. We use probiotics in our processing and finished products to ensure safety and efficacy at every step.

That's just a quick overview of our standards at Beyond Organic. In coming chapters, I will talk more about how you can live beyond organic.

If you're looking to change your diet, change your life, and change your world, then you've come to the right place. I hope that by reading this chapter, you're convinced that:

- CONVENTIONALLY PRODUCED FOOD SHOULD NOT BE A PART OF YOUR MENU

- NATURAL FOOD IS NOT GOOD ENOUGH

- ORGANIC FOODS CAN FALL SHORT

- BEYOND ORGANIC IS HOW YOU WANT TO LIVE

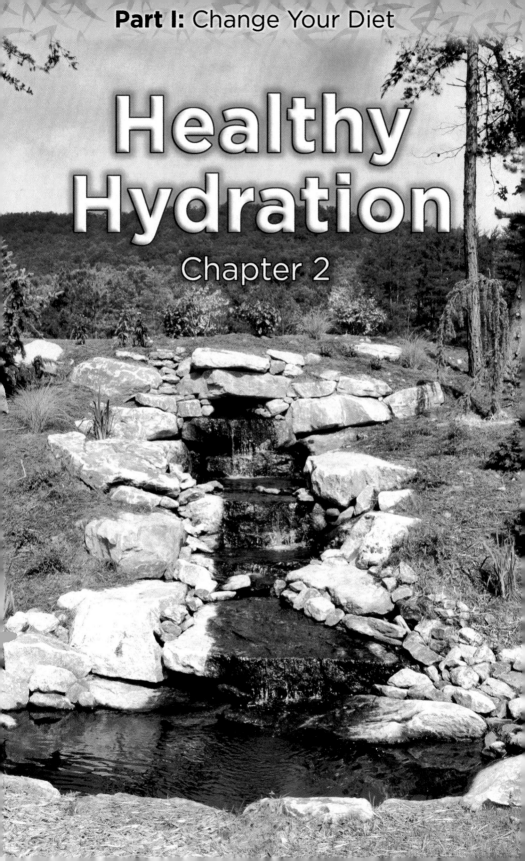

Healthy Hydration

Chapter 2

When I hear the words *spring water*, they often conjure up good memories. I can still see my grandparents' weekend home in my mind's eye, set among the hemlock trees and lush vegetation of Mountaindale, New York, a hamlet ninety miles from New York City near the Catskill Mountains.

The vacation home belonged to Grandpa Jerry and Grandma Ann, who lived in Long Island, where my grandfather was a dentist. Every summer, up until fourth grade, we visited my paternal grandparents in Mountaindale, a resort area populated with small hotels and a Main Street with interesting shops that catered to tourists.

This particular memory begins with Grandma Ann cleaning up in the kitchen after breakfast. That's when Grandpa Jerry—an Americanized version of his given name, Joshua—would call me over and hand me an empty gallon plastic container.

"Jordi, we're going to get some spring water," he'd announce.

As an eight-year-old boy, I knew this was my time to do something special with Grandpa. With empty containers in hand, we'd set off on a short drive, followed by a fifteen-minute walk that would take us to the side of a small mountain, where a fresh spring gushed forth the most refreshing, best-tasting water I'd ever had. We'd fill up our gallon containers and tote them back home.

I didn't know at the time how special spring water was or how healthy it was to drink, but Grandpa Jerry did. I can still remember him handing me a tall, cold glass of his spring water and saying, "See, isn't that refreshing? Drink up, young man!"

I've been drinking a lot of water ever since. I think my one-day record for drinking water is one and one-quarter gallons during a particularly hot and humid summer day here in Florida. I've learned through personal experience that if I fail to drink enough fluids, my body goes into the tank.

The same goes for my wife, Nicki, who fainted and collapsed to the ground one time when we were visiting a health food store on a sizzling afternoon in the Atlanta area. An ambulance rushed her to a nearby hospital, where the ER suggested that one of the culprits was likely dehydration.

We've all dealt with those occasions when our dehydrated bodies leave us feeling light-headed and weak. In those situations, a tall glass of refreshing water is a wonderful balm and the perfect fluid replacement. Only God could come up with a calorie-free and sugar-free substance that regulates body temperature, carries nutrients and oxygen to the cells, cushions joins, protects organs and tissues, trims the waistline, removes toxins, improves the skin, grows hair and nails, and maintains strength and endurance. Water makes up 92 percent of your blood plasma and 50 percent of everything else in the body, but dropping even a couple of percentage points from those figures can lead to catastrophic events.

It was an Iranian physician with the tongue-twisting name of Dr. Fereydoon Batmanghelidj who impressed upon me the importance of water. Author of eight books, including his seminal work, *Your Body's Many Cries for Water*, "Dr. Batman"—as he is often called—said that every twenty-four hours the body recycles the equivalent of forty thousand glasses of water to maintain its normal physiological functions. Without a regular replenishment of water, he wrote, the body can't deliver nutrients to the cells or properly eliminate waste products through the kidneys and bowels. Constipation, the hardship of 20 percent of Americans, is more likely a sign of dehydration than anything else.

Dr. Batman made water the focus of his life's work after he was imprisoned when the Shah of Iran was deposed during the 1979 revolution. Thought to be politically suspect from years of living abroad while studying medicine, Dr. Batmanghelidj was thrown into Evin Prison along with thousands of other political prisoners during the bloody turmoil that swept the streets of Tehran.

The conditions were deplorable for the prisoners, who suffered from the lack of medical attention. When the guards learned that Dr. Batmanghelidj was a physician, they asked him if he could do anything for the prisoners in various states of agony. One complained of excruciating ulcer pain, so much so that two friends had to help him to his feet to move around.

No medicines were available. The only idea Dr. Batmanghelidj came up with was to give the poor soul a couple of glasses of water. When the prisoner's abdominal pain subsided later that day, the Iranian doctor asked him to drink more water. His stomach pains eventually disappeared because the prisoner had been severely dehydrated.

When other prisoners complained of intense stomach pains, Dr. Batmanghelidj diagnosed their afflictions as peptic ulcer disease caused by the stress of being arrested and imprisoned. They, too, were treated with drinking water, and their conditions improved.

Dr. Batmanghelidj continued to "prescribe" water to prisoners with ulcer-like symptoms until his release two years later. Ever the researcher, Dr. Batmanghelidj began writing his clinical observations on the effect of water as a treatment for various stress-induced health problems, leading to his expertise in water and the human body's need for it.

I can remember reading *Your Body's Many Cries for Water* in the late 1990s when I was thirsty for information about the importance of keeping myself thoroughly hydrated. I nodded my head to Dr. Batmanghelidj's assertion that people around the world, especially in Western cultures, did not drink nearly the amount of water they need to keep themselves properly hydrated. Chronic dehydration, he said, was the root cause of painful degenerative diseases, asthma, hypertension, excess body weight, and some emotional problems, including depression.

Dr. Batmanghelidj made a good point when he said that many people confuse hunger and thirst, thinking they're hungry when they're actually dehydrated. The brain generates the sensation of thirst and hunger simultaneously, but many do not recognize the sensation of thirst and assume both "indicators" to be the urge to eat. Thus, they reach for a bag of potato chips when they should reach for a glass of water.

Many people go through the day on automatic pilot like this, with nary a thought about drinking enough water during and between their meals. If you're trying to lose weight and are hungry, before you eat something, drink eight ounces of water. In fact, make it a rule each time you open the fridge or cupboard to drink eight ounces of water. Even if you remember you're hungry, you won't eat as much.

Some believe if they *do* keep a container of water nearby and sip regularly, they'll have to run to the bathroom every twenty minutes. Others sense they need to drink something, but instead of water, they ply their bodies with mocha coffees, flavored sodas, and energy drinks, but those aren't hydrating and could have the opposite effect on your health.

Plain, old-fashioned water is always the right call. Yes, you'll go to the bathroom more often when you're drinking water regularly, but that's more than a good trade-off. Replenishing the body with water is vital because fluids in your body help urine eliminate waste products, keep the digestive system from becoming clogged, dissipate excess heat, and keep you cool on a hot summer day.

I recommend that your daily water consumption be one ounce of pure water for every two pounds of body weight. For example, if you weigh 150 pounds, then you should drink 75 ounces of water daily. If you participate in moderate exercise, you should consume an additional 16 ounces per thirty minutes of active exercise.

Remember, you need to drink water before you're thirsty and not wait until your mouth feels like it's filled with cotton. One great way to tell if you're properly hydrated is the color of your urine. A good rule of thumb is that if your urine is the color of apple juice, you need to drink more. If it's the color of lemonade, you're doing pretty well.

These days, though, you shouldn't drink just any old water, just like you shouldn't eat any old food. When it comes to living a life that is beyond organic, you want to drink the healthiest water possible.

WHICH WATER IS BEST?

The American public, by and large, drinks water right from the tap, although I have a sinking feeling that most people—when they're thirsty—reach into the refrigerator for a soft drink or bottle of juice "drink" sweetened with high fructose corn syrup instead. Those who are more conscious about healthy habits make it a point to drink filtered water or bottled water.

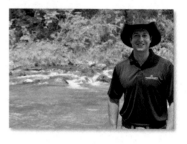

Drinking water straight from the tap is problematic because tap water is municipal water, which must be treated according to federal standards set by the Environmental Protection Agency (EPA) under the 1974 Safe Drinking Water Act. The EPA monitors water supplies for hundreds of organisms, metals, compounds, and chemicals at reservoirs and water treatment plants. Chlorine is added to the water to kill bacteria and aluminum sulfate is added to coagulate organic particles.

While the addition of chlorine to our drinking water has greatly reduced the risk of waterborne diseases, chlorine is a potent toxin. Tap water also has an unpleasant chemical aftertaste, which is why bottled water has become popular and widely purchased in the last twenty-five years. Before the 1980s, I'm told, it was inconceivable. that anyone would *pay* for drinking water, but that feeling has changed because of tap water's poor taste and the word getting out about how our municipal water is "treated" with bacteria-killing chemicals like chlorine and chloramine.

A fizzy French beverage known as Perrier was the first bottled water to make a splash in this country. Advertised as the "Champagne of mineral water," the distinctive green teardrop bottles of Perrier water bubbled into American consciousness and gave birth to what is an $11 billion industry today.

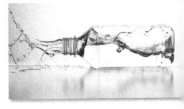

You can see how big bottled water has become by checking out all the brands on store shelves such as Aquafina, Dasani, Evian, Poland Spring, Arrowhead, Deer Park, Sparkletts, Crystal Geyser, Ozarka, and San Pellegrino. Then there are the premium "designer" waters like VOSS, Fiji, and Bling h2o. You may be wondering, *What's the difference?*

I'm not talking about the wide differences in price, which is illustrated by inexpensive and nondescript bottled waters costing a quarter each to premium waters like Bling with their frosted, corked, and hand-labeled Swarovski crystal bottles of Tennessee spring water. Those glitzy bottles of Bling go for $40 a pop.

No, what I'm talking about is the *source* of water.

Most of the best-selling and low-cost brands use **purified water**, which is essentially tap water that goes through a filtering process. Purified water can be produced by carbon filtration, distillation, reverse osmosis, or deionization.

The latter method—deionization—comes from water ionizers that produce a type of water known as **alkaline water.** Proponents of alkaline water say that you can boost your energy level and metabolism, and help your body absorb nutrients better by balancing your body's pH levels. Sounds good, but your body automatically adjusts pH levels in your blood and body fluids no matter what you drink—or eat—since the body must maintain tight biological control of its chemical processes. The bottom line is that not enough research has been done on alkalizing water filters to know how effective they are.

Furthermore, alkaline water filters create water with a high pH level that does not typically occur in nature. The minerals present in alkaline water may not be as absorbable as minerals present in foods, which could lead to a mineral residue left in the body. In Florida, our ground water has a fairly high mineral content, so in order to prevent mineral buildup in our bathtubs and showers, we have a water softener to remove minerals. Consuming highly mineralized (alkaline) water could do the same thing inside your body.

Artesian water comes from a well that taps a confined aquifer, or a water-bearing underground layer of rock or sand. The water level stands at some height above the top of the aquifer. Fiji Water, for instance, comes from a seventeen-mile long aquifer located on Fiji's main island, Vitu Levu. VOSS comes from an artesian aquifer in southern Norway that is pressured enough to allow the water to rise up naturally toward the surface.

Spring water, also known as a rising or resurgence, occurs when waters flows to the surface of the earth from underground without man's intervention. When you consider all the water on Earth, including the mighty oceans and seas that cover 71 percent of our planet, only 2.7 percent is fresh water, and just a fraction of that amount comes purified by the hydrogeologic formations under the earth. Called "living water" by many health experts, spring waters can range from those high in mineral content to those with lower amounts of solids.

As I looked for the purest water to drink, I remembered reading about **distilled water** in Paul Bragg's book, *The Miracle of Fasting*. Distilled water is a type of water that has its impurities removed through steam distillation, a process that involves boiling the water and condensing the steam into a clean container. This is meant to replicate the process in nature where water turns to steam and rises and condenses in clouds and then rains down to earth as essentially distilled water.

Actually, I have bad memories of distilled water. My parents had an old-fashioned water distiller in one corner of our kitchen that sat on top of a short cabinet when I was growing up. The distiller produced water suitable for drinking, cooking, and other household uses. This was back in the late '70s when bottled water wasn't widely available and the tap water was problematic for reasons already stated.

My parents' distiller worked by heating ordinary tap water to 212 degrees Fahrenheit, killing any bacteria or viruses that may have been present in the city water and removing all of the metals and contaminants. I was two years old when I decided to "play" by swinging on the cabinet door that the distiller was sitting on, something my mother had sternly warned me not to do.

Big mistake. Gallons of scalding-hot water cascaded down my face and my torso. I screamed to the high heavens because the boiling water severely burned my skin. My dad immediately rubbed fresh aloe vera on my burned flesh, gave me some homeopathic remedies, and rushed me to the emergency room, where the doctor told my parents that the entire left side of my body would be scarred for life. But thanks to my parents' quick application of aloe vera, homeopathics, and most importantly God's grace, I made a full and complete recovery with only a dime-sized tiny scar on my hip today.

When health pioneer Paul Bragg recommended distilled water as the best source of hydration, I understood why since my health-conscious parents had a distiller in their kitchen. But as I continued my search for the best water to drink, I was influenced by another book called *The True Power of Water* by Japanese researcher Masaru Emoto, who had studied the unique properties of water after a friend introduced him to a type of water that worked miraculously on his foot pain.

His fascination led him to an intense study of water, which over time convinced Emoto that water changed its quality according to "information" that it took in. Emoto took water samples from around the world, slowly froze them, and then photographed them with a high-powered microscope. Each water crystal was unique, just as no two snowflakes are alike. But something greater caught Emoto's eye: clean, pristine water created beautifully formed geometrical crystals, while dirty, polluted water didn't form any crystals at all.

What to make of this? Emoto wasn't sure, so he did some offbeat things. He exposed water to different types of music—classical Bach, Japanese folk music, and heavy metal riffs—to see what would happen to the composition. Distilled water exposed to classical music took the shape of delicate, symmetrical crystalline shapes. Water samples bombarded with heavy metal chords and a big drumbeat did not form crystals at all but displayed chaotic, fragmented structures.

The conclusions that Emoto drew was that the outside world can have a profound effect on water quality because water has "memory" and responds to outside forces and agents—like when water has been treated in a municipal water treatment plant. In other words, water changes properties when man starts messing with it or polluting it.

It's a bit like San Diego's proposed "toilet to tap" recycling program that has festered for decades. The idea of turning raw sewage back into drinking water would seem to go against everything Emoto is talking about when it comes to

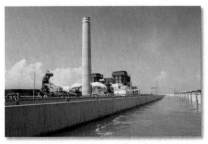

water having a memory. (Maybe that explains why President Nixon, when offered a glass of recycled sewage water at a Chicago treatment plant years ago, smiled respectfully and passed.)

Whether water has a memory or not, God has a process by which He created water for us to drink. Water in oceans, rivers, ponds, and lakes is heated by the sun, which turns it into water vapor, which gets drawn up into the clouds in the form of condensation. When a cloud becomes so full of water that it can't hold any more moisture, it rains. (Paul Bragg always said rainwater is the best form of distilled water that you could ever drink.) The rainwater then travels back into our rivers and oceans, or it soaks down deep into the ground, creating more groundwater.

No new water has been created on the face of the earth since God rested on the seventh day, which is an amazing thought to contemplate when you think about the magnitude of that statement. When God led me to do a search through Scripture to determine what His definition of wealth is and where I should be investing my resources, the first place He led me was water.

Water is absolutely essential to living, and all of the world's great cities were founded near a consistent source of water: Rome and the Tiber River, Paris and the meandering Seine, and London on the Thames. Water has been supremely valuable because without it, humans, animals, and plants wouldn't survive for long. You'd be hard-pressed to live longer than three to five days without drinking water, whereas people have survived forty, sixty, and eighty days without food.

The fact of the matter is that water is more valuable than oil and gold. If you think that is an outrageous statement, consider former World Bank vice president Ismail Seageldin's often-quoted 1995 prophecy that "the wars of this century were fought over oil, but the wars of the next century will be fought over water."

That hasn't happened yet, but if and when it does, it would be further proof that there is nothing new under the sun, as King Solomon said. War and disputes over access to water have occurred time after time throughout the centuries. The Nile, Jordan, and Tigris-Euphrates river systems have been and continue to be flash points. Closer to home, seven Colorado River Basin states (Colorado, Wyoming, New Mexico, Utah, Nevada, Arizona, and California) have bickered for decades on how to share the river's water. Further west, the California water wars from 1910 to 1920 pitted the semi-arid city of Los Angeles against the Owens Valley 200 miles to the northeast, which had plenty of water from winter snows melting in the Sierra Nevada mountains. As the classic 1974 Jack Nicholson film *Chinatown* demonstrated, Los Angeles won.

The California water wars continue even today. In recent years, Central Valley farmers and ranchers have seen their water allotments cut severely because of drought and judicial orders to divert water to the Sacramento Delta to help the delta smelt, a small fish protected by the Endangered Species Act. Forced to let their fields lie fallow or chop down their dying orchards and groves, the agricultural industry has fought back in court and in the court of public opinion, saying that a quarter of the nation's fruits and vegetables are grown in California's Central Valley.

The nation's breadbasket, the livelihood of hard-working farm families, and the desire to protect endangered species—something will have to give in coming years, and that's because there isn't enough water to go around.

At least not enough good water.

WATER THAT REIGNS SUPREME

When I was going through my forty-day health experience in San Diego and thought about one day having my own ranches and farms where I could grow and raise healthy foods, I knew water needed to be part of that mix. While I was looking for land to purchase, the first criteria was that the property must contain a natural water source where the water was not recycled, not polluted, and not former wastewater. I wanted water that was "alive" and highly pure but low in minerals and solids. I desired a combination of all the best properties water could have. What I wanted was a source of living water that retained the properties of distilled water—water that had the highest percentage of H2O.

Why did I feel that way?

Water functions in the body as a delivery system, bringing nutrients into the cells and escorting waste products out of the body. If water is loaded with elements and minerals, then I agree with Paul Bragg's belief that the water is less effective at doing its job. It shouldn't come as a surprise that the best water will always be the purest and highest percentage of H2O.

After all, when it comes to gold, silver, and diamonds there are different measures of quality, and they all begin with purity. For gold, the carat is the measure of the purity. Gold alloys with a 24-carat rating are pure gold; anything less, like 14k gold, is not as pure. Silver that is 99.9 percent solid silver is stamped with a purity mark of "Fine Silver .999." Diamonds are valued by their clarity and color, which are essentially measures of purity as well.

When it came to purity in water, I wanted a natural source with the least amount of solids and the greatest amount of H2O. I wanted water that was free of chlorine, chloramines, and fluoride—chemical agents used to "scrub" municipal tap water. I wanted water that was free of environmental toxins. To me, that was the measure of the healthiest water.

People understand why chlorine is something to avoid when I speak to audiences, but in question-and-answer periods, I'm also asked what I think about mineral water. "Are minerals good in water?" they ask.

I understand where the question is coming from. After all, the health benefits of mineral waters like Perrier and Evian are celebrated around the world. My answer is that minerals are great, but the minerals you find in water are generally in a form unusable in the body because they're minerals that come from rocks. When water runs over rocks, the rock sheds minerals, which become part of the water. While minerals and trace elements like zinc, magnesium, and iron promote overall wellness, they are better when they come from foods.

I decided early on that the best water comes from natural springs. I wanted water that rained down from the heavens, purified by clouds, and landed on the earth, where it seeped through the soil and was purified by the earth only to emerge from the ground naturally as spring water. The water needed to be as pure, and as close to distilled, as possible.

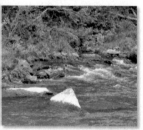
Over the course of several years, I investigated more than one hundred properties and dozens of natural springs around the continental U.S, ranging from Idaho, California, New York, Maine to North Carolina, Missouri, and Georgia. My criteria were precise: I wanted spring water that was low in minerals and solids and came out of the ground without the use of drilling equipment and modern technology.

Since biblical times, families and clans would find a spring coming out of the ground and stay there as long as that spring flowed. They would create their life around a source of natural spring water. My reading of Scripture reminded me that the Lord God, before He created Adam, caused springs to come up from the ground and water all the land. The Hebrews, during the Exodus, journeyed from Gudgodah to Jotbathah—"a land with brooks of water." Elijah was told by the Lord to travel east and hide by Kerith Brook, where he was to drink from the springs and eat what the ravens brought him.

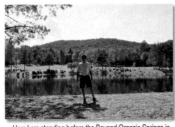

Here I am standing before the Beyond Organic Springs in Blue Ridge, Georgia.

My search for a natural spring led me to Blue Ridge, Georgia, a small town in the Blue Ridge Mountains ten miles from the confluence of the Tennessee and North Carolina borders. Blue Ridge is a popular tourist destination with a quaint downtown populated with several shops and antique stores. Within the town limits was a natural spring that had been providing high-quality bottled water since 1993. Its water had won awards for taste and was known for being pure water—or, as locals called it—sweet water.

After doing my due diligence and water testing, I purchased the property in 2010, and today it is known as Beyond Organic Springs.

The Beyond Organic Springs water source has been around for thousands of years. Due to the exceptional amount of precipitation, the springs produce an abundance of water without depleting water from the surrounding local areas. Even during the recent drought in Atlanta, our water table barely dropped. The unique hydro-geological formations beneath our property purifies the rains from the sky to yield an energized spring water that that has a high percentage of H20, only a tiny amount of minerals, but just enough to provide structure and energy to the water.

When Cline Bowers, former owner of the property and current water manager at Beyond Organic, put a TDS (total dissolved solids) meter into the spring this very morning, it measured at three parts per million, which is nearly as low as distilled water. But unlike distilled water—which takes a lot of water to produce and therefore has issues around sustainability—all of the water produced by the

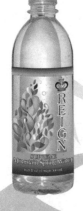

Beyond Organic Springs is bottled for drinking water or flows into a steam to be re-circulated.

As part of my Beyond Organic mission to transform the health of this nation and world one life at a time, we have introduced our own bottled water and decided to call it Reign™ Supreme Mountain Spring Water.

In my mind, the best water in the world is pure spring water coming out of the ground. Since water is the second-most abundant element we need—after oxygen—you need to drink the purest water possible. You get three times the amount of oxygen from the water you drink than from the air you breathe, so if you want to take a big step toward getting healthy, make sure you and your family are adequately hydrated with the best quality water you can find. Remember, hydration is the cornerstone of good health because water is a delivery system designed to usher nutrients into the cells and remove wastes or toxins from the body.

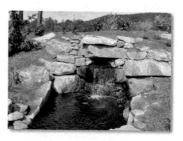

AT BEYOND ORGANIC, WE BELIEVE OUR REIGN MOUNTAIN SPRING WATER REIGNS SUPREME FOR THE FOLLOWING REASONS:

- Reign originates from a pristine spring right here in America, a renewable resource naturally free of contaminants.

- The source of this natural spring water in north Georgia starts with a quartz vein below the earth's crust. The spring bubbles to the surface, where it's filtered through sand and rock, leaving the water pure and natural.

- The spring is protected by 130 certified organic acres.

- The supreme purity of Reign provides maximum hydration and utilization of the body's most important resource—water.

- Reign can also be called the "green water in a blue bottle." Produced right here in the USA, our water is not shipped halfway around the world to your local store or gas station, and we have put in place a program to power our spring through the use of alternative energy.

- Reign Supreme uses biodegradable packaging that's BPA-free.

- Reign Supreme has extensive quality testing going back over a decade."

- Best of all, the spring water that comprises Reign tastes great and has won international awards for flavor.

I believe some of the best spring water in the world comes from our natural source in the Blue Ridge Mountains of north Georgia. So, if you're looking for the purest, God-created water coming out the ground, then you'll want to try Reign Supreme Mountain Spring Water today—before you get thirsty.

THE THIRST FOR SPORTS DRINKS

As I'm writing these words, I've entered a new arena: head football coach.

Of five to seven-year-olds, that is.

Yup, I'm the head coach of my son's Tiny Mite Pop Warner tackle football team in Palm Beach Gardens. We're called the Gators, and our blue-and-orange uniform colors match the colors of the University of Florida football team in Gainesville. For someone who attended rival Florida State and was even part of the cheerleading squad, it's taken some time getting used to wearing a Gator shirt on the sideline.

I don't see myself, however, becoming the next Bear Bryant, the great Alabama coach of the Crimson Tide back in the 1960s and 1970s. Allow me to explain why.

It gets awfully hot and humid here in South Florida, especially in August when team practices begin. My players put on pads and heavy helmets and work hard, but I always make practice fun. This isn't the NFL or even high school football— this is football for kindergarteners and first and second-graders. It has to be fun.

One thing I make sure we do quite often is take hydration breaks. Coach Bryant,

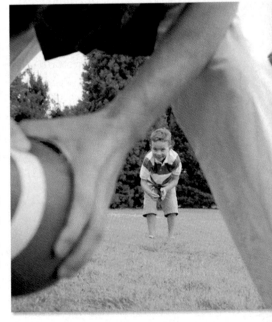

when he was coaching at Alabama, didn't allow his players to take a water break. He was old school all the way. Back in the 1960s, he told his hot, thirsty players to "suck it up" by going through an entire practice without taking a sip of water. To Bear Bryant, this was a test of toughness.

Coach Bryant wasn't making his football players tough; he was unwittingly hurting their bodies. Hard-working athletes out in the hot sun *need* water—and lots of it.

The same goes for five- to seven-year-olds. Some of my boys bring coolers with bottled water, and that's great. Others bring popular sports drinks their moms packed for them.

Now, I understand why millions of kids around the country bring sports drinks to their football practice, their soccer and baseball games, and their tennis matches every single day. Sports drinks dominate all levels of athletics, but my gripe with them is that they are nothing more than a bottled concoction of water (sometimes unpurified), sucrose, glucose, and fructose (sugars); and artificial flavors and colors with some isolated forms of potassium and sodium thrown into the mix. In other words, artificially colored and flavored sugar water with a salty aftertaste.

There is, however, a good reason why these sports drinks contain sodium. During extreme periods of heat and exertion, we can lose our sense of thirst. I've even seen this on our Beyond Organic ranches, where most of our dairy cattle have an inability to sufficiently cool down if they're constantly subjected to temperatures above 70 degrees—which happens almost every hour of every day during the summer.

This past summer, we had several heat waves with periods where the temperature never got below 70 degrees even at night. Our milk production suffered because the cow's sense of thirst and appetite was suppressed. One way we can increase the consumption of water and, subsequently, food the cows consume, is by supplementing our cattle's diets with natural high mineral sea salt.

When our cattle consume salt, believe me, their sense of thirst increases. The same dynamic occurs in humans and forms the basis behind the scientific research studies sponsored by the sports drink industry. The research shows that the inclusion of sodium in these formulations stimulate thirst. The idea is to get athletes thirsty enough to down an entire drink brimming with electrolytes and carbohydrates to replenish their energy-producing stores, so to speak. This was the thinking when the first sports drink was invented back in the late 1960s.

As you have probably figured out already, I'm not a fan of traditional sports drinks. Besides cool water, which my son Joshua freely drinks before, during, and after football practice, there are two other "performance drinks" that are quite effective for athletes and virtually anyone who exerts herself or himself on the playing field or in the gym. These performance drinks are also great for those that want to flood their bodies with nutrients and beneficial compounds.

The first is coconut water, which has been consumed for thousands of years. When I was a kid, we called it coconut milk, but what I'm really talking about is the juice on the inside of the coconut. Coconut water is naturally high in potassium but also contains a small amount of natural sodium and easy-to-digest sugars.

You may or may not have noticed, but sales of coconut water have gone through the roof in the last couple of years. Coconut water has gone from the obscure to a massive success with large corporations like Coke and Pepsi purchasing or launching coconut water brands. Perhaps you've seen the end-cap displays for coconut water in natural food stores or even traditional supermarket chains.

Coconut water is rich in potassium—between 300 and 700 milligrams per serving—and has a nice sweet flavor. This natural sports drink is a staple in tropical regions around the world. I can remember driving the famous "Road to Hana" on the island of Maui and stopping at roadside stands, where native Hawaiians with machetes in their hands were ready to chop open a coconut and pour you a drink. I've come across similar roadside stands in my travels to Malaysia, Indonesia, and the Florida Keys.

You don't have to participate in the Hawaiian Ironman competition to drink coconut water. Many feel like it helps their digestion and elimination because of the high potassium—more potassium than what's found in a banana and around fifteen times more than most sports drinks. I've also heard stories about coconut water being used in Brazilian hospitals in their IVs because the wonderful balance of minerals is a near-perfect fluid electrolyte replacement.

I'm going to make a prediction: it wouldn't surprise me if in the next five to ten years we see a worldwide shortage of coconuts. That's how popular this tropical beverage has become.

There's another performance drink that I want to tell you about, and it's a living cultured beverage that we've created at Beyond Organic that could be *whey* better than what you're currently drinking.

In my search for the perfect performance beverage, not long ago I visited our dairy lab at the Beyond Organic ranch headquarters. I was interested in seeing a production batch of our **GreenFed Raw Cheese**.

During the cheese-making process, I noticed a beautiful golden liquid being separated from the curds.

I knew what it was, but I asked one of the young women anyway. "What is that?" I questioned.

"It's whey," she replied, which instantly reminded me of the little nursery rhyme: *Little Miss Muffet sat on a tuffet, eating her curds and whey . . .*

Most people have heard of whey because they make smoothies and include a dollop of whey protein in their shakes. What most people don't know is that whey has been used as a traditional beverage for thousands of years. Hippocrates and Galen, two founding fathers of medicine, frequently recommended whey to their patients. In Switzerland, whey has been called the "old man's drink" throughout history due to the fact that many believed it made old men feel young again.

As I watched our cheese production process, I mentally reviewed what I knew about whey. This tart, golden liquid—known to the Greek doctors of antiquity as a "healing water"—helped maintain synergistic balance of the inner ecosystem and provided a feeling of youth when consumed. Whey was similar in structure to coconut water but with two distinct advantages:

1. Whey was loaded with B vitamins.

2. Our whey, which comes from GreenFed organically produced milk, not only had naturally occurring sodium, naturally occurring potassium, B vitamins, and other key nutrients, it also contained acidified and organically bound calcium, which was just amazing.

The whey being separated from the curds for cheese was very valuable. My mind started playing around with the possibilities of formulating a beverage that had our Beyond Organic GreenFed whey as a major ingredient.

I shared my idea with our team, and the result is a new beverage that we call **SueroViv™**, which looks like an odd name in English but that's because it's a combination of *suero* (which is Spanish for whey) and *Viv* (which is a French way of saying "life"). So SueroViv means "whey of life."

We took the health benefits of whey to the next level by culturing it with powerful probiotics that create beneficial compounds, including lactic acid. To enhance the hydration experience, we decided to combine whey's healthy attributes with our refreshing Reign Supreme Mountain Spring Water and what I believe to be the ideal sweetener—honey. Then we accented our new drink with organic juices and organic essential oils to produce, in my opinion, the best beverage on the planet.

I compare the slightly sweet and tart taste and the experience of consuming SueroViv to a cross between coconut water and another cultured beverage whose interest has exploded in recent years—kombucha. One major difference is that SueroViv has calcium that neither coconut water nor kombucha bring to the table.

The base of SueroViv is cultured or lacto-fermented whey that was popularized in the U.S. by Swiss naturopath and health legend Dr. Alfred Vogel—who happens to be the developer of Herbamare, my favorite seasoning of all time. I've been using Herbamare liberally since the late 1990s and love it on my foods.

I knew that our Beyond Organic whey would be a great foundation for a healthy sports drink that didn't come with all the baggage that famous commercial brands have. The organic honey used to sweeten the beverage is rich in monosaccharides, meaning it's the simplest form of energy-producing sugar. The gastrointestinal tract finds monosaccharide-rich foods like organic honey easier to digest because this single-molecule carbohydrate can be absorbed through the lining of the small intestine without having to be broken down first. (Note: honey should not be fed to infants under one year of age. SueroViv is great for children over one year of age and adults.)

Honey has been used to enhance sports performance since the original Olympic Games in ancient Greece. Research studies since then have confirmed the use of honey as an "ergogenic aid," meaning a food or ingredient that helps an athlete's performance. One study put thirty-nine weight-trained athletes through an intensive workout who consumed a protein supplement blended with either sugar, maltodextrin, or honey as the carbohydrate source. The "honey group" maintained normal blood sugar levels throughout the two hours following the workout and did not display the typical drop in blood sugar sixty minutes after the other forms of carbohydrates.

Regarding the addition of two more vital ingredients to our formulation of SueroViv—certified organic juices and essential oils—one of the juices is lemon juice, which is a wonderful source of vitamin C and other nutrients. The organic essential oils—distilled from fruits, vegetables, herbs, and spices—not only impart a great flavor but are also the concentrated lifeblood of plants containing thousands of known—as well as those yet to be discovered—beneficial compounds.

Essential oils have been used since biblical times, and if you look at the story of Mary, the sister of Martha, approaching Jesus with an alabaster jar of very expensive ointment (or what we could call perfume today) in John 12, you learn that she poured this essential oil on Jesus' head.

One of the disciples, Judas, was indignant when he saw this happen, complaining about the waste of money. "That perfume was worth a small fortune," Judas said, adding that the essential oil could have been sold and the money given to the poor. Biblical scholars said the fragrant ointment was known as "essence of nard" or spikenard and was imported from the mountains of India, thus making it very expensive—the equivalent of a year's wages, or $40,000 in today's dollars.

So if you think about essential oils and a small alabaster jar being worth a year's wages, you get an idea for how prized these oils were and still are, and that's why we included essential oils in SueroViv, which is a living cultured whey beverage for athletes, active seniors, and everyone in between. SueroViv has about half the sugar (coming from the cultured whey, organic juices, and honey) of store-bought juice and juice drinks, more than 80 milligrams of calcium per 16-ounce bottle, and five to seven times the potassium found in most sports drinks.

I believe SueroViv combines the best of all the cultured and performance beverages available today, and we're excited to introduce this beverage as a *whey* of life to people everywhere.

I'll also be introducing Beyond Organic SueroViv to the Tiny Mite Gators and their parents during our fall season of Pop Warner football. SueroViv comes in three flavors—Citrus, Raspberry Lemonade, and Orange Cinnamon. I think the kids will like the fruity flavors and the taste, and I really do think that SueroViv could be our secret weapon.

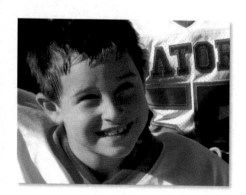 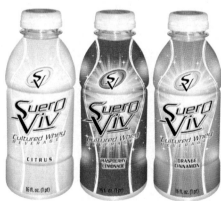

(SSSHH . . . DON'T TELL ANY OF OUR OPPONENTS!)

Probiotics for Life

Chapter 3

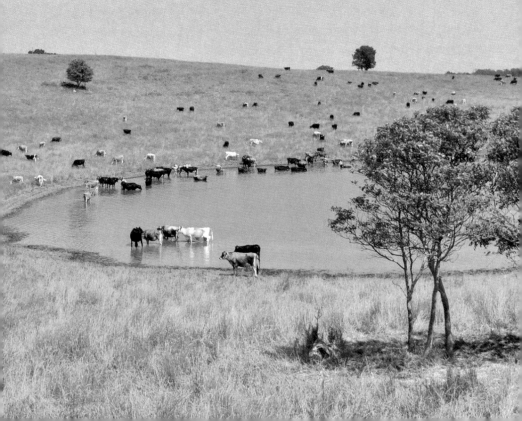

B efore I became deathly ill at the age of nineteen, I never gave a second thought to my digestive system.

Few people do when everything's working right.

Of course, that all changed the summer before my sophomore year of college, when my stomach churned like an overloaded washing machine and my bowels needed instant relief. Up until that time, I figured you ate what you enjoyed eating, drank water with your meals or when you were thirsty, and twenty-four hours later, you took care of business. Like a German Intercity train, everything would roll out of the station on time.

In principle, that's how our digestive systems should work, but according to the latest health statistics, it's apparent that far too many people live with unimaginable digestive distress these days. Dealing with gas, bloating, constipation, debilitating pain, and nausea isn't fun, and it's not a topic you typically share with neighbors or loved ones. Discussing your bathroom habits does not make for scintillating over-the-fence conversation or mealtime chitchat.

Listen, I understand. Many find it embarrassing to bring up "bathroom talk" or bodily functions, but we're going to do that because it's necessary to have a good understanding about the physiological side of digestion and how probiotics can play a key role in your overall health. Pay close attention because as Michael Gershon, M.D., author of *The Second Brain*, once said, "You take care of your gut, and your gut will take care of you."

First of all, digestion is a process that involves the chemical breakdown of the macronutrients (protein, carbohydrates, and fats) found in foods and beverages into smaller and smaller components that the body can absorb, assimilate, and utilize. The digestive system is made up of the digestive tract, which consists of a long tube of organs that runs from the mouth to the rectum and includes the esophagus, stomach, small intestine, and large intestine. Add to that already complicated order the liver, gallbladder, and pancreas, which produce important secretions for digestion that drain into the small intestine. An adult's digestive tract is about thirty feet long, or the length of a ten-yard sideline marker used at my son's Pop Warner football games.

Digestion begins the instant you take a bite of an apple or lift a forkful of food into your mouth, even though digestive secretions can begin when you smell dinner being prepared in the kitchen. Like the choreographed chaos that ensues after a quarterback yells "Hut" to start a play, all sorts of physiological things happen when you begin chewing on food.

Saliva charges out of its three-point stance and floods the mouth when the salivary glands (located under the tongue and near the lower jaw) begin producing saliva. Saliva moistens food so that it will be easier to swallow and contains a digestive enzyme called ptylin, which is a salivary amylase. Ptylin gets to work breaking down the carbohydrates, or starches and sugars, in each bite of food.

Once chewed food enters the esophagus, wavelike contractions known as *peristalsis* push the food down through the esophagus to the stomach. A muscular ring called the lower esophageal sphincter allows food to enter the stomach. Then, the lower esophageal sphincter squeezes shut to prevent food and fluid from going back up into the esophagus.

With age, stress, or poor physical condition, however, the lower esophageal sphincter can weaken, allowing food and acid to go back up the hatch. Result: heartburn and acid reflux. Left untreated, acid reflux can lead to ulcers and bleeding of the esophagus as well as increase the risk of developing cancer of the esophagus.

This juncture where the esophagus and the stomach meet is where digestive distress usually rears its ugly head. Heartburn and acid reflux are quintessential American digestive disorders that have made over-the-counter antacid products fly off the shelves. According to the latest government statistics, 25 million suffer from heartburn daily, while more than 60 million American adults endure occasional occurrences of heartburn. Men and women are affected equally, but the incidence of heartburn increases after age forty.

That's not good news for a nation that loves to celebrate every occasion with food—and lots of it. From football weekends to festive, holiday dinners, we commemorate life's richest moments—and even life's worst times—with the mouth, tongue, and stomach. The problem is that we are indulging rich, processed food six days a week and twice on Sunday while washing everything down with generous amounts of soda, caffeinated beverages, and alcohol.

That can and will spell big-time trouble for your digestive tract.

If the lower esophageal sphincter weakens for some reason, as it sometimes does with those who overeat, ferocious stomach acids can rise up into the esophagus, resulting in a burning sensation behind the breastbone lasting from a few minutes to several hours. That's why heartburn has nothing to do with the heart, even though many experience a quite-noticeable burning sensation in the cardiovascular area. The inflammation or irritation can feel like dancing flames in the upper chest. Some say when they lie down it feels like lava is eroding their tonsils.

For those fortunate enough not to deal with heartburn or acid reflux, let's continue to follow the food as the softened mass reaches the stomach, the J-shaped organ that has three tasks:

- **Store the swallowed food and liquids**

- **Mix the food and liquids with digestive juices produced by the stomach**

- **Slowly empty its contents into the small intestine**

A normal stomach can hold three pints or twenty-four ounces of food, which is enough to fill a large plate. Only a few substances, such as water and alcohol, can be absorbed directly by the stomach; the rest must undergo the "wash-and-spin" cycle that the stomach is known for. The stomach's strong muscular walls churn the food with acids and enzymes, breaking it into smaller pieces and eventually a semi-liquid form called chyme. About four hours after eating a meal, the chyme is released a little bit at a time through the pyloric sphincter, a thickened muscular ring between the stomach and the small intestine.

More digestion and absorption of food happens in the small intestine, which extends to about twenty feet in length, or two-thirds of the entire digestive system. The small intestine's twisting tubes occupy most of the lower abdomen between the stomach and the beginning of the large intestine.

You'd think that the heavy lifting in digestion happens in the large intestine, but that's not the case. Cells that line the small intestine's walls secrete enzymes to finish the breakdown of carbohydrates, fats, and proteins. Any undigested material—such as fiber from fruits and vegetables—travels next to the large intestine.

The large intestine forms an upside down U over the coiled small intestine. With a length of five to six feet—the length of your entire body!—the large intestine is comprised of three parts: the cecum, the colon, and the rectum. The cecum is a pouch at the beginning of the large intestine that allows food to pass from the small intestine to the large intestine. The middle part, the colon, is where fluids and salts are absorbed as the waste material makes its final journey to the rectum. This is where the feces is stored before being expelled from the body through the anus as a bowel movement.

When transit time for feces slows to a snail's pace, however, your body's waste stays in the colon longer, where it putrefies and typically results in toxins entering the bloodstream through the intestinal wall. This can often lead to a condition called **autointoxication**, which is a form of self-poisoning that results in noticeable symptoms such as bloating, indigestion, gas, body odor, and a lengthy list of other maladies.

When the eliminative system of the human body is not in top-notch working order, sluggish and clogged, the digestive tract cannot properly process and eliminate wastes and toxins.

Over time the toxic build-up in the colon can result in major health challenges. Health statistics show that more North Americans are hospitalized due to intestinal tract illnesses than for any other group of disorders. The medical costs of these diseases are estimated to be $20 billion or more per year, and the bloated market for laxatives, antacids, and antihemmorrhoidals tops $2 billion each year.

The idea that chronic constipation leads to autointoxication originated with physicians in ancient Egypt, according to a National Institutes of Health article. The ancient Egyptians believed that an unhealthy element in the bowels was absorbed into the general circulation, where it acted to produce fever and pus. "The ancient Greeks extended the concept of putrefaction to involve not only the residues of food, but also those of bile, phlegm, and blood, incorporating it into their humoral theory of disease," the NIH study declared.

Many factors lead to a constipated colon, which we'll get into shortly. But let's face it: autointoxication occurs because Americans have a love affair with *crap,* as signified by this acronym:

- **Coffee and cruddy foods**
- **Refined sugar and starches**
- **Alcohol**
- **Processed foods**

Autointoxication can also be extenuated by a lack of exercise, which cuts off lymphatic flow. A good workout has a way of stimulating a good bowel movement, although, in my experience, jumping on a mini-trampoline or rebounder for ten to twenty minutes is the best form of exercise to improve lymphatic flow and speed elimination. A brisk morning walk can also do the trick. President Harry Truman was famous for his "morning constitutional" strolls around Lafayette Park next to the White House, accompanied by a single Secret Service agent. (Those simpler days are long gone, of course.)

The body's immune system begins in the digestive tract, where something known as **gut-associated lymphoid tissue, or GALT**, protects the body from invasion. In fact, the intestine possesses the largest mass of lymphoid tissue in the human body and produces 70 percent of the cells within your immune system.

The immune system, which is made up of special cells, proteins, tissues, and organs, protect us against germs and infectious microorganisms every second of every day, around the clock. You could call the immune system the body's main line of defense against bacteria, viruses, fungi, and protozoans that open the door to allergies, asthma, digestive illness, skin disorders, and a whole host of acute conditions and chronic diseases.

There's another thing your digestive system must contend with, and it's the strong link between the emotions and gut health. Yo-yoing emotions and stress can do a number on your gut; just think of the "butterflies" you felt in your stomach on opening night of the school play or taking the field before the first kickoff of the season.

The effect of stress on the human bowel—the stomach, esophagus, small intestine, and colon—has been the life's work of Michael Gershon, M.D., a neurobiologist at New York City's Columbia-Presbyterian Medical Center. His thirty years of research led him to an electrifying discovery: we have two brains— the one inside our craniums and a hidden but powerful brain in the gut known as the enteric nervous system. The presence of a "second brain," Dr. Gershon said, is why we feel queasy when called to perform in public or shoot the game-winning free throw with five seconds left in double overtime.

What happens is that the nervous system in your gut, which contains an independent network of over half of the body's nerve cells, can sense 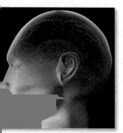 nutrients, measure acids, and trigger peristaltic waves that propel food along the digestive tract. "The brain is not the only place in the body that's full of neurotransmitters," Dr. Gershon explained. "One hundred million neurotransmitters line the length of the gut—approximately the same number found in the brain." These neurotransmitters coordinate with

The brain plays a powerful role with the body's physiological processes.

the immune system to defend your internal environment from invaders.

You need to keep your digestive system—which houses more than two-thirds of the cells that play a key role in your body's immune system—constantly replenished with probiotics. These beneficial or "good" microorganisms promote healthy digestion and normal immune system function.

I believe that being intentional about consuming probiotic-rich foods is part of the "beyond organic" lifestyle because your body needs all the weapons it can get—and in this case, probiotics are weapons of mass construction.

INTRODUCTION TO PROBIOTICS

A couple of years ago, Oprah invited Dr. Mehmet Oz, author of *You: The Owner's Manual* on to her daily television program before Dr. Oz branched off with his own health show. Oprah and Dr. Oz were yapping away when he suddenly mentioned the benefits of including probiotics in your diet.

"Pro-by-what?" asked the famous host.

Even the knowledgeable Oprah hadn't heard of probiotics, which isn't surprising. Not that many folks are aware of what probiotics—whose Latin roots mean "for life"—really are, although that number is increasing thanks to actress Jamie Lee Curtis' advertisements for a probiotic-rich yogurt. As for myself, I've known about probiotics for more than fifteen years. In fact, if you were to ask me what was the most important nutritional component of my health recovery back in San Diego, my answer would be, "Simple—probiotics."

The classic definition for probiotics follows along these lines: **probiotics are the beneficial microorganisms (bacteria and beneficial yeasts) that the body needs to promote healthy digestion, nutrient assimilation, and many other vital processes.** The main job of these beneficial microorganisms is to preserve the natural balance of microflora in the intestines 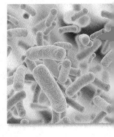 necessary for the proper digestion and assimilation of food.

When healthy intestinal flora—the "good germs"—maintain at least an 85 percent to 15 percent ratio as compared to the "bad microorganisms" in the gut, your body has the tools it needs to experience extraordinary health. When bad microorganisms gain the upper hand, however, the result is a digestive system seriously out of whack. Bellyaches, bloating, and embarrassing flatulence can make life miserable. Women have another area of concern: since live microbial organisms are also present in the vagina, the growth of undesirable microorganisms like candida yeast can cause women painful discomfort.

Probiotics are not to be confused with antibiotics, which are better understood by the public. Antibiotics have been called "wonder drugs" since their discovery in the 1930s because of their ability to cure bacteria-related illnesses such as pneumonia, tuberculosis, and meningitis—deadly diseases that have killed millions throughout history. The best-known antibiotic is penicillin, which has rescued untold millions from deadly infections, especially during wartime, and has been an effective treatment against syphilis and gonorrhea.

One time I happened to walk by a supermarket in Nashville, Tennessee, where a colorful poster had been affixed to the front window.

"Free Antibiotics!" blared the headline.

I peered for a closer look. The small print at the bottom of the poster provided the details: "Just bring in your prescription for oral antibiotics and receive it for FREE, up to a 14-day supply."

The supermarket was trying to drive new business to its pharmacy, but I also knew that many of these antibiotics were oral medicines that physicians routinely prescribe to treat children's ear infections or help adults fight off sinus problems. These antibiotics either annihilate bacteria in the body, or they weaken them so that the immune system can deliver the *coup de grâce*.

There's no doubt that human history would have to be rewritten if antibiotics like penicillin had never been discovered more than eighty years ago. Wounds, gashes, and even simple infections—like an ingrown toenail that can turn septic—are no longer deadly, and pregnant women needn't fear of dying from infection after childbirth. Infants and toddlers screaming for relief from ear infections can be helped by the right antibiotic, although prevention is always the best cure and antibiotic use, while great at relieving symptoms, may not address the root cause of the problem.

For all the good that these wonder drugs do, however, there's a downside to antibiotics that must be reckoned with. Antibiotics can be called molecules of biological warfare, destroying or compromising *all* bacteria, including the good germs. Often times, this action can leave the body temporarily without defenses, especially in the digestive tract.

Many people don't realize that they could be taking in antibiotics—and not even know it—when they eat a hamburger or a helping of cottage cheese. Antibiotics are used to keep infectious diseases down and allow for overcrowded unhealthy living conditions for conventionally raised livestock. These food-producing animals are routinely given antibiotic drugs through their feed, by injection, or even in an ear tag. When you're eating a juicy steak or spaghetti and meatballs from conventionally raised cattle, you may also be consuming antibiotics.

The same goes for dairy products. If you're drinking commercial milk or spooning popular brands of yogurt, you may also be consuming antibiotics. Dairy cows are fed a constant supply of antibiotics from birth until death because of crowded, high-stress living conditions. Every sip of commercial milk can give you the residue of up to twenty different antibiotics, painkillers, and growth hormones, according to a 2011 European study published in the *Journal of Agricultural and Food Chemistry*.

You need to counter the antibiotics you're receiving from conventionally raised meat, poultry, dairy products, eggs, medical prescriptions, and even your drinking water by intentionally looking for ways to consume probiotics, the friendly microorganisms that are good for the gut.

The biological need for probiotics begins the day you are born, a fact we kept in mind when Nicki was pregnant with our first child. Throughout her pregnancy, Nicki made it known that she wanted no part of a home birth like my mother had when I was born in Portland. That meant a hospital setting, which I was fine with.

But both of us went into the experience with our eyes open and a birth plan in hand. We were aware that many obstetricians will steer moms to Cesarean sections because they are practicing defensive medicine and don't want to be sued in case something tragic happens in the birthing room. Nicki and I came to an agreement, however, that we would use a nurse midwife to deliver our first child, and we would only resort to a C-section if *absolutely* necessary.

There were two reasons we felt that way. One, a Cesarean section is major abdominal surgery with high complication rates ranging between 20 percent to 50 percent. The complications include hemorrhaging, infection, damage to other organs, and four to seven times an increased risk of maternal death.

The main reason for our reluctance, though, was that we wanted to give our son—we knew in advance that we were having a boy—his first dose of probiotics.

When labor began, our son would be pushed through the birth canal, where he would be exposed to beneficial bacteria and yeasts as he slipped through. I was aware that bifidobacteria from the mother's birth canal would colonize the infant's internal environment and give the baby's immune system its first infusion of probiotics such as *Bifidobacterium lactis ssp infantis*, *Bifidobacteria bifidum*, and *Bifidobacteria breve*.

The way I saw things, this would be our son's first probiotic bath.

Nicki didn't find the natural route easy. My poor wife agonized through twenty hours of long labor before Joshua Michael Rubin entered the world, collecting his first probiotic boost. Then after he took his first breath of life, Joshua received another ingestion of friendly bacteria when he began to breast feed, receiving in his mother's milk specific oligosaccharides that promoted the growth of bifidobacteria in his squeaky-clean colon.

I'm tremendously grateful for what Nicki endured during a very difficult delivery—and for being committed to breastfeeding our son. We both believed that nothing matched the high-quality nutrients and probiotics found in breast milk.

As Joshua grew, we managed to avoid those common ear infections that send many mothers into pediatricians' offices to receive a prescription for antibiotics. When Joshua was old enough to handle solid foods, we introduced him to egg yolk from pastured-raised chickens, organic avocado, banana, homemade chicken soup, and other fruits, and vegetables, as well as pastured-raised dairy products. Not only were these foods healthier for him and grown without pesticides, but the organically raised meat, produce, and dairy products were sure to be free of antibiotic residues that are commonly found in conventionally grown or raised foods.

Another reason commercially raised livestock are pumped full of antibiotics is so they can fatten as fast as possible. Seventy-five years ago, steers were four or five years old when they were led to the slaughterhouse. That age fell to two or three years in the 1960s. Today, "production" cattle are fattened up in as little as fourteen to sixteen months before being processed into roasts, steaks, and hamburger that are packaged for sale in your local supermarket. Antibiotics help keep cattle free from infections, which allow them to gain weight more efficiently on an unnatural grain diet.

But those antibiotics and other toxins remain part of the meat after the cattle are taken to market, which reminds me of a saying I love to repeat at my seminars: "You've heard it said that you are what you eat, but when it comes to animal food, remember that you are what *they* ate."

Don't believe me? Just ask Alberto Contador, the three-time winner of the Tour de France bike race. Following a stage race during the 2010 Tour, the Spanish rider tested positive for a banned drug—Clenbuterol—that is illegally used in the livestock industry to accelerate growth and increase muscle mass in cattle. The Spanish rider blamed his test result on tainted meat that he and his teammates ate during a rest day in the Tour de France.

Listen, I harbor no sympathies for athletes who test positive for banned substances in their system. (Contador also tested positive for a type of chemical called a plasticizer that is found in plastic IV bags. Evidence of that chemical in an athlete's urine could mean the athlete used a blood transfusion to boost endurance, a practiced banned by the World Anti-Doping Agency.)

I only relay Contador's story to illustrate the idea that if *your* blood was tested after consuming a conventionally raised, grain-fed ribeye or farm-raised "Atlantic salmon," lab technicians would probably find some eyebrow-raising results as well. You would be shocked to learn what cattle producers are putting in animal feed before taking them to market. It's no secret that our nation's livestock are fed with grain containing nitrates and antibiotics and pumped with bacteria-killing medicines to keep them somewhat healthy or even alive.

Then there are the medicines that humans willingly take every day after receiving a prescription for antibiotics from their family physician. All they have to do is step inside a doctor's office complaining of a bacterial infection, sinus problem, or possible STD, and often times they will walk out with a prescription for Amoxicillin, Lephalexin, or Ampicillin in their hands. Many parents don't feel they've done enough for their son or daughter's earache if their pediatrician doesn't write an antibiotic prescription, so they rant and rave until their doctor caves in, often reluctantly.

Other types of pharmaceutical prescriptions leave men and women needing a probiotic boost as well. Birth control pills, along with anti-cholesterol medications, antidepressants, and blood-thinning drugs can leave their digestive tract with a low balance of probiotics, which opens the door to gastrointestinal problems.

Those who wash down their meds with tap water should know that traces of antibiotics, antidepressants, birth control pills, painkillers, and cholesterol-lowering medicines have been detected in water supplies and combined with the chlorine used to treat the water, make for one powerful probiotic destroying duo. People often dispose of unused medicines by flushing them down the toilet, and human waste can contain incompletely metabolized medicines. These trace amounts reach conventional sewage treatment facilities, and from there, the "reclaimed" water can enter waterways, lakes, and even aquifers.

Those who like a latte on the way to work are also in need of a probiotic boost. Caffeine has always been known to stimulate the digestive system because it inhibits an enzyme thought to regulate mucosal secretions in the small intestine. When the secretions go up, the fluid in your bowel rises, and if the amount of fluid in your colon is greater than the amount of fluid you can reabsorb, you better scout out a restroom fast. High levels of caffeine lower the immune system, stress out the adrenal glands, and make the body more susceptible to disease and infection.

Sugar—especially refined sugar—has a way of feeding the "bad" microorganisms in the intestines. One such organism, a yeast called *Candida albicans*, absolutely *loves* sugar. Eating too many sugary foods causes Candida and thrush to thrive and feeds harmful bacteria that irritate the lining of the GI tract.

Starches such as bread, pasta, rice, corn, and potatoes are more difficult to digest as well. What happens in the digestive process is that some undigested carbohydrates remain in the large intestine instead of being safely eliminated from the body. When unabsorbed carbohydrates camp out in the colon, they feed harmful microbes and upset the balance of the intestinal flora and unleash a perfect storm for digestive issues to rear their ugly heads.

There's another perfect storm in the air that we breathe—in our homes. In my home state of Florida, where it's merely warm six months of the year and blazing hot the other half of the year, we breathe recirculated air around the clock because we're usually indoors (except when there's a Tiny Mite football game) or driving around in a car with the air conditioning on.

Today's well-insulated homes and energy-efficient doors and windows trap "used" air that's filled with harmful particles such as carbon dioxide, nitrogen dioxide, and pet dander. Declining indoor air quality has been linked to the rise of asthma and allergies, especially in children, as well as immunologic problems.

Finally, there is a strong link between emotional responses such as anger, bitterness, and resentment and gut health. There's a reason why friends will ask friends, "What's eating you?" When people hold on to a grudge or can't let go of the past, their health takes a hit. These deadly emotions will produce toxins similar to bingeing on a dozen glazed doughnuts.

When you're down in the dumps is not the time to reach for a sugary treat.

It's the time to reach for a probiotic-rich food.

THE HISTORY OF PROBIOTICS

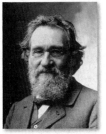

Dr. Elie Metchnikoff is known as the "Father of Probiotics."

I'm a little young to have a "bucket list," but if I did, one of the places I'd love to visit would be the Caucasus Mountains in Bulgaria, a country situated in southeastern Europe and bordering Romania and Serbia. Bulgarian peasants, who live in remote mountain hamlets, reputedly have unusually long life spans. I think it would be interesting to meet these people and learn what they eat to remain so healthy.

My idea came from reading about a Russian microbiologist named Élie Metchnikoff, who studied the remarkable Bulgarians for their longevity a century ago. Born in 1845 in the Ukraine, Metchnikoff earned a glowing reputation for work on immunity from infectious diseases. He, together with Paul Ehrlich, captured the Nobel Prize for Physiology and Medicine in 1908.

Metchnikoff was in his early sixties when he was catapulted to fame. Like anyone getting up there in years, he was contemplating his mortality. For the life of him, so to speak, he couldn't understand why normal life expectancy in humans wasn't 120 years. He was confident that scientific theories and techniques would someday prevent premature old age and senility.

Metchnikoff speculated that senility might be due to illnesses caused by an abnormal ration of intestinal bacteria, which, in turn, were caused by toxins present in the diet. The Russian researcher laid all the blame on the large intestine, which was "the reservoir of the waste of the digestive processes, and the waste stagnating long enough to putrefy," he said. "The products of putrefaction are harmful."

As Metchnikoff continued his investigative inquiry into aging, someone told him to check into the Bulgarian peasants living in the Caucasus Mountains, who tended to live to a ripe old age. They certainly did live a long time—an average of eighty-seven years. This was double the average life expectancy of Europeans in the early 1900s, which stood in the mid-forties at the time. In the Bulgarian steppes, however, living to be 100 years old was more the rule than the exception.

Why did the Bulgarian peasants live so long, especially in an underdeveloped country lacking basic medical care? What Metchnikoff learned was that the Bulgarian peasants consumed large amounts of a cultured dairy beverage known simply as "sour milk."

Back in those days, the Bulgarian peasants didn't have any refrigerators, so they would lug a tin pail of fresh cow's milk to the family cellar. The peasants drank some of the milk, but they left what they didn't immediately consume—which was sometimes quite a bit—in the cellar, where it would culture and thicken over the next several days. The result was a tangy beverage they called "sour milk," whose modern-day equivalents would be the yogurt and kefir found in health food stores and high-end grocery stores today.

The Bulgarians really had a thing for this "sour milk," which became known in Europe as Crème Bulgare. According to Metchnikoff's empirical observations, consuming Crème Bulgare caused the Bulgarian bowels to become acidic and form an inhospitable environment for the unfriendly bacteria, yeasts, viruses, and parasites that would otherwise produce toxins.

For his groundbreaking work, Metchnikoff is known today as the "Father of Probiotics" and is quite the health legend.

Another health legend in my book, a Cleveland dentist named Dr. Weston A. Price, also contributed to my understanding of probiotics. Tired of seeing tooth decay in his patients that kept him drilling like a Texas wildcatter, Dr. Price came up with an idea: why not go out and find the world's healthiest populations and study what they were eating to stay healthy?

Dr. Weston A. Price studied the world's healthiest populations in the 1930s.

He came up with this brainstorm in the early 1930s, when he was sixty years of age and rather well off. For the rest of the decade, Dr. Price and his wife, Florence, traveled around the world on steamships, prop planes, trains, automobiles, canoes, and on foot, befriending and then studying indigenous people whose teeth and gums were untouched by processed foods.

Dr. Price made two trips in 1931 and 1932 to the remote Lötschental Valley in the Swiss Alps—and he had to hike in because the valley was accessible only by foot. He lived among the simple farmers and shepherds who dwelled in centuries-old wooden chalets and studied what they ate. The unaffected townsfolk, who numbered around 2,000, were surrounded on three sides by glaciers and towering granite peaks. They subsisted on what could be grown on small plots of level land in the valley or what they raised from cows and goats grazing on lush alpine slopes in the summertime.

This meant a simple diet: fruits and vegetables from their backyard plots, dairy products from their livestock, eggs from chickens, and *roggenbrot*—or rye bread— from rye grown in the valley. Eating meat was a Sunday-only experience, except when bones and leftover cuts were used to make a hearty soup.

Dairy products like milk, butter, and cream were probiotic-rich sources of vitamins A and D that helped the villagers live incredibly healthy lives. The people of the Lötschental Valley "have neither a physician nor a dentist because they have so little need for them," Dr. Price wrote in his book, *Nutrition and Physical Degeneration*.

I retraced Dr. Price's footsteps in the Lötschental Valley on a 2005 trip to Switzerland, although I didn't have to hike in thanks to an excellent two-lane highway tunnel that bore through the Alps. I became a *roggenbrot* fan and left with a greater appreciation for cultured dairy products and their incredible health benefits.

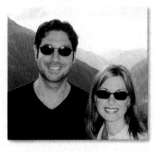

Three years after visiting Switzerland, Dr. Price traveled to the African continent and stayed with a warrior tribe in Kenya and Tanzania known as the Maasai tribe. The American dentist was impressed with their towering stature and physical prowess. The average male stood well over six feet tall with perfect teeth, strong bones, and no intestinal diseases. The tall women gave birth easily to robust babies.

No symptoms associated with autointoxication could be found in the Maasai tribe members, although the same couldn't be said for the white colonists who crossed Dr. Price's path in the backwoods of Africa. They dealt with many of the same health challenges we face today. Then again, they lived off sugar, white flour, canned foods, and processed condensed milk shipped in from home.

Compare that to the Maasai tribe members, who kept things simple. They herded cows, cultured and drank their milk, and even drank the blood of the animals they slaughtered, as well as the meat with all the fat. The Maasai didn't eat much of anything else but were in incredibly great shape, especially compared to the pasty Europeans.

Health pioneers like Dr. Weston A. Price and Élie Metchnikoff blazed a healthy trail that ignited my passion for finding the healthiest, probiotic-rich foods to eat and drink. When I say that probiotics were the most important nutritional component of my health recovery back in San Diego, there was one type of microorganism that stood above the rest and became my true "probiotic hero."

I'm talking about probiotics from the *Bacillus* genus. My road to wellness was paved with probiotic-rich cultured dairy and a powdered compound containing probiotics from the *Bacillus* genus such as *subtilis, licheniformis,* and *coagulans.*

I first heard about *Bacillus coagulans* back in the 1990s when I read abstracts of human clinical studies conducted in India using this probiotic. *Bacillus coagulans* is a spore-forming bacterium that survives the hostile environment of the stomach, colonizes the intestines, and produces lactic acid, which are all components to the success of a good probiotic.

Bacillus coagulans was first isolated in 1932 by German scientists L.M. Horowitz-Wlassowa and N.W. Nowotelnow. Further research confirmed that upon activation of spore formation in the acidic environment of the stomach, *Bacillus coagulans* can germinate and proliferate in the intestines and produce lactic acid, which are critical factors to the success of a probiotic.

Today, one can find foods and supplements containing *Bacillus*-based probiotics, including Primal Defense, which is the dietary supplement that launched Garden of Life. As for me, I consume them daily and recommend them to everyone I meet.

THE TOP PROBIOTIC FOODS

My long journey to restore my body and my life taught me the keys to helping many other people with their health, and my first recommendation invariably is to boost their probiotics.

My list of top probiotic foods starts with cultured or fermented vegetables such as sauerkraut, pickles, pickled carrots, beets, and cucumbers, which supply the body with lots of probiotics. Although these fermented vegetables are often greeted with upturned noses at the dinner table, these foods help reestablish natural balance to your digestive system. Cultured vegetables like sauerkraut are brimming with vitamins, such as vitamin C, and contain almost four times the amount of certain nutrients as unfermented cabbage. The *lactobacilli* in fermented vegetables contain digestive enzymes that help break down food and increase its digestibility.

The following examples of fermented vegetables from foreign lands are cultured foods that contain probiotics, and I encourage you to try them sometime. I have, and I'm better off for having done so. They are:

- **Kimchi from South Korea**
- **Natto, miso, and soy sauce from Japan**
- **Sauerkraut from Germany**

Kimchi, a spicy blend of fermented cabbage and other veggies, has been called South Korea's national dish. Koreans serve kimchi at almost every meal, and few can last more than a couple of days without this condiment before cravings get the better of them. Some like to spice up their Korean version of sauerkraut with other vegetables like onions, garlic, and red hot chili peppers.

The Japanese like to spice up their rice with **natto**, which is made from soaked and fermented soybeans. Long a popular condiment in Japan, natto has a reputation for being an extremely healthy food with health benefits backed by years of research and studies. If you've ever wondered why the Japanese population has one of the highest life expectancy rates in the world, then natto has to take partial credit for the way it supports cardiovascular health, a healthy immune system, and the digestive system. Natto, brimming with bacillus-based probiotics, is considered Japan's "miracle food."

The sticking point is taste and aroma. Natto has a stinky smell that can be a stumbling block for American palates. If you're going to give it a try, then natto is best eaten when served over whole grain rice.

Miso is much better known—and accepted—in this country, where miso soup is often used as a starter in Japanese restaurants. Rich in fiber, protein, vitamins, and minerals, miso soup is an excellent entry point for fermented foods from foreign lands, especially if you're not used to eating cultured foods.

Another Japanese cultured food is actually a condiment that Americans are familiar with is **soy sauce**, which is another form of fermented soybeans. Several microbes, including friendly yeast and *Lactobacillus acidophilus,* are used in the fermentation process of soy sauce, which, when properly prepared and unpasteurized, is a healthy probiotic-rich food. The problem is that commercial soy sauce—the handful of brands that dominate our supermarket shelves—is manufactured using organic acids and not living microbes, presumably to lower the manufacturing costs. That's why I make sure I use a non-pasteurized organic brand of soy sauce made from organic soybeans, mountain spring water, and sea salt. Another cultured soy product worth mentioning is **tempeh**, which is similar to a firm vegetarian burger patty.

If the taste and texture of soy is not your thing, **sauerkraut** might be up your alley, even though this form of pickled cabbage is rarely found on American plates unless it's Oktoberfest. That's a pity because sauerkraut is one of the few foods containing the bacterium *Lactobacilli plantarum*, which is a digestive All-Star that should be penciled into your food lineup whenever possible.

Don't run down to your local supermarket and pull a bottle of commercially prepared sauerkraut off the shelf, however. The Food and Drug Administration recommends that commercial sauerkraut be pasteurized, which effectively destroys all the beneficial bacteria. You should look for raw, unpasteurized sauerkraut in health food stores.

Another raw, unpasteurized condiment that I enjoy is a **"living" salsa** made through a lacto-fermentation process instead of vinegar, which is how most commercial salsa is made in this country.

I also want to give a shout-out to **umeboshi plums**, which are not really plums but are a Japanese fruit that is more related to the apricot. Pickled in a seasoned liquid, these extremely sour and salty fruits are served as side dishes for rice or used in Asian cooking.

After sampling a tangy umeboshi plum, you may want to reach for a probiotic-rich beverage to sip on. I say, "sip" because **kombucha** and **kvass** are two beverages that you don't want to gulp down quickly to cool off on a hot August afternoon.

You may have seen bottles of kombucha in your local natural food grocery, where it's become popular in the last decade. Russian in origin and tart as a Granny Smith apple, kombucha (pronounced *kom-BOO-cha*) is a lacto-fermented beverage with probiotics and enzymes that delivers a cidery flavor and a kick of fizziness.

Kombucha is made from black or green tea and a SCOBY (symbiotic culture of bacteria and yeast)—also known as a kombucha "mushroom" that is a pancake-shaped mass of bacteria and yeast. The mixture ferments for a week or more, resulting in slightly sweet and slightly sour beverage containing a long list of amino acids, B vitamins, and living things like *Acetobacter* bacteria and *Brettanomyces bruxellensis, Candida stellata, Schizosaccharomyces pombe, Torulaspora delbrueckii* and other yeasts.

As I mentioned earlier, kombucha is extremely popular, but you must sip slowly, not sucking down more than four ounces or so at a time. Kombucha has developed a following as more and more health food stores stock this "sparkling Himalayan tonic" in the refrigerated case. In the last few years, though, kombucha has lost a bit of its luster as tests revealed that nearly all major brands contained alcohol and some varieties a significant amount of alcohol—enough to cause some kombucha drinkers to fail breathalyzer tests. If you're trying to avoid alcohol, then it's best to find another cultured beverage to consume.

Kvass, (pronounced *kuh-VAHSS*), is another drink reputed to be Russian in origin. A fermented beverage made from rye, barley, or beets, kvass tastes a bit like beer or ale—but this cultured beverage isn't alcoholic. Those who appreciate kvass say that opening a bottle of kvass releases a fragrant bouquet reminiscent of freshly baked bread cooling on a windowsill.

Kvass is hard to find in this country except in New York City, where there's a large Russian immigrant population. But Kvass can be purchased online and is worth trying—at least one time.

CULTURED DAIRY: SAVING THE BEST FOR LAST

I've traveled to France a few times, and one of the first things that Nicki and I enjoy doing after we arrive in a new city is search for the closest *laiterie*—a store that sells fresh dairy products.

You know how most couples go to France and fall in love? Well, I went to France and fell in love all right—with brebis, which is yogurt made from sheep's milk. Talk about a creamy, delicious cultured dairy product that is nearly impossible to find in the States. I love stocking up on a half-dozen brebis yogurts and taking them back to the refrigerator in our hotel room.

Cultured dairy products like brebis have been around for centuries, from Iran to Greece to Finland, but we get our word *yogurt* from the Turkish word *yoğurt*. Up until Élie Metchnikoff's time, the only people eating cultured yogurt in abundance were farmers and their families in Eastern Europe and Central Asia.

Then Metchnikoff single-handedly started a yogurt craze in Western Europe.

The first industrial production of yogurt was recorded in 1919, in Barcelona, Spain, when an enterprising Spaniard named Isaac Carasso began using bacterial cultures obtained from the Pasteur Institute. In 1929, Carasso opened a plant in Paris and named his company Danone after the name of his son, Daniel. His sales pitch: eat the "Dessert of Happy Digestion."

But commercial yogurt, which came in only two flavors in those early days—plain and plainer—wasn't an overnight success. The tart taste that puckered lips wasn't an immediate hit with city dwellers, who were discovering another form of dairy, thanks to the rising availability of refrigeration. I'm talking about ice cream—*glace* in French and *gelato* in Italian—and its sweet flavors: vanilla, chocolate, strawberry, and pistachio.

In the mid-1950s, though, yogurt finally caught the fancy of the French. A few years later, Carasso gained a beachhead in the United States when he opened a factory in New York. He changed the brand name to Dannon to make it sound more American.

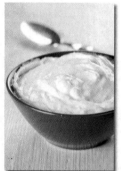

Plain yogurt was still a tough sell until the late 1960s, when yogurt manufacturers, like Dannon, tore a page from the ice cream playbook: *Let's make more flavors and make it sweeter!* They added natural and artificial fruit flavors as well as sugar, and *voilá,* instead of a pasteurized tangy product languishing in a specialty market, yogurt with "fruit on the bottom" became a sweet sensation with a pleasing tart aftertaste. Suddenly, you had yogurt manufacturers falling all over themselves to create new flavors like maple syrup, blueberry cheesecake, apple cinnamon, and piña colada.

The healthiest yogurt doesn't come with sugary "fruit on the bottom."

You won't find piña colada yogurt in our refrigerator, however. I think a healthier alternative is plain sheep's milk yogurt with honey and fruit added, which has been a big hit around our house. Another cultured dairy product that I'm a huge fan of is kefir, which I learned to drink during my San Diego health experience.

Sold in ready-to-drink quart bottles, this tart-tasting, thick beverage contains naturally occurring bacteria and yeast that work synergistically to provide health benefits superior to yogurt. Kefir is also a great base ingredient to build smoothies around: just add eight ounces of kefir into a blender, an assortment of frozen berries or fruits, a spoonful of honey, and you're well on the way to whipping up a delicious, satisfying smoothie.

Yogurt and kefir are wonderful examples of cultured dairy, but the commercial versions have always left me wanting. I prefer whole milk organic kefir, plain and tart—in other words, without added flavorings. But purchasing grass-fed, organic yogurt and kefir from true whole milk has been a challenge and a logistical difficulty. At times I've had to drive to a parking lot behind a Palm Beach strip mall to purchase my cultured dairy from a local farmer who drives into town in a white van with picnic coolers topped off with fresh-from-the-pasture milk, yogurt, and kefir. Customers, in turn, bring their own coolers and cash.

These type of transactions have inherent challenges and are not likely to work long term. As I continued on my new journey to create some of the world's healthiest foods, I knew I wanted to produce some form of cultured dairy that would be "beyond organic." Then I remembered a cultured dairy drink that I had tried in South Africa called *maas.*

Five years ago, I traveled to South Africa to speak at two conferences, and while in Johannesburg, Nicki and I met up with Carol Green, a talented executive chef from South Africa. Carol had traveled to the States on several occasions to help me tape cooking segments for my syndicated television show, *Extraordinary Health*. She wanted to show us around Johannesburg and help us get a lay of the land.

We visited several health food stores in Jo'burg as well as a couple of grocery stores. It was in the latter that she introduced us to *maas*, a traditional food inspired by the Maasai tribe that was also called *amasai*. My ears perked up because I had heard of the Maasai tribe from my reading of Dr. Price's book.

Maas, Carol explained, was widely consumed in South Africa, and its preparation has been handed down generation after generation. The traditional method to make it was to start with a calabash, or a dried gourd from a tree. You drop a few cups of rice or corn with hot water into the calabash and shake it around to remove all the loose seeds. Then you rinse out the gourd a few more times.

Next, you pour in fresh milk and allow the dairy to "improve" or culture for about three days, depending on the temperature and the taste you want. The first batch will probably not taste good and will need to be thrown out until the calabash is seasoned.

The next time around, when the *maas* is ready, you pour out two-thirds and refill the gourd with more milk. You leave everything to ferment for many hours until it's ready.

I liked the *maas* I tried in South Africa very much, and when I purchased our land in southern Missouri, I wondered if there was some way to replicate or produce a cultured dairy product like *maas*. Our research-and-development team put their heads together, and I believe that we have created a beverage that will soon be the next generation of cultured diary.

IT'S CALLED BEYOND ORGANIC AMASAI.

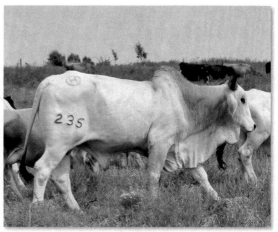

Just as yogurt became popular in the 1960s in this country, just as kefir made a splash ten years ago, Amasai is the next innovation in cultured beverages. With the taste, nutrient density, and acceptability of a cow's milk product coupled with the tolerability of a sheep or goat's milk product, I believe Amasai has all the earmarks of a sensational cultured beverage.

I feel confident making this bold statement because of the type of cattle that we use to produce Amasai. Our cattle have, in many ways, the same genetic makeup—or genotype—as the African cattle herded and milked by the Maasai tribe. These cattle originated out of the "cradle of civilization"—India, Africa, and the Middle East—and differ from 99.9 percent of the dairy-producing cattle in the U.S. today. **The cows we milk to create our Amasai genetically resemble the cattle that have nourished civilizations since the days of the Bible.**

We don't believe there is anything in America like our cultured dairy produced by our selective breeding and feeding program. That's one of the main reasons why our Amasai is such a powerful food.

We use an "old school" approach to breeding cattle at Beyond Organic Ranch.

A TART BUT SMOOTH TASTE

Beyond Organic Amasai, delivered from our farm to your family, is a beverage that you can pour into a glass and drink. It's like a smoothie, but you can also use it as an ingredient in many beverages and foods. (See the Beyond Organic Recipes in the Appendix for Amasai-containing smoothies, meals, snacks, and desserts.)

I think it tastes great, but I'll admit that I'm slightly biased. The taste is tart yet smooth, kind of a cross between yogurt, kefir, and sour cream. I really don't know how else to describe it except to say that I think I know *why* Amasai tastes so good.

We use true whole milk to produce Amasai—something you can hardly find in a natural food store or supermarket these days. Nearly all commercial and organic whole milk is 3.5 to 3.7 percent fat, but our fat percentage varies between 4.2 to 4.9 percent fat.

I know what you're thinking: *Isn't that too much fat?*

Far from it. First of all, you're receiving everything that's coming out of the cow, so you can't get more natural than that. As I've often said, if God wanted milk to be skimmed, He would have put a cream separator on the cow's udder.

Since we're not skimming any fat, the result is a healthy balance of fats and proteins with natural levels of fat-soluble vitamins like A, D, K, and E, which our bodies need in a great way. The GreenFed aspect of Amasai—the green grazing and feeding program—and the Olde World culturing technique inspired by the traditional recipe of the Maasai tribe, helps us offer a unique and delicious beverage cultured with over thirty different probiotics.

In addition, we create a safe and healthy product by employing a long-term, low-temperature pasteurization of our fresh milk prior to culturing, which leaves delicate proteins in their whole, undenatured state. Pasteurization—named after the 19th century French scientist Louis Pasteur—kills any contaminating organisms through a process of quickly raising the temperature of the milk to 180 degrees Fahrenheit and keeping it there for a number of seconds to kill off bacteria and pathogenic microorganisms.

Public health drove the need for pasteurization in the early decades of the 20th century. Before pasteurization, you literally put your life—or your children's lives—at risk when you served industrially produced milk because cows were routinely fed a mixture of waste grain from distilleries. The cows became diseased and emaciated, and coupled with poor sanitation and zero refrigeration, commercial milk killed thousands of adults, youngsters, and babies each year. Pasteurization was viewed as the solution to the growing "milk problem."

The problem with high-temperature pasteurization is that heating the milk to that elevated a temperature kills probiotics, destroys enzymes, and alters the protein and fat in milk. "In spite of modern techniques of pasteurization, high-temperature pasteurized milk is dead milk that will rot on standing," contends William Campbell Douglass II, M.D. and author of *The Milk Book.*

I sought a different path that would ensure product safety for Amasai while not destroying what's so good and healthy about our cultured dairy beverage. Our long-term, low-temperature pasteurization method provides that pathway, taking up to 180 times longer than high-temperature pasteurization or ultra-heat treatment that is commonly used today. This allows for the proteins and certain microbes to remain intact to be gently pre-digested by the probiotics. This measure of safety allows Amasai to be sold legally in all 50 states. In addition, our Olde World culturing process, which takes two-and-a-half to four times longer than modern yogurt, ensures that there are more than thirty live probiotic cultures that create a wide array of beneficial compounds, including organic acids and enzymes.

The question of pasteurization was also on the forefront of our minds when we started making a cheese that can only be described as "beyond organic." The result is our **Beyond Organic GreenFed Raw Cheese** containing enzymes and probiotics and never heated above cow body temperature, which is around 101 degrees Fahrenheit. This means our cheese is "really raw" as compared to cheeses labeled as raw, even though those cheese makers are legally allowed to heat the milk to just under pasteurization temperature—a process that negatively impacts important probiotics and enzymes—and continue to call it "raw." We believe our healthy milk from our genetically selected cows and artisanal production methods make a considerable different in quality and taste. Our Beyond Organic GreenFed Raw Cheese is both delicious and nutritious.

No discussion on probiotic cultured foods and beverages would be complete without discussing **SueroViv™**, the cultured whey beverage that I introduced in the last chapter. In fact, this living beverage not only contains probiotics but also enzymes, vitamins, minerals, and electrolytes.

As someone who experienced the life-transforming power of cultured dairy foods and beverages while on the road back to good health, I'm greatly excited about Beyond Organic's Amasai, GreenFed Raw Cheese, and SueroViv.

You should be, too, especially if you need a probiotic boost.

THE TOP 10 PROBIOTIC FOODS

1. AMASAI not only contains probiotics, but this cultured beverage also contains pre-digested proteins that make it highly digestible.

2. REALLY RAW CHEESE such as Beyond Organic Raw Cheese is a source of probiotics and nutrients. With its portability, ease of storage, and calcium and fat-soluble vitamins, raw cheese is an awesome probiotic-rich food.

3. CULTURED WHEY, which is found in SueroViv, contains vitamins, minerals, enzymes, and probiotic microorganisms.

4. CULTURED VEGGIES such as kimchi, organic soy sauce, and properly prepared sauerkraut, add spice and vigor to meals. These condiments, popular outside our country, really need to be included more in the American diet.

5. KVASS, a Russian staple of refreshment for centuries, has a malty taste with a sweet finish and light sparkle. This probiotic beverage of the first rank is slowly finding its ways into finer natural foods stores but is readily available online.

6. NATTO, a fermented soybean paste with an unappetizing smell, is full of *Bacillus subtilis* spores as well as other wonderful probiotic nutrients. You'll have to shop at Asian markets or well-stocked natural food stores to find this amazing Japanese import.

7. PROBIOTIC SALSA may resemble commercial salsa, but that's where the similarity ends. Rejuvenative Foods makes my favorite "living" salsa.

8. KEFIR will always have a place in my heart after I drank quart after quart of this thick probiotic beverage during my health comeback in San Diego.

9. KOMBUCHA is much more widely available than its Russian cousin, kvass. This fizzy fermented beverage is made from black or green tea and a fungus culture.

10. YOGURT deserves to be on any Top 10 list, especially if you can find sheep's milk or goat's milk yogurt.

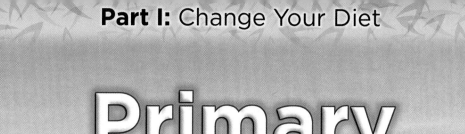

Primary
Protein
Chapter 4

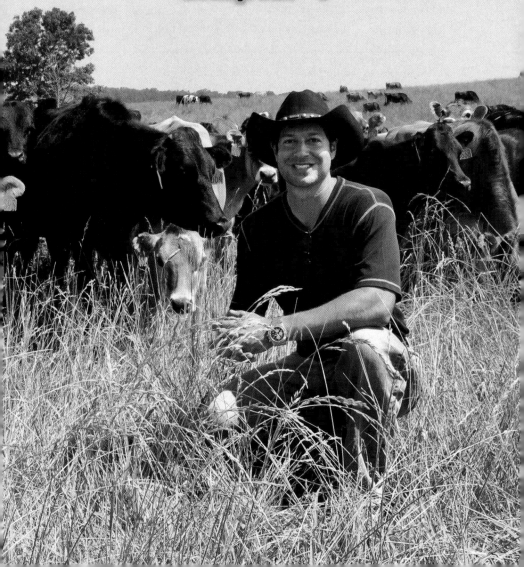

Whether you're reading *Live Beyond Organic* in paperback form or viewing pixels on a Kindle or iPad screen, I want you to stop and look at your arms and hands for a moment, even down to the tips of your fingernails.

What you're seeing beyond your flesh, bones, and sinews is **protein**—the major constituent of every living cell and body fluid, except for bile and urine. Responsible for building and repairing tissue, protein ranks as the most important nutrient that your body needs—even more important than carbohydrates and fats. If you don't consume enough protein, your body will wither and become very weak—so feeble that you wouldn't have the energy to hold this book or e-reader in your hands.

The word protein is derived from the Latin term *proteus*, which means "of primary importance" or "that which comes first." Proteins are the essential building blocks of the body, the foundation that the body relies upon to transport oxygen, contract muscles, transport electrons, and replace tissues. Most muscles, organs, and hormones are comprised of protein. Since the human body simply does not store proteins for later use, as it does with carbs and fats, you have to continually replenish the body's stores by consuming various protein-containing foods.

When you eat protein-rich foods such as meat, poultry, fish, dairy products, eggs, and beans, the digestive juices in your stomach and intestines go to work. They break down the proteins in food into basic units called amino acids, which can then be reused to make the proteins your body needs to maintain muscles, bones, blood, and body organs.

All proteins are combinations of twenty-two amino acids, eight of which are "essential" nutrients for adults (nine for children). Your body can make fourteen of these amino acids without you ever knowing it, but the other eight amino acids *must* be supplied by a healthy diet that includes protein-rich foods.

These eight essential amino acids, which come from animal sources such as beef, chicken, fish, eggs, and dairy, are known as "complete" sources of protein because they supply all the essential amino acids in the appropriate ratio. These amino acids are considered "essential" because the body cannot create them—they must be derived from the diet. On the other hand, vegetarian sources are incomplete proteins because they do not supply all the essential amino acids. This doesn't mean, however, that vegetarians or vegans can't survive because you can combine several top-quality vegetable proteins together to form a complete protein, but that takes work and some knowhow.

That's why I remind those choosing not to eat meat and dairy products to be very intentional about what's on their menu. Protein is *that* important. Besides driving the engine of growth and development within your body, protein does the following tasks without complaint:

- **Provides the body with energy**
- **Manufactures hormones, antibodies, enzymes, and tissues**
- **Helps maintain the proper acid-alkaline balance in your body**

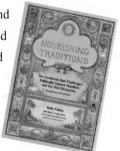

The body's other main sources of macronutrients, fats, and carbohydrates, are unable to do what protein does handily—build strong bodies, burn fat, repair the daily wear of vital muscles, and replace body chemicals. While carbs fuel the body and fats are a vital source of energy, protein wears many hats. Sally Fallon, author of *Nourishing Traditions*, said the human body assembles and utilizes about 50,000 different proteins to form organs, nerves, muscles and flesh, which is why proteins are called the building blocks of human life.

Many Americans naturally add protein to their three square meals each day. Scrambled eggs and toast in the morning. A sandwich filled with chunks of turkey for lunch. Hamburgers or grilled chicken for dinner. Since providing your body with a healthy source of protein is vital, the question becomes: *What are the best, most effective sources of protein?*

You're going to find the most complete, healthy sources of protein from:

- **Organically raised, pasture-fed cattle, sheep, goats, buffalo, and venison**
- **Pastured poultry and eggs**
- **Cultured dairy products derived from cow's milk, goat's milk, and sheep's milk.**

And don't forget about wild-caught fish with scales and fins caught from oceans and rivers, which also provide the eight essential amino acids along with healthy fats.

These protein-rich foods can sustain you for a long time, which contrasts with the quick and relatively short energy provided by grains and fruits since they are high in starches and sugars. While you'll hear people argue about whether meat or dairy products are healthy to eat, I can assure you that these foods are wonderful, or Jesus wouldn't have consumed them, nor Abraham, Isaac, Jacob, David, and Solomon. Throughout the Bible, whenever there was a feast, they killed the fatted calf or lamb. Throughout the march of history in biblical times, they consumed healthy dairy products. And today we can as well.

At the risk of further offending my vegetarian and vegan friends, I must clearly state that animal foods are the best sources of protein. What vegetarians must do—especially the strict ones—is exercise constant vigilance. While nuts, seeds, legumes, cereal grains, and fermented soy products are decent protein sources, vegetarians have to be careful to give their bodies enough protein to provide essential amino acids like methionine, cysteine, and cystine, which are crucial to the brain and nervous system. Lacto-ovo vegetarians have an easier time of it because they can consume high-quality protein sources such as eggs and cultured dairy.

The bottom line is that it's crucial for vegetarians and vegans to be proactive about what they choose to eat. But for the rest of this chapter, I will assume that you consume meat and dairy products as I do and will share information accordingly. Since it's vital that you give your body a variety of protein sources throughout the day, the first category we'll start with is cultured dairy products.

CULTURED GREENFED DAIRY

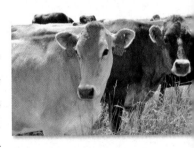

Thanks to nearly twenty years of the *Got Milk?* advertising campaign, some people think they have to walk around with a milk mustache. Others in natural health circles think milk is white poison.

For my health, a type of milk—the right kind— helped save my life. I've seen healthy dairy and cultured dairy products do the same for many others. But there's an issue in many people's minds with dairy, and that's tolerance. For a variety of reasons, many people stay away from dairy because of a lactose intolerance, casein sensitivity, or they think there's too much fat in whole milk dairy products.

Let's take the fat issue first. When people talk about dairy, I hear them say all the time, "Isn't that fattening?" They obviously heard somewhere that dairy has too much fat.

Folks, I can guarantee you that I probably eat more fat than anybody in the state of Florida, and I'm incredibly healthy and at my ideal weight.

I'll be frank here: you've been lied to about fat being bad. I hear people say all the time that you should drink low fat or skim milk instead, but that's not natural and not right. Milk doesn't come out of the cow's udder in low fat or skim versions, does it? Of course not. There's a process involved to take the fat out of rich, nutritious milk. Since that takes some doing, why is skim milk sold for the same price as whole milk at the store?

That's a good question. When you see identical prices, you might be thinking, *Wait a minute. How can skim milk cost the same as whole? And why would the dairy industry promote its consumption so strongly?*

Because the dairy industry knows that when you consume low fat or skim milk products, you're going to crave fat *even more*. That happens because your body needs fat, and if you don't get it with skim milk over your cereal, then you'll crave it in the form of butter, cream cheese, and ice cream later in the day. In other words, they'll make more money selling you that other stuff since the skim products weren't doing it for you.

You really have to wonder why you can't find a single yogurt made from whole milk in the grocery store today. But promoting this agenda of skim milk means that the milk producers can create a culture of people looking to satisfy their body's natural desire for fat.

So I have a question for you: If fat and cream are so bad for you, why do we call the top athletes, the top performers, or the top competitors the "cream of the crop"?

Few can explain that idiom, even though it's still used these days. I'll give it a shot. When milk comes from the herd after the spring calving, the fat percentage is how you judge how successful the dairy farmer was. When we say, "The cream always rises to the top," we mean that those who are the best and most distinguished rise to the top, just as cream—the richest part of the milk—rises to the top of the milk pail.

And yet, as a culture, we're drinking low fat and skim milk much more than whole milk because of the perception that fat is somehow bad for you. That's a perception I hope to change.

As for the tolerance issue, I was fairly intolerant to dairy at one time. Being of Jewish ancestry, I think I know why. Among Americans, those of Jewish descent,

African-Americans, and people who descend from the Middle East and India seem to be the least tolerant of dairy. Yet in the Middle East, the subcontinent of India, and the continent of Africa, people groups originated in areas where their diet was based around dairy.

So what gives?

Several years ago, I learned of what is believed to be a small genetic mutation that occurred up to two thousand years ago that is often found in modern dairy cows populating North America, Europe, and Australia. This genetic mutation may play a role in the widespread dairy intolerance among a large swath of our population.

As I discussed in my last chapter, we have a selective breeding program using ancient genetics and Olde World production methods that produce dairy products that are not only healthy, but according to many satisfied users, highly tolerable—even in cases when they wouldn't do well with regular dairy. This is due in part to the culturing and subsequent pre-digestion of the nutrients contained in our dairy as well as the ancient genetic breeding program we employ.

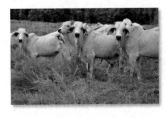

Our Beyond Organic cows are genetically patterned after the "sacred" cows from India and cattle from the Maasai tribe of Africa. The Maasai, who are not known for eating greens, vegetables, or fruits, are feared for their strength and military exploits. Their diet consists of freshly killed meat and a cultured dairy product called *maas*, which is cow's milk that has been fermented for several days in a gourd.

As our guide and host Carol Green explained to me during my trip to the southernmost tip of the African continent, *maas* has become widely popular in South Africa. Cultured with a particular type of probiotics, easily digestible for virtually everyone, the creamy *maas* has been a huge hit throughout the countryside and South Africa's big cities.

Maas, as I've said, was the inspiration for Beyond Organic's Amasai. One reason why our cultured beverage is such a healthy protein-rich food is because we feed our cows the way they were created to be fed—with greens, not grain. Ruminant animals such as cows, goats, and sheep were not designed by the Creator to eat grain—but conventional dairy operations feed their livestock grain because it's easy (just pen up the animals and set out the feed), it's affordable (there's an economy of scale to factory farms), and it's subsidized (the U.S. government dispenses up to

$30 billion a year in farm subsidies, part of which is used to produce cheap grain from genetically modified seed).

Munching on clumps of green forage is what cows are born to do. Essentially, these animals have three stomachs—the alimentary canal, the stomach, and a secondary cud receptacle—to "wash and rinse" their vegetarian diet. Their green food is incredibly healthy, containing twenty-three times as much vitamin A as carrots, twenty-two times as much vitamin B2 as

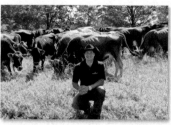

I love hanging out with some of my new "lady friends" at lunch time.

lettuce, nine times more thiamin than green leafy vegetables, and fourteen times more vitamin C than citrus fruits by weight. We are the beneficiaries because cows convert these vitamin- and mineral-rich green foods into milk, which, in my opinion, is the closest thing we have to a perfect food on this planet.

When Dr. William Campbell Douglass said in *The Milk Book* that proteins from cultured dairy were the finest proteins one can consume, he was making that statement based on the knowledge that billions of live, friendly bacteria in yogurt, kefir, and amasai not only predigest any fat, sugar, and protein, but they also create beneficial compounds within the dairy. But the good news doesn't stop there: these microorganisms actually *manufacture* nutrients.

Unfortunately, it's a big challenge to find cultured dairy from pasture-fed animals, something I found out more than fifteen years ago in San Diego. They're hard to find and even if you can, there's little chance that the milk was produced from cattle with the ancient genetics and Olde World production methods we use at Beyond Organic. Some of the most popular brands of kefir in natural food stores come from conventionally raised cows, and even "organic kefir" comes from grain-fed cattle and only in a "low fat" version—meaning the levels of fat-soluble vitamins are less than optimal.

The point I want to reiterate is that cultured dairy, from GreenFed cows, will give you some of the best proteins available anywhere. You get a little more than eight grams of protein with one cup of Beyond Organic's Amasai. You receive seven grams of protein from eating just once ounce of Beyond Organic's GreenFed Raw Cheese.

These cultured dairy products are also great sources of sulfur-based proteins because of the high levels of amino acids such as methionine, glycine, cysteine, and cystine. Sulfur-based proteins aid assimilation, and when ample amounts of these sulfur-rich proteins are found in the blood and tissues, you're more likely to be healthy.

WHERE'S THE HEALTHY BEEF?

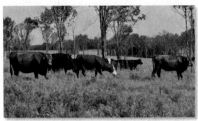

This is where cattle belong—foraging on open, green pasture.

A little more than a century ago, a muckraking journalist named Upton Sinclair worked undercover in the meatpacking plants of the Chicago stockyards and wrote about his experiences in a 1906 novel named *The Jungle*.

The book's main thrust was a pro-Socialist agenda, but Sinclair's page-after-page description of the horrid conditions he found in the meatpacking industry astonished the nation. He described how dead rats were shoveled into sausage-grinding machines, how bribed inspectors looked the other way when diseased cows were slaughtered for beef, and how filthy entrails were swept off the floor and sold as "potted ham."

An aroused public—whipped up by the newspapers of the day—demanded sweeping reforms in the meatpacking industry. President Theodore Roosevelt, the original Rough Rider, swung into action and called upon Congress to establish the Food and Drug Administration, which instituted federal inspection standards for the first time.

I thought of Sinclair when we were putting together our herds on our southern Missouri ranches. We purchased various cows from around the country, and some arrived with staph infections. We were told that we could not treat the staph infections without the use of antibiotics, but as we huddled with our veterinarians, I learned that there was a strong chance that even if the infections subsided, these cows could present with staph infections again in the future—and pass them along to the rest of the herd.

That was not a risk we were willing to take, so we decided to get rid of the suspect cows, which were taken to the cattle "sale barn."

We sold these cattle at a considerable loss—pennies per pound, I'm afraid. Out of integrity, we made it known at the sale that these cows had staph infections. Afterward, I asked one of our stockmen, "Who buys these cows anyway?"

The stockman gave me a knowing look. "A distributor bought them, who'll have no problem selling them as quickly as possible to fast food chains," he said. "How else can they sell hamburgers for 99 cents the last twenty years?"

We will not process any sickly cattle at Beyond Organic, and the reason is a variation of the Golden Rule: *I will not sell what I would not eat.*

If you're seeking to produce beef that will receive the USDA "organic" stamp of approval, the rules are complex. The USDA says cows on organic farms should have "access to pasture" and eat grass. If the weather doesn't allow that, then their diets can be made up of dried grass or hay.

The phrase "access to pasture" is subject to interpretation. The rules don't specify how long or how often cows should have "access" to a pasture, nor what percentage of their food has to come from pasture. The rules state that cattle must be on pasture for at least 120 days a year, or four months, but that doesn't have to be continuous. The rest of the time, at least 30 percent of "dry matter" of their diet must come from grass. The other 70 percent? That can be grain-based feed.

At Beyond Organic, we have higher standards, and our goal is for our beef cattle to be out in the pasture *all the time*. We will never feed them grain. But the real difference in our "beyond organic" standards is how the cattle finish.

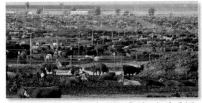

This sad photo illustrates the miserable reality of modern feedlots in today's beef industry.

As I mentioned in Chapter 1, it's not how you start but how you finish when it comes to producing the healthiest beef. In the conventional world, cattle go the feedlot ninety days before they're processed, where they are fed—almost exclusively—grain that's been laced with growth-promoting chemicals as well as other byproducts you don't want to hear about. This growth-spurt formula is the backbone of the U.S. beef industry. A feedlot cow can grow to slaughter weight up to a year faster than a cow fed only forage such as grass and hay.

In the organic world, though, there's some wiggle room.

According to USDA organic standards, producers of organic beef can put their animals in feedlots for the last four months of their lives. In other words, cattle can be bunched up in pens and fed *organic grain* while they stand in one place, packing on the pounds before their date with destiny. It's anyone's guess as to how many organic beef producers are taking advantage of this loophole.

I know that people swoon over Kobe beef from Japan, saying that the flavor, tenderness, and fatty, well-marbled texture can't be beat. Well, Kobe cattle are routinely sent to the feedlot for 180 days of "finishing," where they are fed grain—and beer. The Kobe cattle are supposedly rubbed and massaged before they're turned into steaks, sukiyaki, shabu shabu, sashimi, and teppanyaki. The same goes for Wagyu beef as well. To me, that's like super feedlot beef.

We have a different finishing program for our cattle that is, essentially, the "anti-feedlot." We take our animals and finish them on organic greens in our open pasture. During our finishing process the cattle are put on a three-day, specially designed bovine detox program, if they need it. The bovine detox program involves a combination of minerals and other compounds that help remove toxins from the body.

With the help of ear tags and a computerized tracking system, we can track where each cow is in the finishing process. While our beef cattle do not qualify as USDA certified organic (since many are not born on our ranches), while under our care the cows graze on chemical-free organic pastures and are not treated with any chemicals or medications.

In addition to our unique GreenFinishing program, we employ biblical slaughter methods in our beef processing. The Bible says, "The life is in the blood" (Leviticus 17:11), so it is important to remove as much blood as possible. Our processing procedures adhere to animal kindness standards. Most organic and grass-fed producers slaughter cattle with trauma to the head, which may result in pooling of the blood and an increase in adrenaline, which impact the quality of the meat. Whereas most kosher beef producers slaughter correctly, they feed the animals grain and may use antibiotics and hormones. We strive to finish and process our cattle in accordance with biblical principles.

We go to all this effort so that we can produce one of the best sources of protein on the planet. Our GreenFinished Beef has:

- **Vitamin E, beta-carotene, and vitamin C**
- **A healthy ratio of omega-6 to omega-3 fatty acids and conjugated linoleic acid (CLA)**

CLA is a fatty acid that has been the subject of research the last several years for its ability to influence human health. GreenFinished beef may have three to five times more CLA than grain-finished animals. But one of the greatest benefits of our GreenFinished Beef is its great taste, and taste is important. In fact, I've had plenty of people over the years approach me at my seminars and say, "I want to eat grass-fed beef, but it's tough and tastes like cardboard."

I understand where they are coming from, and I like the taste of a good steak myself. First, we learned that different breeds have different amounts of fat when they are on a green diet, so we have worked hard to raise cattle that excel at marbling on a no-grain diet. As any steak connoisseur will tell you, marbling has a big impact on the juiciness and flavor of the meat.

Marbling is the small streaks of fat that are found within the muscle—not the fat that surrounds the organs, lungs, and kidneys. That's the type of fat that the Hebrews were told *not* to eat as commanded in Leviticus and Deuteronomy. In general, the more marbling in a cut of beef, the better the cut of meat, although meat with excessive marbling can be too much of a good thing and makes the cut greasy.

We wanted to have the right amount of marbled fat in our meat at Beyond Organic, and I believe we have succeeded on that front while delivering beneficial omega-3 fatty acids and CLA.

If and when you try our GreenFinished Beef, I want you to be able to tell your friends and neighbors, "That was the best-tasting beef I've ever had."

NOTHING FISHY ABOUT WILD-CAUGHT

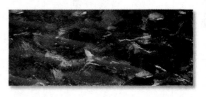

Wild-caught fish is an absolutely incredible food and should be consumed liberally. Fish caught in the wild, instead of those raised on fish farms (like salmon, trout, and tilapia) provide an excellent source of protein and omega-3 fatty acids—the fats we lack the most in our diets. Omega-3s balance the overabundance of omega-6 fatty acids, which are found in processed foods and refined grains.

Most people consume too many omega-6 fatty acids in comparison to omega-3s because they don't eat foods such as wild-caught fish and eggs from pasture-raised poultry. Instead, they consume an abundance of grains, seeds, and their oils, including safflower, corn, and soybean oils, which are all high in omega-6 fatty acids. A diet heavy in omega-6s—processed and sugary foods—impacts your health for the worse by increasing levels of inflammatory compounds.

.Vild-caught tuna and sockeye salmon are my personal favorites, and many restaurants that specialize in seafood should have wild-caught versions on the menu. Ocean-caught fish provides a rich source of vitamins and minerals, and salmon contains the powerful antioxidant astaxanthin.

If you're trying to lose weight, then you probably know that many popular diets include canned tuna and salad as a lunchtime or dinner staple. Look for tuna canned in spring water with a high level of fat. This indicates not only a high level of omega-3 fats, but also a lower amount of heavy metals including mercury. This is due to the fact that smaller, younger tuna have higher levels of good fats and lower levels of toxins.

When raised right in the wild, fish are an incredibly nutrient-dense food. According to the research of Dr. Weston A. Price, traditional people groups around the world prized seafood above every other food, and they went to great lengths to obtain wild-caught fish by making sure they lived near oceans, lakes, and streams.

If they didn't live close to these bodies of water, they were willing to travel long distances to find those fish because they knew what a difference consuming that rich protein made in their health.

GOBBLING UP WILD POULTRY

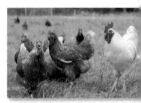

Eating—let alone finding—wild poultry is rare. Even organic chickens are fed predominantly corn and soy, so they're not hunting and pecking for worms and grubs as they should. Plus, there isn't much of a market for game birds like quail, pheasant, wild geese, wild turkey, and wild ducks. And who can—or wants to—hunt for wild game these days?

"Chickens, like cows, thrive on pasture."

There's a huge demand for poultry, though. Chicken is the country's most popular meat and the foundation of lunch and dinner for umpteen millions each day. Chicken is cheap, tastes good, and adapts well to sauces and spices. To keep up with the heavy demand, ten *billion* chickens are raised and killed for food every year in the United States. Thinking about all the nuggets, wings, and drumsticks eaten each day makes my head spin, just as thinking about the tons of chicken dipped into batter and dropped into vats of boiling oil saddens me.

It's no secret that commercial chickens are raised in horrible and inhumane conditions—stuffed into floor-to-ceiling cages inside stuffy enclosed barns.

They do not go outside for the duration of their short dreary lives, and their "living space" is the size of a standard sheet of printing paper. They are raised to gain weight as quickly as possible, fed antibiotics to fend off illness, and live no more than two months before ending up in a refrigerator case.

While commercially produced chickens are raised entirely indoors with tens of thousands of other chickens in close quarters, never seeing the sun or pasture, organic or "free range" chickens may have life only marginally better. I say that because there's no standard definition or industry guideline on how long chickens need to be outdoors on pasture.

In addition, the USDA definition of "free-range" is in the eyes of the beholder. Some poultry producers interpret "access to pasture" as a small "doggie door" at the end of a hundred-foot shed filled with uncaged birds moving around the litter-covered floor. Many never bother to push through the door and go outside.

Others feel like the spirit of the rules means that the birds have to get outside in the open air and sunshine, but their "free range" extends no further than a dirt patch, where some sort of feed has been set out for them to pluck on. Meanwhile, consumers have certain expectations for what a "certified organic" sticker on the whole fryer packaging means, and they would be surprised to learn that their organic chicken was cooped up most of the day, pecking at grain.

I think there's a way to raise poultry that is "beyond organic." I've seen it done right. A few years ago while I was on my Perfect Weight America tour, I visited Coyote Creek Farm in Elgin, Texas.

The farm was owned by Jeremiah Cunningham, a 74-year-old cancer survivor who got into organic farming after reading my first book, *Patient, Heal Thyself*, released in 2002. When I asked Jeremiah what he decided to do after he learned he had cancer, he said with the most deadpan Texas twang, "I read your book, and then I began raising chickens the right way. I also went out and bought me some cows."

"Wow," I replied. "Most people read my books and go out and buy some supplements and carrot juice, but you really took the bull by the horns."

Jeremiah shared a laugh. He was six feet, six inches tall, had a full head of hair, and looked like a strong farm boy.

When we toured the farm, Jeremiah told me that he was quite conscious about the soil quality of his ninety acres of certified organic land. They sprayed ıst tea four to six times a year to foster healthy microorganisms, and they also fed the "biology" of the soil by spreading hydrolyzed fish, molasses, and humic acid twice a year.

What Jeremiah was really proud of, though, was his chicken flock—more than 7,000 chickens. His pastured chickens got as much as 30 percent of their diet from the pasture, where they ate grass, worms, grubs, and other little creatures. His high-quality omega-3 eggs were phenomenal. In fact, I took twenty-four dozen Coyote Creek eggs back to the tour bus, and then I cracked three eggs into a small glass and drank them raw—just like Rocky did in the movie—in front of our film crew guys. That got their attention!

At our Beyond Organic ranch, we're working on producing our own poultry on a large scale, but we're not there yet. Our goal is to produce chickens that are truly "free-range and pastured" without using soy-based feed. Look for Beyond Organic Chicken sometime in the future.

In the meantime, let me add a few more thoughts about poultry.

First of all, the "white meat,"—the chicken or turkey breast that everyone loves to go after—is the least nutritious part of the bird. The dark meat found in the thighs and legs are more nutritious, in terms of nutrients, than the light meat.

The best way to consume poultry is in a soup or stock. I've recommended in many of my books for people with real sensitive systems or health challenges to go on a chicken soup cleanse, meaning that they should make their own chicken soup and then consume it exclusively for two, three, five, or seven days at a time.

The recuperative effects of chicken soup date back for centuries and start with the stock, which is also called broth. Stock—which is made up of chicken meat, bones and all—contains generous amounts of natural gelatin, an odorless, tasteless substance extracted by boiling bones and animal tissues like cartilage.

My Grandma Rose was practically raised on homemade chicken soup. She grew up the sixth of seven children on a Polish farm. Her parents could afford only one chicken a week as their meat, so to stretch a single chicken to feed a family of nine, her mother made a big pot of chicken soup. The heat extracted all the nutrients and compounds from the carcass, and when combined with all the vegetables, spices, and sea salt, they would eat heartily and nutritiously at least one night a week unless there was leftovers.

I encourage you to make your own chicken soup. Check out the recipe on page 262, which is easy to follow.

THE EGG-CEPTIONAL EGG

God created the perfect protein in the humble egg.

Within the thin shell is a nutrient-dense food that packs six grams of protein, as well as vitamin B-12, vitamin E, lutein, riboflavin, folic acid, calcium, zinc, iron, essential fatty acids, and all eight essential amino acids. All this in a nifty sixty-eight calorie package.

Eggs have some of the highest-quality protein of any food, yet up until a few years ago, eggs were disparaged in the popular culture. We were told that eggs were bad, bad, bad for you—cholesterol bombs. And if you scramble eggs in the morning, make sure you get rid of the yolks.

The whole egg white craze was a huge mistake. If you take the yolk out, you lose two-and-a-half grams of your six grams of protein—more than 40 percent—as well as important branch-chain amino acids. Virtually all the vitamins and nutrients are in the yolk, so cracking open an egg and tossing the yolk into the kitchen sink is folly.

Unfortunately, we can't produce eggs at Beyond Organic that can be shipped across the country, although I do have our pastured eggs with beautiful bright orange yolks shipped directly to me from the ranch every week or so. After consuming Beyond Organic eggs, believe me, it's hard to eat any other kind. We will be increasing the size of our egg operation to use them in our prepared meals that we're planning to offer in the future.

The Rubins are an egg-eating family. We probably go through a dozen eggs each morning, from the sunny side-up eggs Samuel eats to the raw smoothies we serve to the kids and consume ourselves.

Now that's what I call the breakfast of champions.

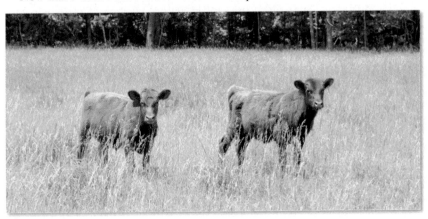

THE TOP 10 PROTEIN FOODS

1. AMASAI, GreenFed, low-temperature processed, cultured with over thirty probiotics and supplying eight grams of protein per one cup, is inspired by a traditional recipe from Africa's Maasai tribe.

2. WILD-CAUGHT FISH, especially those from pristine sources in Alaska and the north Atlantic, are a rich source of omega-3 fats, key amino acids, potassium, vitamins, and minerals.

3. GREENFINISHED BEEF Is minimally processed from cattle that intensely graze on grasses and greens such as forbs, herbs, and legumes—and no grain.

4. REALLY RAW CHEESE—meaning never heated above cow body temperature (around 101.5 degrees Fahrenheit)—is much different than pasteurized cheese, and tastes great, too. Give GreenFed Raw Cheese a try. You will receive seven grams of protein in each one-ounce serving.

5. LAMB has a distinctive but pleasing gamy taste that is high in vitamin B12 which supports the production of red blood cells and allows nerves to function properly and carnitine which promotes a healthy cardiovascular system.

6. BISON is low in saturated fat, just 2 to 3 percent compared to the 40 percent found in corn-bed beef.

7. VENISON AND ELK meats are wonderful, nutritious, and worth getting out of your comfort zone and trying sometime. I'll predict that you'll love these healthy and worthwhile wild pasture-fed meats.

8. WILD POULTRY—chicken, turkey, and pheasant, for example—is especially healthy for you when eaten in a homemade soup.

9. PASTURED EGGS are unsung heroes that provide outstanding nutrition.

10. RAW LEAFY GREENS, especially micro veggies, have a very good balance of raw proteins. As you can see, this is the only vegetarian food in this Top 10 list, but raw leafy greens and their juice have low molecular weight proteins, which promote excellent health in the body.

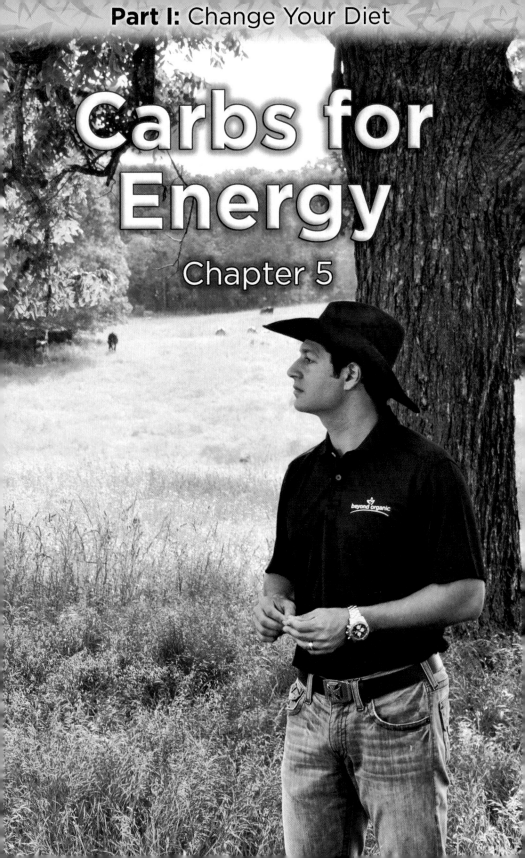

Carbs for Energy

Chapter 5

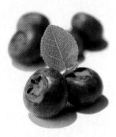

My seven-year-old son, Joshua, loves hiking, and recently we climbed to the top of North Carolina's Yellow Mountain, which offers a magnificent 360-degree view of the Great Smoky Mountains from the 5,127-foot summit. Joshua was a trouper, never complaining, as we marched through the picturesque highlands.

Along the way, I spotted some wild blueberries among the bushes lining the trail to the top. Seeing this as one of those teachable moments, I guided my son for a closer look.

"Look, Joshua. Wild blueberries. Don't they look different than the ones we have at home?"

My son peered for a closer look. The blueberries on the branches were small—no bigger than the white pearls seen on a woman's necklace. Their pigment was a deep blue, almost purple.

"Go ahead and pick one," I said.

Joshua cautiously tugged on a few wild blueberries and held them in the palm of small hand. Then I plucked a few myself.

"You can eat them," I said.

Joshua popped the blueberries into his mouth, and the look on his face was priceless.

"These taste awesome!" he exclaimed. "These are the most amazing things I've ever tasted."

While picking wild blueberries and eating them on the trail is certainly the "beyond organic" way of doing things, I'm not suggesting that you should fly to North Carolina's Great Smoky Mountains or the lowbush areas of Maine, where the wild blueberry is the official fruit of the Pine Tree State, to get your fix of blueberries.

What I'm saying is that this story about Joshua and I eating wild blueberries illustrates how excited we were to discover a whole different level of freshness and flavor in a simple blueberry we found out in the wild—and it also shows how disconnected we are from food in its most natural state these days. Let's face it: nearly all city folks like us parade through life without consuming anything grown in the wild.

When it comes to living beyond organic, getting a taste of foods in their ideal state is certainly at the top of the menu. Blueberries are considered a carbohydrate-rich food, and while the carbohydrates found in fruits and vegetables are one of the three macronutrients found in food—protein and fat are the other two—they are not essential.

Many people may not understand what I'm about to say, but you could live just fine by eating only fats and protein. Anthropologists tell us that the Eskimos—prior to their interaction with white explorers and whalers—survived for centuries eating only animal foods rich in fats and proteins, thriving on the flesh of walruses, whales, seals, and salmon. That was just about the only available food they could find or hunt for on the frozen tundra above the Arctic Circle, yet despite their unvarying diets, the Eskimos were among the healthiest people on Earth.

However, I hasten to add that while carbohydrates are not essential, I do believe they are beneficial. I feel this way for three reasons:

1. Carbohydrate-rich foods are an important source of **energy**, especially for those called to perform such as athletes. That's why you hear the phrase "carb-loading" on the night before a big race or an Ironman competition.

2. Carbohydrate-rich foods are the go-to place for **antioxidants**, which are compounds that preserve and protect the body from free-radical damage. Without going into a long explanation, free radicals are something you don't want running rampant within your system. Free radicals are oxygen molecules with a single electron, but these unstable molecules are known to attack the immune system's cells. The antioxidants in blueberries, for example, neutralize free radicals, which is a great thing for the body.

3. Carbohydrate-rich foods provide the body with **fiber**—or what Grandma called "roughage." Fiber is the indigestible remnants of plant cells found in vegetables, fruits, whole grains, nuts, seeds, and beans. These high-fiber foods help keep you regular. As fiber works its way through the digestive tract, it increases the elimination of waste matter in the large intestine and gives you an urge to have a bowel movement. That's why I've always said that eating fiber can turn a frown right side up for those walking around with constipation.

When it comes to carbs, my focus has always been on choosing the best carbohydrate foods—those that are high in fiber, high in antioxidants, and low in sugar.

To zero in on those superior carbohydrate foods, there are three types of carbohydrates that you need to think about, and they are all fifty-cent words: monosaccharides, disaccharides, and polysaccharides. If you remember your Latin prefixes, then you'll know that "mono" means single or one, which in this context means that monosaccharides are comprised of a single sugar. Most fruits, vegetables, natural cheeses, cultured dairy, nuts, and raw honey contain carbohydrates predominantly in the form of monosaccharides. The gastrointestinal tract finds monosaccharide foods easier to digest because these single-molecule carbohydrates can be absorbed through the lining of the small intestine without having to be broken down first.

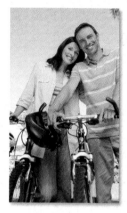

Disaccharides, with the Latin prefix of *di* meaning two, refers to any substance that is composed of *two* molecules of sugar that are linked together. Examples of disaccharides are sugar, sugar, and sugar. Okay, I'm exaggerating, but any sort of food with refined white or brown sugar—ranging from cookies, cupcakes, and pies to ketchup, peanut butter, and teriyaki sauce—contain disaccharide carbohydrates. Processed grains like boxed cereals, breads, bagels, dinner rolls, muffins, and cinnamon rolls are comprised of starches that are disaccharides. Milk sugar, or lactose, is the disaccharide found in certain dairy products such as fluid milk and ice cream.

Polysaccharides, as you would expect with a prefix of *poly*, which means many, have many sugar molecules. Most fiber-rich foods contain polysaccharide sugars. To simplify things for the rest of this chapter, though, I will refer to carbohydrates with multiple sugars, such as disaccharides and polysaccharides, as simply disaccharides.

Disaccharides are *much* more difficult to digest and stack up in the gut like an army of toy soldiers marching into a blind alley. When unabsorbed carbohydrates remain in the large intestine undigested, they feed potentially harmful bacteria and other microorganisms and upset the balance of the intestinal flora—prompting digestive problems to strike.

Eating excessive amounts of disaccharide-rich foods can also lead to malabsorption in the gastrointestinal tract, which means that food travels too rapidly through the digestive tract. The "end" result: bouts of occasional diarrhea and/or constipation as well as loss of nutrients that can lead to stunted growth and development. Since the gastrointestinal tract has less time to break down the starch and sugars, their absorption into the bloodstream is severely impaired.

But the right kind of carbs—monosaccharides—give you the horsepower your system needs to drive chemical processes throughout the body. When the digestive system breaks down carbohydrates into glucose, the body is supplied with the energy for cellular processes such as thinking, breathing, or moving an arm or a leg.

As you would imagine, monosaccharide-containing carbohydrates are the ones I tend to gravitate toward. I'll talk first about fruits and then move on to veggies, nuts, seeds, legumes, grains, and sweeteners.

FRUITS ARE FUN

When Joshua and I picked a few wild blueberries on our trek up Yellow Mountain, I couldn't get over how much smaller and more compact they were compared to the organic blueberries we serve at home, which were probably double in size and plumper and juicier. I'll note something else: the wild blueberries were not as sweet as the ones we buy in stores, but the wild blueberry taste was more intense, more tangy than cultivated blueberries with a thicker skin. That's why Joshua exclaimed how good they were.

I chalked up the taste intensity to the high-altitude and intense sunshine in the North Carolina mountains, which produces very nutrient-dense wild blueberries with great subtlety and depth of flavor, although I did detect a slightly gritty aftertaste. Cultivated blueberries, on the other hand, have a smooth interior but not as much depth of flavor.

Don't get me wrong: I'm not down on organic blueberries or any other type of organically grown fruit. I *love* organic fruit. When compared to conventionally grown fruit, organic fruit is tastier and packs more nutritional punch. *The Journal of Applied Nutrition,* over a two-year period, purchased both organically and conventionally grown fruits and vegetables such as apples, pears, potatoes, wheat, and sweet corn in the western suburbs of Chicago and analyzed these foods for their mineral contents. On a per-weight basis, the average levels of essential minerals were much higher for the organically grown fruits and veggies—more calcium, more chromium, more phosphorous, more potassium, more zinc, and less mercury, which is a toxin.

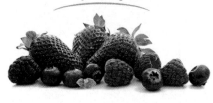

You have to figure the antioxidant levels are higher in wild fruit, but that's not the reason why I told the wild blueberry story with Joshua. I merely wanted to point out the differences between picking your own blueberries on a hike versus picking up a pint carton of blueberries at your natural health food store. Both kinds are excellent for your health. That's why blueberries are my favorite fruit and thus my favorite carbohydrate.

Blueberries rank at the top of the list of high-antioxidant foods based on the ORAC (Oxygen Radical Absorbance Capacity) test, which measures the total antioxidant power of foods. Researchers at Tufts University in Boston developed a way to analyze the ORAC units per 100 grams, or about three-and-a-half ounces, in fruits and vegetables.

HERE'S THE ORAC NUMBERS FOR COMMONLY EATEN FRUITS (I'LL SHARE THE ORAC NUMBERS FOR VEGETABLES IN THE NEXT SECTION):

FRUITS:

- **Blueberries (2400)**
- **Strawberries (1540)**
- **Plums (949)**
- **Red Grapes (739)**
- **Kiwi Fruit (602)**

- **Blackberries (2036)**
- **Raspberries (1220)**
- **Oranges (750)**
- **Cherries (670)**
- **Pink Grapefruit (483)**

As you can see, blueberries sit atop the leader board when it comes to antioxidant power, which is another reason why blueberries should become as popular in your home as they are in mine.

Since I'm a berry lover, I like many other varieties as well, including blackberries, raspberries, strawberries, boysenberries, and huckleberries. Two other lesser-consumed berries are a wonderful source of nutrients and antioxidants. The first is black raspberries, which are affectionately known as "blackcaps" by growers. Native to North America, black raspberries have a distinct and moderately tart flavor with an extremely high level of phenolic compounds (such as eliagic acid, gallic acid, and rutin) compared to other berries.

The other is Jaboticaba, which is a grapelike berry that grows on the bark of trees. I first learned about Jaboticaba while visiting a small farm on the island of Hawaii. Nicki was pregnant with Joshua at the time, and we visited a man named John who farmed twelve acres and had hundreds of exotic species of fruits and veggies growing on his land.

We had to hike up a steep hill to get to his property. John, who is a bit eccentric, lived in a tree house, Swiss Family Robinson style. Out of all the exotic fruits I saw, Jaboticaba interested me the most. Based on its thick outer skin and deep purple color, I predict that Jaboticaba will one day be the next "superberry."

There are some other interesting berries out there as well. Aronia berries or chokeberries are native to the Eastern Seaboard, and their hardy shrubs produce bitter dark purple fruit clusters with a high concentration of flavonoids and antioxidants. Aronia berries have been an integral part of the Native American diet for hundreds of years.

Another extremely popular antioxidant-rich berry I have to mention is acai (pronounced ah-SIGH-eee) berries, which are inch-long, reddish, purple fruit coming from the acai palm trees native to Central and South America. Each time I travel to Southern California, I marvel at the acai berry "cafes" that have sprung up to sell "acai bowls," which are thick, smoothie-like masses of blended acai berries smothered with granola and organic toppings.

Another fruit that hasn't been discovered yet in health circles is the Muscadine grape, which is native to the southeastern United States. The Muscadine—also known as a scuppernong—is much higher in antioxidants than many other fruits and contains high levels of resveratrol, one of the compounds in red wine thought to reduce the growth of abnormal cells and promote healthy cardiovascular function.

There's one more thing that I feel strongly about when it comes to the consumption of fruit, no matter how good it tastes or how healthy it is for you. I recommend that you eat no more than two servings a day, and when you do eat fruit, you should also consume foods containing healthy fats to help slow down the absorption of sugar.

Some great foods that you could eat with your fruit are GreenFed raw cheese, almonds, almond butter (great with slices of apple), avocado, coconut, and Amasai.

VEGGIE TALES

I like keeping things simple: while my favorite fruits are berries, my favorite veggies are greens. Why? Because these low-calorie vegetables are the most nutrient dense foods that you can consume. Bite for bite, they contain fewer calories than other carbohydrate-containing foods and have high levels of vitamins, essential fatty acids, fiber, and minerals.

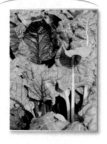

I'll never forget the time when I was with Jerry Frye, the rancher whom I bought our first Missouri property from. We were out in the fields, and Jerry knelt down in the pasture of mixed species of forage. He plucked several blades of grass, a few herbs, some forbs and legumes, and held them up. "Ah, tiny solar panels, capturing the power of the sun to transfer its energy to us," he said. In fact, that's where I first understood the term GreenFed. I'll never look at pasture the same way again.

At the end of the day, green leafy vegetables are alive with the sun's radiant energy and one of the richest sources of biophotons, which is essentially how energy is transferred. While all veggies are good, greens are the best. Greens contain large amounts of beta-carotene and folic acid, which support cardiovascular health.

THE LEAFY GREEN VEGETABLES WITH THE HIGHEST LEVELS OF ANTIOXIDANTS ARE KALE AND SPINACH, WHICH RESIDE AT THE TOP OF THE ORAC RANKINGS FOR VEGETABLES:

- **Kale (1770)**
- **Brussels Sprouts (980)**
- **Broccoli (890)**
- **Red Bell Pepper (710)**
- **Corn (400)**
- **Spinach (1260)**
- **Alfalfa Sprouts (930)**
- **Beets (840)**
- **Onion (450)**
- **Eggplant (390)**

Kale and spinach are slightly bitter-tasting greens, so some people don't adjust to the taste. But if you can get used to their unique flavor and add them to your salads and juices, then you'll really give your body a huge antioxidant leap. The most well-known antioxidants are vitamins E and C and carotenoids such as beta-carotene, lycopene, and lutein. Through scientific research, we've learned that:

- VITAMIN E is a fat-soluble vitamin present in leafy green vegetables, spinach, broccoli, and asparagus.

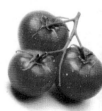

- VITAMIN C is a water-soluble vitamin present in green peppers, cabbage, spinach, broccoli, and kale.

- BETA-CAROTENE is a precursor to vitamin A (which means the body converts beta-carotene to vitamin A) and is present in spinach, carrots, squash, broccoli, yams, and tomatoes.

- LYCOPENE is a carotenoid found in tomatoes, watermelon, and pink grapefruit.

- LUTEIN is found in a variety of fruits and vegetables including kale and spinach, peaches, and oranges.

For all the wonderful things that green leafy veggies do for the body, I believe I've found something even better, and that's micro veggies.

Never heard of micro veggies?

I hadn't either until a few months ago when I met a farmer who grows micro veggies hydroponically, meaning he grows certain vegetables in a temperature-controlled setting using water, nutrients, and natural sunlight. The result is a tiny form of edible greens produced from the seeds of vegetables, herbs, or other plants. These micro veggies range in size from one to two inches long, including the stem and leaves.

What amazes me about micro veggies is the surprisingly intense flavors considering their small size. A micro-onion, for example, looks no bigger than a sprig of rosemary, but when you pop that into your mouth, you feel like you've just eaten an entire onion. *Shazam!* That's the feeling you get when you take a bite of a micro veggie.

One great thing about micro veggies is that they have been tested to contain higher nutrients and lower levels of pathogenic microorganisms, including bacteria, than organic vegetables because of the controlled environment that micro veggies are grown in. When I said that micro veggies are grown hydroponically, I was referring to a method of growing vegetables and produce without the use of soil and in a controlled indoor environment. The roots of the plants are suspended in nutrient-rich water, usually inside an enclosed greenhouse. These growing techniques mean that these micro plants can grow year-round. I urge you to seek out hydroponically grown micro veggies.

Micro veggies such as broccoli and pea shoots can deliver health benefits far beyond the usual range of vitamins and minerals found in other vegetables. For example, broccoli sprouts are young broccoli plants that look more like regular sprouts than broccoli, and research scientists at Johns Hopkins and other universities believe that micro broccoli can control the growth of unhealthy cells.

Micro broccoli and other micro cruciferous vegetables such as red cabbage, purple radish, and kale have a compound called sulforaphane, which has shown immune-boosting properties in university studies. The tiny micro veggies have more than fifty times the amount of sulforaphane found in mature broccoli.

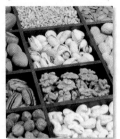

Since learning about the powerful nutrition in these small micro veggies, I've begun consuming them daily, and I think you should too.

REACHING FOR NUTS, SEEDS, AND LEGUMES

Nuts, seeds, and legumes are not only a good source of carbohydrates in a monosaccharide form, but they are also a good source of protein—that is why they often make up a large part of a vegetarian diet.

Whether you're a vegetarian or an omnivore like me, the key is thinking about eating more seeds than nuts because I believe seeds are more digestible and more nutritious. Then again, it's hard to tell what's a seed or a nut sometimes. Almonds are the king of nuts and a personal favorite of mine, but I would put almonds more in the seed category because they are actually the seeds of the almond tree, a tree that bears pink and white flowers.

Cashews and peanuts, two of the most popular American pre-dinner snacks, are technically legumes and not nuts.

LEGUMES COME FROM PLANTS THAT BEAR THEIR FRUIT IN PODS, WHICH ARE CASING WITH TWO HALVES, OR HINGES. A GREEN PEA PLANT IS PERHAPS THE MOST RECOGNIZABLE LEGUME, BUT OTHER LEGUMES INCLUDE:

- **Lentils**
- **Kidney beans**
- **Black Beans**
- **Lima Beans**
- **Green Beans**
- **Cacao (chocolate)**

What I suggest is that you soak nuts, seeds, and legumes prior to consumption, a process that greatly helps digestion. When soaked or allowed to germinate, these abundant sources of nutrition transform into nutritional powerhouses with vitamin C and various B vitamins—B2, B5, and B6. If you don't soak raw nuts, seeds, or legumes because you don't want to go to the trouble, you could purchase raw nut and seed butters instead, which, due to their fiber being broken down through grinding, can be easier to digest.

It's not that difficult to soak your favorite nuts, seeds, or legumes, however. Just place them in a bowl of water and let them sit overnight. The next morning, you can put them on a cookie sheet and place the sheet in the oven at the lowest setting for the rest of the day. When they come out of the oven, they taste almost like they were dry roasted, although they weren't. One thing you won't find in our pantry are honey-roasted nuts or any nuts or seeds roasted in oil.

In the nuts and seeds area, I'm a big fan of chia, hemp, and flaxseeds. Chia is an edible seed that grows abundantly in desert plants found in southern Mexico and parts of South America. Chia seeds are rich in alpha-linolenic acid (ALA), which gives chia's fiber-rich seeds the highest percentage of omega-3 fatty acids of any plant, including another favorite of mine, flaxseeds. We keep flaxseed crackers around the house for the kids, which they love to snack on.

BE CAREFUL WITH GRAINS AND STARCHES

While I believe that grains don't need to be a big part of your diet, there are certain grains that I enjoy eating, especially at dinner time. My favorite grains, however, aren't really grains at all.

Quinoa is considered to be a healthy whole grain, but it's actually a seed. Let's not split hairs, though. Native to the Andes, quinoa is mild and slightly nutty, with a beautiful, pillowy texture that reminds me of couscous. Quinoa is a non-gluten leafy grain (like amaranth, millet, and buckwheat) and is not a grassy grain (like barley, oats, rice, and wheat).

Amaranth, which is technically considered a fruit, was a major food of the Aztecs and almost disappeared as a crop in the Americas until research began on this "lost grain" back in the 1970s. Amaranth seeds are super tiny and are unusually high in protein for a non-legume. Even better, the protein is well balanced in amino acids and gaining a following in natural food stores.

Millet and buckwheat are worthy of your attention as well. Millet, thought to be one of the first grains cultivated by man, was a staple in many lands until the advent of rice and maize (corn). Buckwheat, technically, is a fruit like amaranth but is high in protein and contains the eight essential amino acids. Having a distinct, pleasant, rich flavor all its own, 100 percent buckwheat flour makes delicious pancakes.

I can't remember the last time we had pancakes in our home because as a rule, we minimize our grain consumption in the Rubin household. But if I do consume grains, then I will search out heirloom whole grains and make them more digestible by soaking them prior to consumption. We like to soak "grains" like quinoa and amaranth in water, apple cider vinegar, or amasai. Doing so makes them much more digestible.

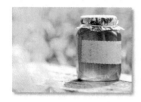 We're also not big bread eaters in the Rubin home. The only breads we allow in the house are whole grain, yeast-free sourdough bread and sprouted whole grain bread, which, through fermentation or germination, have been partially pre-digested and contain a larger percentage of monosaccharides than typical whole grain breads.

Starches such as rice, potatoes, corn, and gluten-filled grains must be approached with caution as they contain primarily disaccharides, meaning the body has more difficulty breaking them down in the digestive tract.

THE SWEET TASTE OF SWEETENERS

Americans love their sweets.

From a bowl of sugary cereal for breakfast to the glazed doughnut at morning break to the cookies and syrupy soft drinks at lunchtime to the vending machine candy bar in the afternoon to the big bowl of Rocky Road ice cream after dinner, piling on sweet after sweet from morning to night raises blood sugar levels dramatically, which causes the body to produce excess insulin in the bloodstream. When blood sugars are high, cells burn sugar instead of fat, which is how fat accumulates in the body. And Americans are accumulating too much fat on their bones.

So perhaps you can understand my reluctance to deliver a full-throated endorsement of various sweeteners, which seems a bit like pouring kerosene on the raging fire of obesity. I will grant you that the desire to eat something sweet—a "treat" as many call it—is strong, and I like the occasional sweet as much as the next guy. When the urge to eat something sweet approaches, though, I recommend using raw, unheated honey.

Honey is God's created sweetener—and unlike sugar, honey is a monosaccharide carbohydrate, which means that it doesn't have to be broken down by the digestive tract. Raw, unheated honey is the only nearly 100 percent predigested food source in nature. It's great topically, meaning that it can be applied to wounds. It's great orally, with people reporting that consuming local honey can bring giving relief to seasonal allergy symptoms. It's great tasting and can sweeten teas, juices, or just about any food.

I understand that if you're going to bake, honey can be more difficult to work with. Substitute sweeteners would be organic cane juice, evaporated cane juice, organic cane sugar, and organic maple syrup, although I would rate this bunch "average" on the health scale. But they are positively superior to commercial white sugar, which should be avoided at all costs.

I'm hearing good things about a sweetener made from coconut sap called coconut sugar or coconut nectar. This type of sweetener is not made from coconut meat but from tapping the coconut tree and draining the sap in a process similar to producing maple syrup, although coconut nectar does not require heating as maple syrup does. Coconut sugar is naturally low on the Glycemic Index (GI), which is a plus.

I'm not in favor of the popular sweetener agave nectar or sugar alcohols such as maltitol, xylitol, and sorbitol. Agave nectar, which comes as syrup, is actually a highly refined sweetener that has more concentrated fructose than high-fructose corn syrup, according to my friends at the Weston A. Price Foundation.

Sugar alcohols are problematic as well because part of their chemical structure resembles sugar, and a part resembles alcohol—hence the confusing name of sugar alcohol. These sweeteners are routinely used in chewing gum, candy, fruit spreads, and even toothpaste and cough syrup. Sure, sugar alcohols taste like sugar, but the body doesn't break down or absorb sugar alcohols very well, and they also seem to have a laxative effect on the body.

There's another no-calorie sweetener that I'm not doing cartwheels over, and that's Stevia. It's not that Stevia is horrible for you by any means, but it's my sense that when you eat something sweet in nature, then the body expects energy in the form of sugars. When consuming calorie-free sweeteners, the body isn't fooled and will make up the calories somewhere else.

Finally, let me say a few words about artificial sweeteners—those blue, pink, and yellow packets found on restaurant tables. Researchers at Purdue University say that these sugar substitutes can interfere with the body's natural ability to count calories based on a food's sweetness. In other words, drinking an iced tea with an artificial sweetener instead of two heaping teaspoons of white sugar will reduce your caloric intake, but it could also trick the body into thinking that other sweet items don't have as many calories either.

Besides, artificial sweeteners such as aspartame, saccharin, and sucralose have sparked debate for decades because they can be highly addictive and trigger toxic substances to cross the blood-brain barrier, causing neurological problems.

THE TOP 10 CARBOHYDRATE FOODS

1. WILD BLUEBERRIES are in a league of their own. Since wild blueberries are difficult to find, difficult to gather, and not in season very long, organic blueberries will have to stand in. Their antioxidant levels are off the chart, or at least at the top of it.

2. BLACK RASPBERRIES have higher levels of antioxidants than other raspberries. We're starting to see black raspberries, which are mainly grown in the Pacific Northwest, become more available every summer.

3. MICRO CRUCIFEROUS VEGGIES such as purple radish, red cabbage, broccoli, and kale are worth seeking out. Watch out—their flavor and nutrient levels are rather intense!

4. GREEN PEAS may be overlooked by many, but they contain a unique assortment of health-protective phytonutrients, which provide key antioxidant benefits.

5. CHIA AND FLAXSEEDS are wonderful sources of fiber, essential fatty acids, and powerful phytochemicals, which support bowel health and promote healthy cellular structure.

6. HEMP SEEDS have plentiful amounts of an omega-3 fatty acid known as alpha linolenic acid (ALA) as well as omega-6 fatty acids (linoleic acid), which are key players in immune system health, vision, cell membranes, and the production of hormone-like compounds.

7. ALMONDS, one of those perfect snack foods, are higher in fiber than all other nuts and contain 50 percent more total fiber than peanuts as well as healthy omega-9 oleic fatty acids.

8. QUINOA AND AMARANTH are ancient grains worthy of making a 21st century comeback. Give them a try.

9. RAW UNHEATED HONEY is the best sweetener you can have, and being unheated means it preserves its rich storehouse of naturally occurring enzymes and bee pollen.

10. POMEGRANATES deserve a mention, even though I haven't talked about them up to now. The Bible refers to the pomegranate, which has 613 seeds (the same number of laws in the Bible's Torah or first five books), as the fruit of royalty. It is renowned for its antioxidant qualities.

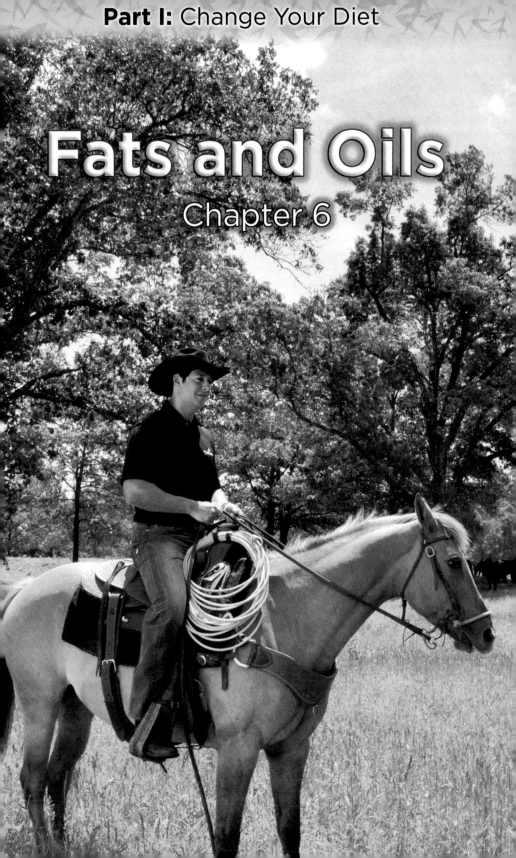

Fats and Oils
Chapter 6

B ack in the summer of 2008, I wanted to get into top physical shape—to really see how strong I could get in a short period of time.

I was turning thirty-three, and while I was in excellent condition, I was inspired to really push myself. To do so, I needed a plan and a couple of buddies for accountability, so for four or five mornings a week, we gathered at 6:30 a.m. in my home gym and plowed through a grueling hour of exercises using Russian kettlebells.

Kettlebells are traditional Russian cast iron weights that look like cannonballs with handles, and they come in various sizes. Swinging and lifting kettlebells was one of those old-school workouts that really got the heart pumping and the muscles fatigued. The results were immediate and impressive.

I also went on a high-fat, high-protein diet to add bulk to my frame. I'm talking about raw eggs tossed in a blender, ceviche (raw sockeye salmon mixed with citrus juices), and even a form of raw beef known as carpaccio, which was raw steak with raw mustard sauce. I ate avocados like they were going out of style, drank raw cream by the pint, and ate raw butter mixed with honey. Let me tell you, I was in the best shape of my life after three months of an intense, predominantly raw diet and exercise program.

I know that if I carried the same plate of high-fat foods into a weight-loss clinic, I'd be run out on a rail. The prevailing message permeating throughout the diet-to-lose-weight culture is that the saturated fats found in meat, dairy, and coconut products are bad for you—something to avoid at all costs. "It's fat that's making you fat" has been a mantra that's been repeated *ad nauseum* by dozens of diet authors, and it has been rehashed so often on TV shows and in magazine articles that the statement has hardened into a concrete fact.

I have a problem with that way of thinking, and it's because the good fats found in pasture-fed meat, wild-caught fish, pasture-fed dairy, unprocessed oils, and other higher fat foods have gotten mistakenly lumped together with the unhealthy fats and oils found in a large percentage of the processed foods sold in grocery stores or prepared in restaurants and fast food joints.

The well-meaning folks who say "fat is making you fat" have it all wrong. Sure, eating the wrong fats can add pounds to your midsection, clog your arteries, and put you at risk for developing life-threatening disease, but when the right fats are consumed, your body receives a concentrated source of energy, nutrients, and source material for cell membranes and various hormones. You *need* the good fats because they play a vital role in the health of your bones, support the immune system, and guard against harmful microorganisms in the digestive tract. Without fats providing satiety, you would go hungry within an hour of finishing a meal, and foods wouldn't taste nearly as good. Who would have thought that fats were so important—or good for you?

BUT YOU HAVE TO CONSUME THE RIGHT FATS, INCLUDING:

- Omega-3 polyunsaturated fats found in cold-water fish, eggs from pastured chickens, and chia, hemp, and flaxseeds, and you can even find omega-3 fats in pasture-fed meat and dairy products

- Omega-9 monounsaturated fatty acids found in avocados, almonds, olive oil, and macadamia nuts

- Omega-6 fats such as gamma linolenic acid (GLA) from unprocessed oils (borage and evening primrose) and nuts and seeds like sunflower, pecans, walnuts, and borage

- Healthy saturated fats containing short- and medium-chain fatty acids found in pasture-fed dairy and coconut and palm oil

- Surprisingly good for you is the trans-fatty acid conjugated linoleic acid (CLA), which is found in pasture-fed meats and dairy products

I'll make more recommendations about the foods containing these important fats and their benefits for the body, but first I need to talk about the difference between omega-3 and omega-6 fatty acids, which are known collectively as essential fatty acids (EFAs).

Omega-3s as well as omega-6s are EFAs that the body must have because they regulate functions such as heart rate and blood pressure, maintain body temperature, insulate nerves, and cushion and protect body tissues. They are essential to health because the body cannot naturally manufacture its own omega-3 or omega-6 fatty acids, which means the body must get them from food sources.

Breaking things down even further, omega-3 fatty acids are a type of fat that supports cardiovascular function, healthy inflammation, and brain function. They manufacture and repair cell membranes and hormones, balance the nervous system, and help expel harmful waste products. Omega-6 fatty acids support skin health and a healthy immune system, so both omega-6 and omega-3 fatty acids are vital to good health.

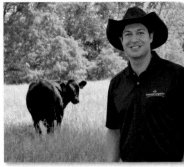

As you can see, GreenFed cows are not shy of the camera.

The problem is that with our modern diet, we get too little of one (omega-3s) and way too much of the other (omega-6s). The main source of omega-3 fatty acids is the flesh of cold water fish like salmon, sardines, mackerel, herring, and tuna, as well as eggs laid by pasture-raised hens who feed on worms, grubs, and insects. You can also find small but significant amounts of omega-3 fats in pasture-fed dairy and beef.

Plant-based omega-3s are found in chia, hemp, and flaxseed as well as green leafy vegetables. Unfortunately, that's not a long list of foods to draw from. Many Americans don't go out of their way to eat fish, especially wild-caught where omega-3 fatty acids are abundant, nor do they eat eggs from pastured hens, which are nearly impossible to find. We're not big salad eaters or snackers on flaxseed crackers.

Omega-6s fatty acids, on the other hand, are plentiful in our diets—for all the wrong reasons. Sure, they are found in nuts and seeds, but most people receive their omega-6 fatty acids from refined vegetable oils like sunflower, safflower, corn, cottonseed, and soybean oils, which, in turn, are found in processed foods and grains. If you're consuming the Standard American Diet (SAD)—breakfast cereals, doughnuts, chicken nuggets, French fries, pizza, cakes, and pies—then you're receiving a ton of omega-6 fatty acids.

That's not good for your health. Excess omega-6s are stored in the body as fat, which contributes greatly to our nationwide obesity problem today. Over the long term, too many omega-6s can imbalance blood pressure, impact brain health, damage the immune system, and even cause dry skin.

Since the typical American diet is weighted heavily toward omega-6 fatty acids instead of omega-3s, most folks have a ratio of 20 omega-6s to one omega-3, or a 20:1 ratio. New research suggests that ratio may be as high as 32:1. Either way, that ratio is dangerously out of proportion. According to the diet of our ancestors, the proper dietary ratio should be between a 4:1 and a 1:1 ratio of omega-6s to omega-3 fatty acids.

I'll never forget during my Perfect Weight America bus tour when families let me come into their homes and do a "Perfect Weight Makeover." This meant I was given free rein to enter their kitchens and pantries and toss out all the food that didn't meet the standard—frozen

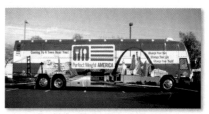

"I can't believe I lived on this bus for 26 weeks."

chicken pot pies, frozen pizza, store-bought cookies, salty crackers, sugary cereals, tubs of ice cream, boxes of candy bars, bags of white sugar, salad dressings, and unhealthy sauces and condiments. I dumped everything into black trash bags that were carried out to their garbage cans.

Then I escorted the shell-shocked family to a nearby natural food grocery, where I showed them how to shop for pasture-raised beef, free-range chicken, organic fruits and vegetables, whole grains, organic condiments, and even healthy snacks. These "makeover" families were universally grateful to get a new start on life while their crummy processed foods made a one-way trip to the landfill.

One thing I pointed out to these families was the importance of eating foods high in omega-3 fatty acids, like wild-caught salmon and other cold-water fish because I had seen firsthand that their diet centered around processed foods, which meant their omega-6 to omega-3 ratio had to be in the 20:1 or 32:1 area. I can remember telling some of these makeover families, "Wild-caught fish is an absolutely incredible food and should be consumed as often as possible." I also recommended pasture-raised beef and pastured eggs.

I also pointed out that consuming conventionally raised eggs would only hurt their omega-6 to omega-3 ratio. I'd seen test results for eggs produced at one of those factory farms where tens of thousands of chickens were confined in the tiniest space possible and not allowed outside for fresh air, and they delivered eggs that had a 20:1 omega-6 to omega-3 ratio, which was way out of balance.

That's why it's important to purchase eggs from pastured chickens, the ones that have free access to pasture land, where they hop around and eat what they find in nature. Sure, pastured eggs cost considerably more than conventional eggs, but the benefits far outweigh the extra dollars they cost. You would be consuming eggs with a proper omega fatty acid ratio of 4:1, maybe even as low as 1:1.

I was interested in what the omega-6 to omega-3 ratios would be for our dairy products at Beyond Organic, so I had our Amasai, raw cheese, and beef tested by an independent laboratory. I am happy to report that our GreenFed dairy products tested out on average between 1.5:1 to 1.2:1 omega-6 to omega-3s, which are right where we want them to be.

I also told the makeover families about the importance of consuming pasture-raised beef from animals like the ones we raise at Beyond Organic. The omega-3 fats in pasture-raised animals are reported to be roughly *seven* times more than the omega-3 fatty acids found in grain-fed animals finished in a feedlot. When our Beyond Organic beef was tested, we learned that our GreenFed meat came in at an approximate ratio of 2.3:1 omega-6 to omega-3 fatty acids.

THE MYTH THAT FATS AREN'T GOOD FOR YOU

It's a good thing I love avocados—I try to include one in my salad every single day—because avocados are a great source of **monounsaturated fats.**

What are monounsaturated fats? Sally Fallon, in her excellent book, *Nourishing Traditions: The Cookbook that Challenges Politically Correct Nutrition and the Diet Dictocrats*, described monounsaturated fatty acids as having one double bond in the form of two carbon atoms double-bonded to each other and therefore lacking two hydrogen atoms.

That's a lot of technical talk, but monounsaturated fats are found in olives, olive oil, macadamia nuts, almonds, and the aforementioned avocados. Studies show that eating foods rich in monounsaturated fats supports healthy cholesterol levels and cardiovascular health.

Yet if you take a man-on-the-street poll, most people would tell you that eating foods high in dietary fat leads to the development of high cholesterol levels and cardiovascular disease. This opinion stems from an entrenched, widely held belief in modern medicine that a high cholesterol diet promotes coronary heart disease, and the best way to *prevent* heart disease is for patients to restrict their diet to low-fat, high-fiber foods. The "diet-heart" connection, as it's known in the hallways of our nation's medical schools, is one of the most deeply ingrained beliefs in conventional medicine.

Dr. Uffe Ravnskov, a Swedish medical physician, took a contrarian view. He had seen patients who had the fear of God put into them from other doctors about the "dangers" of eating red meat, butter, eggs, and cheese since they contained monounsaturated and saturated fats. Dr. Ravnskov's patients came to him complaining of ill health, lack of appetite, and little stamina or zest for life, despite following a doctor's orders to restrict their diet to low-fat, high-fiber foods such as grains, beans, legumes, fruit, and vegetables.

Dr. Ravnskov, who had also earned a Ph.D. for his scientific studies at the Departments of Nephrology and Clinical Chemistry at the University Hospital in Lund, Sweden, before starting his private practice, decided to look closer at peer-reviewed studies in top American medical journals as well as the Framingham Heart Study, a sixty-year-long project of the National Heart, Lung, and Blood Institute that sought to identify the common factors or characteristics that contribute to cardiovascular disease. A major finding of the Framingham Heart Study was that cholesterol-level abnormalities were found to increase the risk of heart disease.

Dr. Ravnskov studied the data and said he couldn't find conclusive proof regarding the connection between high cholesterol and cardiovascular disease. He further stated that there was no evidence that too much fat in the diet promoted heart attacks.

The Swedish doctor put down his findings in a book called *The Cholesterol Myths*, which I read, and his work confirmed my suspicions that the oft-recommended low-fat, high-fiber diet touted for preventing high cholesterol would never be a hoped-for panacea. Too many doctors are recommending that people stay away from certain traditional foods that can actually be quite beneficial to overall health.

The reason why Dr. Ravnskov said it's a myth that high blood cholesterol promotes coronary heart disease was because studies like the Framingham Heart Study showed that people with low blood cholesterol levels were just as prone to coronary heart disease as people with high cholesterol levels. Besides, cholesterol was not some deadly poison but a vital substance found in every cell membrane, said Dr. Ravnskov. We *need* cholesterol, and because we do, we should eat foods with healthy fats that supply the body with cholesterol.

Saturated fats are considered the worst offenders by those who subscribe to the "diet-heart" connection that Dr. Ravnskov was fighting against. The reality, however, is just the opposite: the saturated fats found in beef and dairy products can be some of the best fats for you—as long as you are consuming foods from pasture-fed animals.

HERE ARE SOME EXAMPLES OF FOODS THAT CONTAIN HEALTHY SATURATED FATS:

- Butter from pasture-fed cows
- Cheese from pasture-fed cows
- Coconut and palm oils (look for extra virgin)
- Whole milk dairy from pasture-fed cows
- Beef, venison, buffalo, and lamb (when green finished)
- Pastured eggs
- Chicken, duck, and turkey (pastured, free-range)

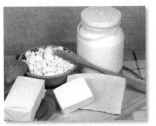

Dietary fats such as saturated fats come in forms of triglycerides, each containing three fatty acid chains. Short-chain and medium-chain fatty acids found in foods such as true whole milk dairy, coconut and palm oils can be excellent for health.

Butter is a prime example of food containing short-chain fatty acids, including one called butyric acid, which makes butter easy to digest. Udo Erasmus, in his book *Fats That Heal, Fats That Kill*, decided to do a comparison of butter and margarine by using a simple scoring system. He examined all the good points as well as bad points of butter and margarine and awarded 1 point for each positive factor and -1 point for each negative factor.

I won't go through Erasmus' entire scorecard but will share some highlights:

- Butter received points for having about 500 different saturated and monounsaturated fatty acids that were relatively stable to light, heat, and oxygen.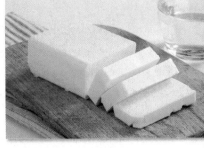

- Margarine contained few short-chain, easily digestive fatty acids, no cholesterol (which the body needs, remember), plenty of *trans* fatty acids (a byproduct of hydrogenation, which produces non-natural chemicals), and traces of aluminum. Margarine wasn't suitable for frying like butter was and ended with a negative -11 score.

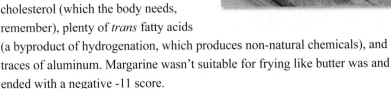

I concur with Erasmus and believe that butter from pasture-fed cows is a beneficial dairy product that gives food a luxurious "mouth feel" and flavor.

"Butter is better," stated Dr. Mary Enig, the author of *Know Your Fats: The Complete Primer for Understanding the Nutrition of Fats, Oils, and Cholesterol.* Dr. Enig, who's in her early eighties today but still going strong, is a research scientist and nutritionist who was a contributing editor for Sally Fallon's book, *Nourishing Traditions: The Cookbook that Challenges Politically Correct Nutrition and the Diet Dictocrats.* Their thought-provoking, groundbreaking book contained the startling message that animal fats and cholesterol were *not* villains but were necessary for normal growth, proper function of the brain and nervous system, protection from disease, and maintaining optimum energy levels.

Dr. Enig, who made it her life's goal to fight a misinformation campaign from "Diet Dictocrats" who assert that naturally saturated fats from animal sources are the root cause of heart disease and cancer, said, "Butter bore the brunt of the attack and was accused of terrible crimes. The Diet Dictocrats told us it was better to switch to polyunsaturated margarine, and most Americans did. Butter all but disappeared from our tables, shunned as a miscreant."

Butter is making a comeback, thanks to voices like Dr. Enig's. Butter is the best and most easily absorbed source of vitamin A, which plays a strong antioxidant role. The notion that butter causes weight gain is another sad misconception, said Dr. Enig. "The short- and medium-chain fatty acids in butter are not stored in the adipose tissue, but are used for quick energy," she said. Fat tissue in humans is composed mainly of longer-chain fatty acids, which comes from refined polyunsaturated oils made from grains and seeds high in omega-6 fatty acids—yet another reason why butter is an excellent form of saturated fat.

Pasture-fed beef, also high in omega-3 fatty acids and important vitamins like vitamin B12 and E, has something extra going for it: **conjugated linoleic acid** (CLA), a fatty acid that has been studied by researchers at the University of Wisconsin School of Medicine. CLA is a nutrient the body cannot produce and is also known as rumenic acid because it is made in the rumen of cud-chewing animals through microbial action.

A few years ago, CLA received media attention when it was identified as a component of red meat and dairy from pasture-fed animals that promotes good health. CLA is found in meat and milk, but it's most highly concentrated in milk fat—yet another reason to forget about skim or low fat dairy products. Furthermore, the full fat or whole milk dairy from pasture-fed cows can contain as much as five times more

CLA than milk from standard grain-fed cows, and pasture-fed beef has three to five times more CLA than grain-fed cattle.

Here's another interesting point about pasture-fed beef: although the total saturated fat is similar between pasture-fed and grain-fed beef, there are differences in the type of fatty acids present in the meat. Pasture-fed beef has lower amounts of cholesterol-raising myristic and palmitic saturated fatty acids and more stearic acid than grain-fed beef, and pasture-fed meat is also lower in calories than grain-fed meat, contains more healthy omega-3 fats, more vitamins A and E, higher levels of antioxidants, and many times the beta-carotene.

A six-ounce cut of pasture-fed beef tenderloin may have 92 fewer calories than the same cut from a grain-fed cow. Given that the average per-capita consumption of beef is 67 pounds a year, switching to pasture-fed beef could save you 16,642 calories a year.

LAST CALL ON OMEGA-3S

Omega-3 fats are long-chain, **polyunsaturated fats**. I've talked about monounsaturated and saturated fats; now I'd like to switch gears and talk about omega-3-rich polyunsaturated fats.

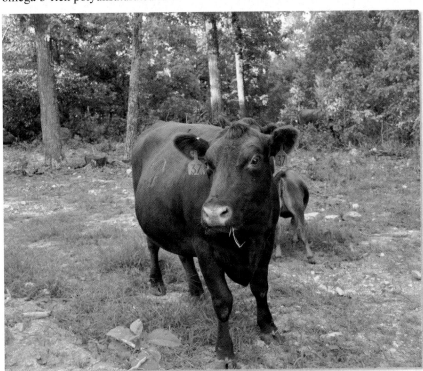

First of all, there are two principal types: vegetable-derived and animal-derived. The vegetable-derived come in the form of alpha-linolenic acids (ALA), and the most well-known animal forms are eicosapentaenoic acid (EPA) and docosahexaenoic acid (DHA). Both play important roles in the function of our bodies.

These fatty acids help with forming neural transmitters, which are vital for brain function. EPA and DHA are converted into hormone-like substances called prostaglandins, which regulate cell activity and healthy cardiovascular function. DHA plays a key role during fetal development and early infancy. Those who are up there in years need EPA and DHA to bolster cognitive function and mental focus, as well as maintain the immune system. EPA and DHA also insulate the body against heat loss, prevent skin from drying and flaking, and cushion tissues and organs, and these important fats are found mainly in cold-water fish and pastured eggs.

Plant-based omega-3s are found in abundance in chia, hemp, and flaxseeds, and, to a lesser extent, pumpkin seeds in the form of alpha-linolenic acid (ALA), which is a key player in immune system health, vision, cell membranes, and the production of hormone-like compounds.

I remember hearing about flaxseed when I was a little kid from my Grandma Rose. She told me stories about the small family farm she grew up on sixty kilometers west of Warsaw, where her father operated a mill that pressed poppy seeds and flaxseeds into oil. A big taste treat in those days was to take the pressed seeds and patty them into hard cakes, which were dipped into *schmaltz*, or the rendered fat from chicken soup.

Eighty, ninety years ago, a poor Jewish family living in the Polish countryside knew nothing about omega-3 fatty acids or beneficial fiber present in flaxseeds, but they somehow knew that flaxseeds were healthy for you.

Thanks to modern science, we know better today—or should. Don't believe the conventional wisdom that says fat is what is making you fat or that fat is bad for you. Of the three macronutrients—protein, carbohydrates, and fat—fat is the one most likely to determine whether you have poor health or good health.

In fact, if someone approaches me after a seminar and says he or she is having a health challenge, one of my first questions is: "What types of fats are in your diet?"

Answering that question correctly could mean the difference between life and death.

THE TOP 10 FOOD SOURCES OF HEALTHY FATS

1. COCONUT contains beneficial medium-chain fatty acids. Consume the meat, oil, and cream. I use extra-virgin coconut oil for cooking, baking, and frying, and I also use raw coconut cream in my smoothies.

2. PASTURE-FED DAIRY contains the right balance of fats that your body needs, so there's no reason to go to low-fat or skim versions. Seek out really GreenFed raw cheese, Amasai, and butter.

3. PASTURE-FED RED MEAT should be regularly on your menu as well, which would mean GreenFinished beef, lamb, venison and bison. These type of pastured meats offer a good balance of omega-6 to omega-3 fatty acid as well as conjugated linoleic acid (CLA).

4. AVOCADOS are great in salads and a wonderful source of monounsaturated fats as well as vitamin E, potassium, and fiber.

5. WILD-CAUGHT FISH such as salmon, mackerel, herring, sardines, and tuna are superior sources of omega-3 fatty acids. If you're shopping for canned tuna, look for higher-end tuna packed in spring water with six-to-eight grams of fat.

6. CHIA AND FLAXSEED are excellent sources of alpha-linolenic acid (ALA), which is a type of omega-3 fatty acid healthy for the entire body.

7. HEMP SEED is another fine source of ALA as well as the important omega-6 fatty acid known as gamma linoleic acid (GLA).

8. NUTS AND SEEDS, including sunflower, walnuts, and pecans, are good sources of omega-3 and 6 fatty acids.

9. EXTRA-VIRGIN OLIVE OIL is a wonderful source of monounsaturated fats and antioxidants. Use extra-virgin olive oil when making homemade salad dressing but not in cooking since key nutrients and compounds break down under high heat.

10. EXTRA-VIRGIN RED PALM OIL is an excellent source of saturated fats, mainly comprised of medium-chain fatty acids and contains beta-carotene and vitamin E. Watch out, though. Red palm oil stains, so you don't want to spill it.

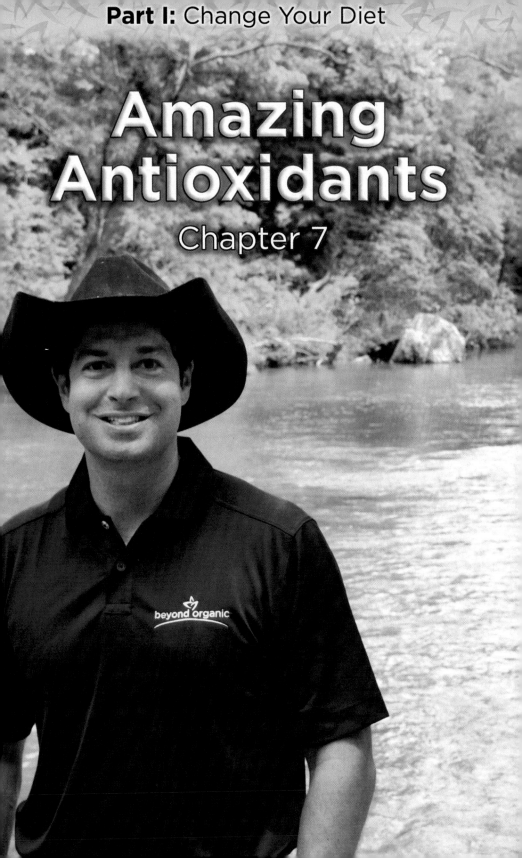

Amazing Antioxidants

Chapter 7

A couple of years ago, my wife, Nicki, and I were looking for a special way to celebrate our tenth wedding anniversary. We initially considered the usual "second honeymoon" ideas—the romantic beaches of Hawaii; the high-energy stimulation of New York City and Broadway; or an ooh-la-la week taking in the memorable sights of Paris—but the more Nicki and I discussed our options, the more we thought about shaking things up.

So Nicki started surfing the Internet. She discovered a long trek across the Sahara desert with the nomads, but the idea of sitting on a camel for ten hours a day, wondering if bandits with long swords would slit your throat, convinced me to squash that idea.

Then Nicki proposed staying in a tree house tucked away in the western cape of South Africa. That idea sounded promising until I learned that it would take us nearly forty-five hours—door-to-door—to get there.

Then Nicki found an interesting opportunity in another foreign country—but on our own continent. The place was called Clayoquot Wilderness Resort on the western flank of Vancouver Island, the British Columbia isle west of the Canadian mainland. From our home in South Florida, this eco-retreat still looked half a world away, and in many ways, it was. Billed as a "temperate rainforest" with its own biosphere, the Clayoquot Wilderness Resort offered a "discreet paradox of individual pampering and remote, untamed wilderness," according to its promotional literature. (Clayoquot is pronounced *clay-kwat*, dropping the "o" syllable.)

Guests stayed in elegant white canvas tents furnished with a soft Adirondack-style bed, a pair of oil lamps, antique dresser, and a private outdoor composting toilet. The prospector-style quarters were built on raised wooden platforms and connected by cedar boardwalks under a canopy of towering old-growth trees. Experienced chefs prepared "modern natural" cuisine that belonged in *Bon Appétit* pictorials. Three massage tents, two wood-fired cedar hot tubs, and a wood-fired cedar sauna beckoned with the allure of rest and relaxation.

They called it *glamping*—glamorous camping.

As a product of American suburbia, the idea of "roughing it" in comfort and style while kayaking in the Clayoquot Sound, whale watching in the Pacific, riding horses through pristine meadows, and hiking into the rainforest was very tempting. We stepped outside our comfort zone and booked a weeklong stay in late August and early September 2009.

Soon after our arrival, Nicki and I went on a mountain bike tour with a guide, who pointed out the wild huckleberries and salmonberries on the trail. I had to try some. The salmonberries looked like raspberries and tasted just as good. I was quite happy that my body was receiving wonderful antioxidants from freshly picked berries in the Canadian wilderness.

During one of the camp dinners, we met some nice folks who told us about the wild salmon they caught on a fishing trip organized by the Clayoquot staff. They mentioned that their catch was being processed by a local fishery and shipped back home. The salmon could be either canned or smoked and then transported frozen in temperature-controlled packaging with dry ice.

I loved the idea of catching my own wild salmon in the Canadian straits and having my bounty shipped to Florida. Where do I sign up?

My first fishing trip took me up the sound into inland waters, where Nicki and I dropped fishing lines into the clear cold water. I caught five salmon between six and nine pounds but had to toss two back because they were protected Coho salmon from a nearby hatchery, identifiable by the notch in their fin. A few days later, we took a second fishing trip, but this time we ventured into deeper ocean waters, where I caught my biggest fish, a king salmon.

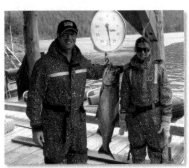

Just in case you didn't believe me, here is proof of my fishing "expertise"

What an awesome experience! That king salmon gave me quite a fight, and the battle was extremely excruciating on my forearms as it took me a good twenty minutes to land the fish. The lunker weighed twenty-five pounds and had to be three feet long. I reeled in four other nice-sized salmon as well.

All eight fish were canned or smoked in various flavors in Canada prior to their shipment to Florida. My family and I could have eaten all of the wild-caught salmon within a month of coming home, but I decided that we'd dole it out as a special treat or when we had friends over to the house. It's been a lot of fun setting small pieces of smoked salmon on an hors d'oeuvre plate and letting everyone try a piece while I say something like, *Well, everybody, this is from the king salmon I caught off Vancouver Island . . .*

My friends find that funny because they know I'm not much of a fisherman and this could be the only time I catch wild salmon—or any other fish, for that matter—in my lifetime.

I still have some canned Clayoquot wild salmon in our pantry more than two years after our anniversary trip. I'm so hooked on the great taste and bountiful nutrients of wild fish that I have packages of wild sockeye salmon shipped to my Florida home every other month directly from a small sustainable fishery in Alaska. I would say that I eat wild sockeye salmon five to seven times a week for two reasons:

1. The high amount of omega-3 fatty acids, whose benefits I discussed in the previous chapter.

2. A powerful antioxidant contained in salmon that I'm going to talk about in *this* chapter.

Antioxidants are substances mainly found in the pigments that color fruits and vegetables, but surprisingly there are antioxidants in the flesh of wild-caught fish and other animal foods such as pastured eggs and even GreenFed beef.

In fact, there are two classes of antioxidants: those best absorbed in the presence of fat, known as **fat-soluble antioxidants**; and those best absorbed in the presence of water, known as **water-soluble antioxidants**. The difference between the two types of antioxidants can be significant, but both are tremendously beneficial for the body.

Let's start with water-soluble antioxidants first, which are found mainly in the pigments that color fruits and vegetables. These antioxidants are also known as phytochemicals, which offer antioxidant protection against free radicals running rampant within your molecular system. As I mentioned in Chapter 5, free radicals are unstable molecules generated within the body that can cause cell damage, which can lead to health challenges if left unchecked. These unstable molecules love to attack the healthy cells of the body.

Thankfully, there's an antidote to the voracious electron appetite of free radicals, and that's water-soluble antioxidants. Since these antioxidants do a great job of neutralizing free radicals, you should have a steady supply of antioxidants coming into the body—through fresh foods like fruits, vegetables, and botanicals such as herbs—or free radicals will gain the upper hand. That's not good for your short-term or long-term health. It should be noted that in addition to water-soluble antioxidants, many vegetables and fruits contain fat-soluble antioxidants such as beta carotene and lycopene.

Here's an analogy to describe what antioxidants do to those mayhem-minded free radicals roaming around your body. I want you to think of a lit fire, burning and crackling inside a fireplace. Sparks come off the fire, which is why prudent folks place a screen in front of the fireplace—to catch any loose sparks. Your body is like that raging fire, setting off sparks, or free radicals, but those sparks won't harm anything if you put a screen in front of them. Consuming antioxidant-rich fruits and vegetables is like setting a screen before a roaring fireplace.

Pigments with health-promoting properties color every fruit and vegetable on display at your local health food store or farmer's market. Green vegetables owe their color to chlorophyll. Tomatoes and watermelons are red because of a carotenoid antioxidant known as lycopene. Blueberries—the Rubin household favorite—are

colored by the phytochemical anthocyanin, which is also found in "red" fruits like strawberries, raspberries, and red grapes. Water-soluble antioxidants such as anthocyanin are nature's way of fighting off potentially dangerous molecules in your body.

Fat-soluble antioxidants found in wild-caught fish (astaxanthin), eggs (lutein), and seaweed (fucoxanthin) actively seek out and destroy rogue cells in the human body as well as neutralizing fat-soluble toxins and supporting the replenishment and health of the particular individual cell. Since they promote the health of cells on the cellular level, fat-soluble antioxidants are extremely important to your body.

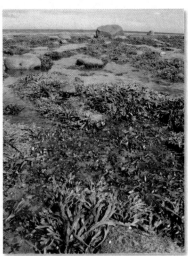
Brown seaweed is naturally high in antioxidant nutrients.

The antioxidant contained in the flesh of wild-caught fish is called astaxanthin, a powerful antioxidant that's known as the "King of the Carotenoids." The reason for this moniker is because astaxanthin has been shown to increase strength and endurance and boost the immune system—to name just a couple of health benefits backed up by clinical research. Astaxanthin is what gives the flesh of sockeye salmon its rich red color as well as the distinctive red shells for sea creatures like lobsters and crabs.

Here's another reason why I've never been a fan of farm-raised fish. When "Atlantic salmon" spend all their lives swimming in concrete tanks, fattening up on fish meal, the result is an absence of natural pigmentation in their flesh. Normally, when salmon are in their natural habitat, like in the waters off Vancouver Island, they obtain their coloration from natural food sources, including algae and crustaceans, but when raised in holding tanks, their meat turns out whitish or even gray. Since the unattractive look of off-white "salmon" meat makes for a tough sale in the supermarket meat case, fish farmers add a form of synthetic astaxanthin to the fish feed to give the meat a more orangey color.

I'm not fooled, and I hope you aren't either.

Another type of antioxidants that I want to tell you about are the **intracellular antioxidants** or antioxidant enzymes known as glutathione, superoxide dismutase (SOD), and catalase. As research continues to unveil the importance of antioxidants, none may be as important as glutathione. While glutathione is produced by the body, the consumption of high-quality amino acids such as cysteine, glycine, and glutamic acid in its tri-peptide form is considered to be a pre-cursor to glutathione production. Certain foods such as minimally processed high-quality dairy products contain these amino acids.

Here's some background on why glutathione is so significant.

I've told you how antioxidants work at the cellular level to combat free radicals that damage cells. If you had to define one reason why toxins are bad, it may be because they lead to oxidative stress within the body, causing a proliferation of free radicals.

Where the human body is concerned, glutathione is at its highest concentration in the liver. As the collection point of toxins, the liver is prone to oxidative stress and damage from free radicals. Although the liver has the ability to manufacture glutathione, that won't happen if you're not supplying the body with high-quality, naturally processed foods such as pasture-fed dairy.

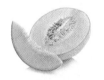 Superoxide dismutase, or SOD, and catalase can be obtained from raw produce, especially from green foods such as sprouts or micro veggies. SOD and catalase are also found in melons such as cantaloupe. SOD converts superoxide radicals into hydrogen peroxide, which is then turned into water and oxygen by another intracellular antioxidant enzyme catalase. This incredible physiological process lessens the oxidative stress on and within cells.

Antioxidants—whether they are water soluble, fat soluble, or intracellular—are wonderful things. We'll spend the rest of this chapter describing the antioxidants found in select healthy foods.

THE ANTIOXIDANTS IN FRUITS

HERE'S A LIST OF MY FAVORITE ANTIOXIDANTS AND THE FRUITS THEY'RE FOUND IN:

- POLYPHENOLS, which help reduce cellular damage and oxidative stress, are found in tea, herbal infusions, and many fruits. Tea comes in several forms, but black, green, white, and rooibos, or red tea, are the most popular. Black tea is the tea people are most familiar with. In the South, iced tea and "sweet tea" are made from black tea, which has approximately 20 percent of the caffeine found in a cup of coffee.

Green tea is the most popular tea around the world, mainly because it's the beverage of choice in Asia. Green tea has half the caffeine as black tea and healthy antioxidants like epigallocatechin gallate, or EGCG, which supports the flow of blood through the vessels and is good for cardiovascular health. EGCG is a powerful antioxidant or "anti-rust" agent that supports immune system health.

White tea is the purest and least processed of all teas. This loose-leaf tea has very little caffeine and generous amounts of polyphenols. Rooibos tea, a red tea made from a South African red bush, is a naturally caffeine-free tea that promotes digestion, supports your immune system, and promotes healthy, skin, teeth, and bones.

- ANTHOCYANIN is the antioxidant that gives blueberries their deep-blue, purplish color and makes them a phytonutrient superstar. Low in calories and rich in nutrients, blueberries are getting a lot of attention in university laboratories, where the antioxidant anthocyanin is being studied for its positive impact on health. You could almost call anthocyanin a "crime fighter" for the way it takes on free radicals in the body, protects the cardiovascular system by reducing the oxidation of LDL cholesterol in your bloodstream, prevents blood cells from sticking together, improves elasticity in your blood vessels, and prevents your arteries from constricting.

Blueberries may have the highest concentration of anthocyanins, but they aren't the only place where you can get these valuable antioxidants. They can also be found in herbs, grains, and many fruits and vegetables, but the best anthocyanin-rich foods—besides blueberries—are blackberries, raspberries, strawberries, cherries, plums, eggplant, cabbage, and red onions.

And here's some good information to file away: recent research shows that fresh blueberries can be frozen without damaging their delicate antioxidants, so go ahead and buy frozen organic blueberries to enjoy in and out of season!

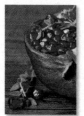

- ELLAGIC ACID, another phytochemical or beneficial plant compound, is found in generous amounts in raspberries and pomegranates and to a lesser extent in strawberries, cranberries, walnuts, and pecans. This antioxidant is reputed to support healthy cellular development and retard the growth of unhealthy cells.

   My go-to source for ellagic acid is pomegranates, which can help cleanse the body of harmful toxins and has more antioxidants than green tea and red wine combined. High in fiber and fat-free, a great way to include pomegranates in your diet is to sprinkle pomegranate seeds onto your salad. In Song of Solomon, when Solomon was praising his bride, he described her as an "orchard of pomegranates with choice fruits."

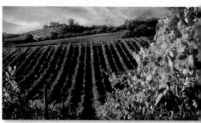

- RESVERATROL has been all the rage, and it seems to be a big topic of discussion on major health shows—probably because resveratrol is found in red wine.

Hey, honey, let's crack open that bottle of merlot. I want some of them resveratrol antioxidants. Shall we have a toast?

I can understand the desire of some to find another justification to drinking wine, although that's never been a consideration for me since I don't drink. Sure, red wine can provide the antioxidant resveratrol, but red grapes, blueberries, and pomegranate are good sources as well.

That said, resveratrol supports healthy blood sugar levels, supports the health of the immune system, and helps negate the effects of a calorie-laden diet. Resveratrol's cholesterol-supporting benefits make it ideal for those concerned about heart health and may help explain the "French Paradox."

Anyone who's vacationed in France, which I've been fortunate to do, has seen firsthand how any self-respecting Frenchman wearing a blue beret wouldn't think of sitting down in a restaurant without ordering a glass of Bordeaux. The French have the highest per-capita consumption of wine in the world, eat a diet loaded with butter, cheese, cream, meats, and rich pâtés like *foie gras*, and many smoke, but they have a much lower rate of coronary heart disease than Americans and deadly heart attacks claim half the victims in France as they do in the United States.

That's why this phenomenon is known as the "French Paradox," and many believe a big reason is the resveratrol in their diet.

- HYDROXYTYROSOL is one of the most beneficial components in olives and extra virgin olive oil and is an extremely rare—and difficult to pronounce—polyphenol. Researchers are discovering that hydroxytyrosol is a highly potent antioxidant associated with healthier breast tissue, colon function, and cardiovascular health. After ellagic acid, hydroxytyrosol is believed to be one of the most powerful antioxidants and one of the strongest free radical-scavenging compounds available.

In nature, hydroxytyrosol is found in olive leaves, olive fruit, and olive oil. Olive oil has been prized for centuries and even used as currency for trade. Biblical kings in Israel placed great worth on their olive orchards, guarding them fiercely against anyone who would harm their harvest. Much of the shipping in the Mediterranean at that time involved the trading of olive trees, olive, and oil.

Extra virgin olive oil, as you are aware, makes for a wonderful and healthy salad dressing when mixed with a bit of balsamic vinegar and lemon juice. And with each bite of delicious salad, your body will receive hydroxytyrosol.

- LYCOPENE is the reason behind the red color of certain fruits and vegetables—like watermelons and tomatoes. Because lycopene is in tomatoes, and because tomatoes and tomato sauce are popular in the American diet—think garden salads, ketchup, tomato sauce, and salsa—lycopene has become a great topic of research and discussion.

Researchers are trying to pin down how lycopene protects cells from free radical damage and the DNA inside of white blood cells. Another fascinating area of research is lycopene's support of the immune system and prostate health.

According to Ohio State researchers, when tomatoes are eaten in a salad, the lycopene molecules are in a linear configuration, a structure that hinders the molecule's absorption through the intestinal walls and into the bloodstream unless the body can successfully bend these molecules to make them easier to be absorbed into the blood and transported to other tissue.

When the tomatoes are *cooked*, however, as in a tomato sauce, those lycopene molecules are already bent prior to ingestion, which increases the amount of lycopene into the bloodstream. Lycopene is a fat-soluble antioxidant and is best absorbed when consumed along with a healthy fat or oil. Caprese salad, anyone?

Maybe the Italians knew something when they started making pasta and pizza centuries ago.

- I doubt you've heard of this next antioxidant, E M B L I C A N, or the berry that contains it in significant amounts—Amla berry, which is also known as Indian gooseberry. This fruit ripens on Amla trees in wet, hilly forest in the Indian subcontinent, where the amla tree is considered to be sacred. The berries, while nourishing, taste rather sour.

The emblican antioxidant is prevalent in the Indian gooseberry, a botanical that is known for its rejuvenating and anti-aging effects. This berry works to inhibit the aging effects of ultraviolet light by preventing the breakdown of collagen. The result is smoother, suppler skin. Another cool fact is unlike most antioxidants that die off after fighting free radicals, emblican can regenerate itself and live to fight another day.

THE ANTIOXIDANTS IN MICRO VEGGIES

I introduced **sulforaphanes** in Chapter 5, the chapter on carbohydrates. Sulforaphanes are nifty antioxidants found in a variety of micro veggies, the young seedlings of broccoli, cabbages, radishes, mustards, beets, and other greens.

Micro veggies are grown hydroponically or in a few inches of potting soil. Take micro broccoli, for instance. With a few spritzes from a misting bottle, the seeds sprout within two days, throwing down roots. A week later, tiny leaves are lush and ready for "harvesting." You can clip a small leaf at the bottom of the stem, plop the whole thing into your mouth, and taste broccoli distilled to its tender green essence.

Sulforaphane is a compound most associated with broccoli. Research has shown that sulforaphane activates a protein called Nrf2 in your arteries, which supports heart health and healthy levels of inflammatory chemicals. Kale is another green cruciferous vegetable that contains high levels of sulforaphane.

Chlorophyll is another wonderful antioxidant that's common in micro veggies and all other green plants. In fact, it's chlorophyll that gives lettuce, kale, and wheatgrass its luscious green color. Chlorophyll is very similar in structure to the protein hemoglobin, which may explain why consuming green leafy vegetables can increase the blood's capacity to deliver oxygen and other nutrients to the cells of the body.

The main element in chlorophyll is magnesium, and every cell in your body needs magnesium, as it performs more than three hundred biochemical reactions in the body. Bone health, for example, is supported by the magnesium contained in green leafy veggies. By eating micro veggies and leafy green salads regularly, your body receives magnesium along with chlorophyll, which can also help cleanse the body of accumulated toxins.

Along with chlorophyll in green foods, you'll find that **superoxide dismutase (SOD)** plays a role in supporting healthy inflammation throughout the body and in slowing down the cell deterioration process of tissues and organs.

- Working with SOD is C A T A L A S E, an antioxidant enzyme that loves to take on free radicals in the body. According to some recent scientific studies, low levels of catalase may play a role in the graying process of human hair, so that's one more incentive for Nicki and me to keep eating our green salads during the day!

THE ANTIOXIDANT IN PASTURED DAIRY

Remember when I talked about the cheese-making process and the curds and whey in Chapter 2? Certain amino acids found in the whey portion of dairy stimulate the body's production of **glutathione**, a major antioxidant indispensable for the healthy functioning of all body cells, with special protective roles for the liver, the cardiovascular and immune systems, and red blood cells. Laboratory studies have demonstrated that glutathione has the potential to improve many aspects of our health.

All the more reason to seek out pastured dairy, which is also rich in vitamins including vitamin E, beta-carotene, and vitamin C.

THE ANTIOXIDANT IN SALMON

Astaxanthin is what gives salmon and other sea-faring creatures such as lobsters and crabs their red pigment. Closely related to beta-carotene, astaxanthin provides antioxidant benefits and therefore may play a role in defending cell membranes from free radical attack. Astaxanthin may also enhance joint function and mobility, while supporting the body's normal recovery from muscle overuse. Additionally, astaxanthin supports eye health, skin health, and healthy immune function.

THE ANTIOXIDANTS IN SEAWEED

About thirteen years ago, I was introduced to the Russian biochemist Dr. Zakir Ramazanov, whose specialty was identifying and concentrating phytonutrients and antioxidants found in land and ocean plants. For instance, the Georgian scientist applied innovative technology to the extraction of lycopene, beta-carotene, and lutein from tomatoes, mushrooms, and algae; the extraction of antioxidants from fruits and vegetables; and the intensive biotechnological cultivation of health-promoting marine plants or seaweed.

But Dr. Ramazanov's real passion was research into sea vegetables, particularly brown seaweed, because epidemiological data from some of the longest living and healthiest cultures on the planet—most notably the Japanese—showed that the human consumption of brown seaweed portended tremendous health benefits. Dr. Ramazanov informed me early on—this had to be around 2002 or so—that he was having success concentrating a carotenoid called **fucoxanthin** from brown seaweed.

Dr. Ramazanov believed fucoxanthin could regulate a protein called uncoupling protein 1, or UCP1, which controls the amount of fat stored in cells of the body. UCP1, which regulates the activity of a key gene responsible for maintaining the body's temperature, is found in white adipose tissue, or visceral fat. What Dr. Ramazanov and his team surmised was that fucoxanthin possessed strong thermogenic—or fat-burning—properties.

Long story short, we decided at Garden of Life to use fucoxanthin as the foundation for a nutritional supplement called fücoTHIN, which went on to become the No. 1-selling weight-loss product in the Natural Products Industry.

If you're looking to lose a few pounds, then fucoxanthin—a powerful antioxidant—could help you naturally burn fat with no nervousness, jitters, or lost sleep.

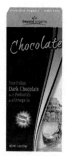

THE ANTIOXIDANT IN CHOCOLATE

"Chocolate is no ordinary food," writer Geneeth Roth explained one time. "It is not something you can take or leave, something you like only moderately. You don't like chocolate. You don't even love chocolate. Chocolate is something you have an affair with."

Well, I wouldn't go that far, but chocolate is delicious and can even be healthy, as long as you don't go overboard. Dark chocolate, preferably made from organic ingredients, is better for you than lighter milk chocolate because it has higher concentrations of **theobromine**, an antioxidant. The compounds in dark chocolate also releases both serotonin and endorphins.

Many chocolate lovers will be very happy to learn that we're offering Beyond Organic dark chocolate bars that are crafted by fifth-generation Italian chocolatiers containing probiotics and the superfood flaxseed. Our Beyond Organic dark chocolate is GMO-free and USDA certified organic.

I bet you can't stop at one small piece.

THE ANTIOXIDANTS IN COFFEE

Even though just about everybody knows about Starbucks, not many know that coffee is a fruit. Actually, there's a cherry on the outside, and what we call the coffee bean is really a seed on the inside. The seed starts out green and increases in caffeine as it matures. Believe it or not, coffee is the number-one source of antioxidants in this country, but I'm not sure that's a good thing. The reason for this finding by a research team at the University of Scranton in Pennsylvania is because Americans drink so much coffee and don't eat enough wild-caught fish, dairy, fruits, and vegetables, which are so much better for you.

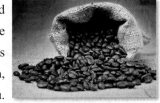

Coffee's notable antioxidants are **chlorogenic acid** and **caffeic acid**, which help support healthy blood sugar levels and cardiovascular health. I don't recommend drinking coffee more than occasionally, but if you consume coffee made from organic beans, grind it yourself, and use a healthy sweetener such as honey and real cream, you could actually receive some health benefits from your cup of Joe.

THE ANTIOXIDANTS IN TEA

Tea is the number-two source of antioxidants in this country, but that's because we drink so much tea and not enough other antioxidant-rich foods that I've already mentioned.

Tea does have wonderful **polyphenols**, which is why I recommend green and white tea from organic sources. Some of the best natural, organic teas I've found are imported from the pristine Wuyi Mountains of China, where tea leaves are harvested by hand and not subjected to pesticides and chemical fertilizers.

THE ANTIOXIDANTS IN SPICES

How strongly and how quickly a particular antioxidant can "neutralize" an oxidizing agent is expressed by the ORAC value (Oxygen Radical Absorbance Capacity) that I introduced in Chapter 5.

Two of my favorite spices—cinnamon and oregano—rank second and third, respectively, in the ORAC list of the Top 10 antioxidant spices. (Cloves top the list.) The sweet, warm taste of cinnamon is a spice derived from the bark of a small evergreen tree native to Sri Lanka. Its antioxidant properties are much more powerful than those in six other antioxidant spices such as anise, ginger, licorice, mint, nutmeg, and vanilla. As for oregano, this popular herb used in Italian and Greek cooking is high in antioxidant activity and supports healthy inflammation response in the body.

Spices such as cinnamon, oregano, rosemary, and thyme have volatile oils that are very high in antioxidant activity.

THE ANTIOXIDANTS IN ESSENTIAL OILS

I believe significant health benefits can be derived from consuming essential oils both orally and topically. Consuming essential oils of ginger, orange, lemon, cinnamon, thyme, rosemary, and oregano are great for your body. You can also inhale essential oils by rubbing a few drops of myrtle, coriander, hyssop, galbanum, or frankincense onto the palms, then cup your hands over your mouth and nose and inhale. Taking a deep breath will soothe the mind, invigorate the spirit, and give you an antioxidant boost.

I've rubbed some of these essential oils on the soles of my feet, and I've been amazed that I can taste cinnamon or peppermint oil on the tip of my tongue within twenty minutes. This is because when you take spices and botanicals and distill the oils, you're concentrating many of the antioxidants by a factor of one hundred times or more.

Whether you consume essential oils in foods or beverages, rub these oils into your skin or add them to your bath, you'll experience a renewed sense of health.

THE TOP 10 DIETARY SOURCES OF ANTIOXIDANTS

1. BLUEBERRIES, filled with water-soluble antioxidants, top my list once again. The list of blueberries' health benefits gets longer every year as more studies uncover the power of these great-tasting berries. The latest show that they support brain health and have been shown to increase short-term memory in animal studies.

2. WILD-CAUGHT SALMON contain a powerful fat-soluble antioxidant known as astaxanthin that is known to be hundreds of times more potent than typical antioxidants such as vitamin C, vitamin E, and beta-carotene.

3. COFFEE, especially the green coffee seed, is even higher in antioxidants than tea.

4. GRAPES contain resveratrol, as well as hundreds of other antioxidants. It's important to note that the seeds and skin contain the richest source of antioxidants, so don't buy the seedless variety!

5. DARK CHOCOLATE (or cacao) contains potent antioxidants that support cardiovascular health in the same way that green tea and blueberries do because chocolate comes from cacao beans that are full of natural plant compounds.

6. TEA is the poster child for polyphenolic antioxidants. Green tea has a tremendous amount of antioxidants, including one called ECGC. White and rooibos (red) tea are even higher in antioxidant compounds.

7. MICRO VEGGIES contain the antioxidant chlorophyll, and because they are germinated and harvested at a very young stage, they contain SOD and catalase, which are antioxidant enzymes.

8. CINNAMON, one of my favorite spices, is loaded with antioxidants and has been shown to support healthy blood sugar levels.

9. AMLA BERRIES, OR INDIAN GOOSEBERRIES, help regenerate your body's own antioxidants. One of those is SOD, which is important for skin health.

10. POMEGRANATES, the royal biblical fruit, contain ellagic acid and other powerful antioxidants. They're great exclamation points to any fruit or vegetable salad.

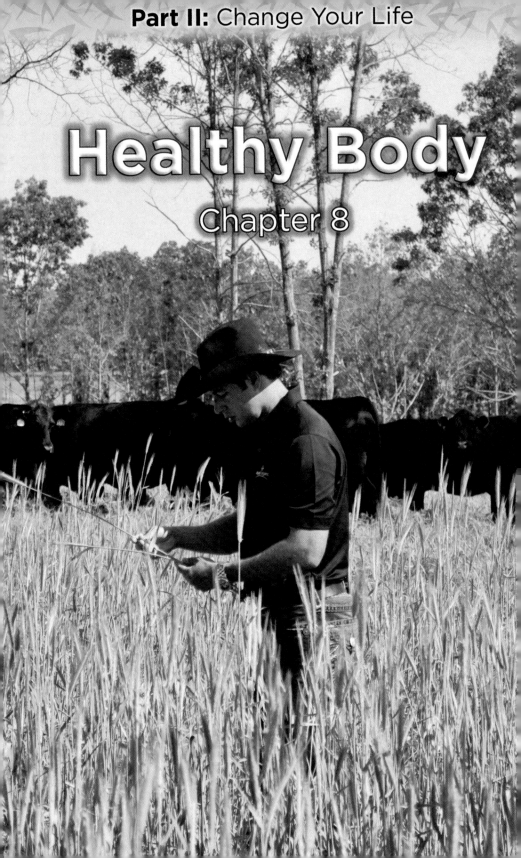

Healthy Body

Chapter 8

Recently, a friend of mine said I *had* to meet John Brookfield, the creator of an exercise program called Battling Ropes.

"He's an elite strength athlete and coach, and he's done incredible feats like pulling eighteen-wheel trucks and ripping card decks in two with his bare hands. He'd like to tell you what Battling Ropes is all about."

I had the opportunity to speak with John and learn that he was a man of faith who believed that his Battling Ropes exercise program was inspired by God. That certainly got my attention. I also learned that John had appeared on TV shows like *Good Morning America, The Today Show,* and *Regis and Kathie Lee,* where he performed amazing feats of strength, like ripping fifty-five decks of cards in half in less than a minute.

I immediately connected with John and liked him a lot. He said he spent nearly a year working in his backyard on a new exercise system that involved heavy, braided ropes that were fifty or more feet long and two inches in diameter. The basic exercise involved stretching the rope so that any slack was taken out of the rope. With a partner standing on one end of the rope (or after securing the other end of the rope around a pole), you whip the rope up and down powerfully and quickly. This movement creates a wave action, or "tsunami" effect, toward the rope's anchor point.

With enough force, one could create a series of waves or tsunamis going all the way to the end of the rope. The goal was to maintain constant velocity and power output until your arms weakened and couldn't keep the waves going any longer.

When I first tried the Battling Ropes system, the basic exercises looked deceptively easy to do, but I found them hard and taxing on my arms, shoulders, and even my back. Unfortunately, I could keep the waves going for only thirty seconds or so. But I enjoyed the workouts, and so did Joshua. In fact, I've learned that when you're engaging in an exercise program where you actually look forward to the next workout, you're very likely to experience great results.

For years, I've been an avid fan of exercise. Ever since I became a certified personal trainer and fitness instructor after my health recovery, I've been drawn to "functional fitness"—a form of exercise that helps the body stay strong, agile, and flexible with movements and exercises that resemble real-life activities. I found functional fitness to be a welcome antidote to the "one plate more" philosophy with free weights or heavy squats with barbells.

John explained that he felt like the Lord gave him the idea for using the tsunami-like wave motion with ropes to develop grip strength and superior cardio conditioning without suffering joint impact. When I asked him where the "battling ropes" name came from, John said the name stemmed from a warrior-minded desire to let participants engage in exercise that could improve performance in their sport or battlefield. He added that he had trained hundreds of elite military soldiers and top athletes. The NFL's Tampa Bay Buccaneers have adopted Battling Ropes as part of their training regimen.

I was impressed after watching the DVDs John was kind enough to send me. I also received a fifty-foot rope, which I put to good use with Joshua. We both discovered that you needed mental toughness as well as physical stamina to perform the Battling Ropes exercises.

With some practice, we were able to make the tsunami-like waves. Working the arms to keep the waves going quickly turned into lung-bursting exercise. (Just type "John Brookfield Battling Ropes" into your search engine and you can see videos on how it's done.)

Joshua, being much smaller, initially had a hard time getting his rope to make waves. But he was a gamer and kept improving each time he gave it a try. As for myself, I quickly got the hang of things, but let me tell you: making the tsunami-like waves wore me out quicker than I thought it would.

I told Joshua that our goal was to do the Battling Ropes for fifteen seconds before taking a break and letting the other one try. Naturally, I had the stamina to go longer and do more "reps" than Joshua did, but that didn't diminish the fun we enjoyed from getting a good workout in a short amount of time. I felt that ten or fifteen minutes in the driveway with the rope wrapped around the pole of our basketball hoop was enough to give me a quality workout before switching to other forms of exercise or practicing football drills with Joshua.

No matter what type of exercise program you undertake, physical fitness is essential to good health and is one of the best things you can do for your body, mind, and spirit. Exercise does a body good; pumping those legs and arms speeds up the heart and makes you breathe faster, which helps transfer oxygen from your lungs to your blood and increases the body's natural immune system function. Exercise stimulates the important white blood cells in the body to move from the organs into the bloodstream, where they can mount a defense against invaders and toxins inside the body.

Exercise contributes to positive mental health as well. New research suggests that physical exercise encourages healthy brains to function at their optimal levels. You even get a self-esteem boost and feel better about yourself. Perhaps the greatest benefit from consistent exercise is stress reduction.

I saw this happen time and time again whenever I worked with clients as a personal trainer, which is why I believe exercise is a critical body therapy that's nearly as important as the foods you eat on your journey to living beyond organic.

In this chapter, I'll be passing on some of my favorite ways to improve the health of your body not by what you take in, but by what you put out, so to speak.

HERE COMES THE SUN

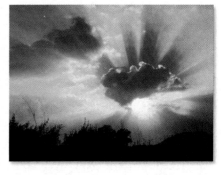

One thing I liked about the Battling Ropes exercises that I did with Joshua—beyond the father-son bonding—was performing those sweat-inducing exercises *outside* . . . under a hot Florida sun.

Getting sunlight is extremely important for our bodies because of the way the skin synthesizes vitamin D from the ultraviolet rays of sunlight. Vitamin D, which is actually a hormone, keeps bones healthy, plays a role in immune system health and blood cell formation, and is also needed for adequate blood levels of insulin.

This topic of vitamin D is very important to me because I'm convinced that exposing our skin to sunlight is something that's not done nearly as often as it should be in this country. Only 23 percent of Americans reach the vitamin D levels needed for optimal health, according to recent research led by Dr. Neil Binkley at the University of Wisconsin. This finding suggests that a strong majority of the American population is vitamin D deficient, leaving us at increased risk from bone disorders and many other diseases.

Exposure to the sun is the most significant source of vitamin D. When your face and your arms and legs are exposed to sunlight, the skin—with the help of the kidneys—miraculously turns those ultraviolet B rays into a hormone that's critically needed by the body. Higher levels of vitamin D may reduce the risk of developing neurological and autoimmune diseases.

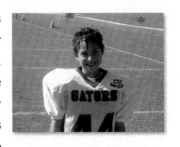

When Joshua and I are outside working the ropes or passing the football to each other, I know that our faces and limbs are taking in this important hormone. Listen, I know we're fortunate to live in the Sunshine State, where it's sunny and warm nearly year-round. For those living in the northern climes of the country, sunlight exposure from November to February is insufficient to produce significant vitamin D synthesis in the skin.

A deficiency of vitamin D carries health consequences and can lead to mental and behavioral issues, fatigue, unhealthy weight loss, blood sugar disturbances, heart health challenges, and bone loss.

But what about skin cancer, Jordan? Are you putting sunscreen on yourself and Joshua?

I have a couple of thoughts here. I understand that conventional wisdom says that being out in the sun is bad for you. Parents fear skin cancer, and I agree: the rates of melanoma and other skin cancers are far too high today.

But U.S. government surveys show that we spend 90 percent of our time indoors or in a car, so we're not outside very much in the sunshine, which means we are missing out on the vitamin D that the body needs. As for the skin cancer issue, I have a question: Our ancestors toiled outside from sunup to sundown, but they didn't get skin cancer at nearly the same rates as today. So what gives?

I believe we're seeing higher cancer rates these days because we lack adequate nutrients in our diets, don't eat enough antioxidant-rich fruits, vegetables, and healthy fats, and don't synthesize enough vitamin D through exposure to the sun. In addition, environmental toxins surely contribute to the rising rates of cancer.

Because the body derives vitamin D—which supports immune health and keeps bones healthy—from the sun, I believe it's imperative to get outside and soak up some rays. Fifteen, twenty minutes every other day is usually enough to meet your vitamin D requirements, according to the National Institutes of Health (NIH).

If you or your children stay out in the sun longer than that, then a toxin-free sunscreen is in order. You can apply a natural sunscreen with an SPF of at least 15 to protect the skin, but you should know that any sunscreen greater than SPF 8 will block vitamin D conversion and absorption. What I recommend is rubbing on some extra-virgin coconut oil before you go outside in the sun, which helps you take in vitamin D and has a minor protective element. Then after a quarter of an hour—maybe longer depending on the time of day, the time of year, and the intensity of the sun—you rub some sunscreen on your skin.

It's good to get a little color from the sun, but you don't want to burn.

SLEEPING IN

I don't sleep enough.

I have no problem admitting that I don't sleep as much as I should. With three small children ranging in ages from seven to four, there seems to be no way to get enough rest, and that goes for Nicki, too. While I write this book, our youngest daughter Alexis sneaks into our bedroom nearly every night to sleep with us. She'll grow out of this phase someday, but for now, Nicki and I have to deal with sporadic and uncomfortable sleep.

Precious slumber is something I need to focus on with much greater effort. I understand that sleep plays a major role in preparing the body and the brain for an alert, productive, and healthy tomorrow. A good night's rest revitalizes tired bodies, gives us more energy, and helps us think more clearly throughout the day.

Sleep experts say the magic number to shoot for is eight hours each night, but the National Sleep Foundation says we're lucky to get seven hours, which is 20 percent less than our great-grandparents slept. Then again, our ancestors didn't have radios, TVs, personal computers, or iPads vying for their attention a century ago, but all that stimulating electronic media and entertainment are here to stay. We all have to make the choice to shut things down and go to bed.

Another modern-day peril to good sleep is travel. I'm on the road a great deal and have always found changing time zones and sleeping in hotels to be difficult. When flying home from the West Coast, I often take red-eye flights so that I won't miss another day with my family. I don't get any beauty rest during the night flight; I barely close my eyes while twisted like a pretzel in my cramped airline seat. After arriving in West Palm Beach early in the morning, I somehow power through the day, but I'm exhausted by the effort and pretty pooped by the evening.

I know I have to "catch up" on my first night back and maybe for another couple of nights after that, which is always easier said than done in our household. What I have found is that the old saying stating that one hour of sleep *before* midnight is equal to several hours of sleep after midnight is grounded in truth.

What Nicki and I will not do is take sleeping medications like you see advertised on TV. They are extremely sedating and often leave you feeling even *more* groggy in the morning. I've found exercise, consuming a cultured dairy product before bed, and forms of hydrotherapy (which I'll talk about shortly in this chapter) to be a good approach to getting a good night's rest.

But everyone finds out what works for them. Nicki also likes to exercise sometimes before going to bed, saying that makes her sleep better. Other times she'll read or listen to books on tape by her favorite Christian authors.

Whatever approach you like to end the day with and fall quickly and timely to sleep, I say go for it. If you can sleep more than me, then more power to you.

THE VALUE OF RESTING ONE DAY A WEEK

Sleep happens each night—unless you're on a crowded red-eye flight—but the rest I'm talking about should happen one day a week.

A time of rest should come on the weekend, but Saturdays and Sundays have become crowded with kids' sports, errands, shopping, church services, and more shopping. It used to be that "weekends" meant a time to kick back, but it seems like our weekends are wall-to-wall, shop-until-you-drop extravaganzas.

When God created the earth and the heavens in six days, we were told that He rested on the seventh day. God wasn't worn out by His labors, but I believe He rested to give us an example and to remind us that we were designed to work six days and rest on the seventh.

We need to follow that example, and once again, that's a huge challenge for me. As I write this book, I am making a concerted effort to keep the Sabbath, which happens to be the fourth of the 10 Commandments. By not working and focusing on God and family, I know that my Sabbath will become a day looked forward to by me and my family and best of all, will honor God.

To know the physical importance of resting one day per week, look to elite athletes, who understand that their bodies need to recuperate. Triathletes are religious about not doing any swimming, biking, or running one day a week so that their muscles can heal from the exertions of the previous six days. NFL football players always get a day off after the big game on Sunday, but football coaches never take *any* days off during the season. Guess who complains about burnout?

Having all stores open seven days a week—some twenty-four hours—

doesn't help matters. When I was in Europe, I was struck by how all the shops and department stores close on Sundays—even supermarkets. If you need food for Sunday, you better get to the grocery store before five o'clock on Saturday afternoon!

A rest-filled day gives us a break from life's constant stresses. I've long felt that if you give God that one day of rest each week, then He'll do greater things with the other six days than you can in seven days.

CLEANSING WITH HYDROTHERAPY

Although at this point my schedule may not be filled with enough sleep or rest, I have discovered a way to slow down for a short time during the day. Some time during the daylight hours, I'll slip into my far infrared sauna in our master bathroom. (I recommend the far infrared saunas from a company called Sunlighten.) During my sauna session, I'll read the Bible, pray, drink several glasses of Reign, and enjoy my quiet time while sweating out the toxins.

Then I hop into our steam shower, where a humidifying steam generator produces water vapor and really opens up my pores. I finish with my shower.

Each of the aforementioned activities—sauna, steam, and shower—are examples of hydrotherapy, which is the use of heat, steam, and water for therapeutic reasons. For instance, one form of hydrotherapy could be as simple as sitting in a hot tub and allowing the water jets to massage and knead sore muscles and tender areas of the body, especially the lower back. Or you could lie down in an infrared sauna and crank up the thermostat past 150 degrees Fahrenheit and allow the infrared heat to calm the body and slow down the activity of the internal organs.

The use of hot and cold water is another form of hydrotherapy. The next time you're taking a shower, start with your normal hot water, but after several minutes, switch to cold water—as cold as you can stand. Cold water stimulates the body and boosts oxygen use in the cells. Hot water dilates blood vessels, which improves blood circulation, speeds the elimination of toxins, and transports more oxygen to the brain.

I really like taking a sauna and a steam before I shave because I know my skin pores will be open, causing the hair follicles to be more relaxed. In the old barbershop days, when people used to get a shave and a hair cut for two bits (25 cents), the barber would put a hot towel on the man's face before taking a straight-edge razor to his beard. The same principle is at work here.

If I can offer one more tip about showering, it would be this: watch how you soap up after you've been outside in the sun. Vitamin D experts point to research showing that the body needs up to forty-eight hours to absorb the majority of the vitamin D that was generated from outdoor sun exposure. That means if you go for an energetic Sunday afternoon walk on a hot day and come home and jump in the shower because you're sweaty, you very well could wash away much of the vitamin D that your skin is in the process of absorbing, thus decreasing the benefits of your sun exposure.

This doesn't mean I don't want you to shower. What you don't want to do is wash away the oils on your skin, so just lather up where the sun don't shine, so to speak—the underarms and groin area. This way you avoid soaping up the larger areas of the body that were exposed to sunlight and are still synthesizing the ultraviolet rays.

ANOTHER GREAT FORM OF EXERCISE

Another exercise genius that I've spent some quality time with is Pavel Tsatsouline, a Pied Piper for Russian kettlebells who trained Red Army Special Forces back in the day. Pavel, a Russian, immigrated to the United States determined to put kettlebells on the map, and I'd say

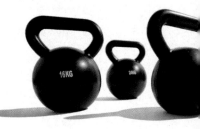

he's making great progress as the kettlebell craze is in high gear here in the States.

Kettlebells are different from free weights because their handles give them a displaced center of gravity. They come in various weights from 10 to 26 pounds for women and 26 to 106 pounds for men.

Proponents say that it's not a matter of *if* kettlebells will work for you; it's a matter of *how* to work with them to fit your needs. Kettlebells deliver all-around fitness in a hurry and when used properly, can replace the following list of hardware: barbells, dumbbells, lever bars, medicine balls, and cardio equipment.

Russian kettlebells are definitely on the radar screens of fitness buffs these days. These hunks of iron on a handle have become ferociously effective for developing explosive strength, dramatic power, and tip-top conditioning. I've been using them for four years and can attest to significant gains in cardio conditioning, muscle tone, and strength. I have two sets of kettlebells at my home given to me by my friend John DuCane of Dragon Door, and I use them as my go-to workout tool.

Technique is very important when training with Russian kettlebells. A beginning exercise is holding a kettlebell by the horns, chest-height, and performing front squats called goblet squats, keeping your weight on your heels. A primary kettlebell exercise is the KB Swing, which as Pavel says, "is the closest thing to throwing a punch." For a fun way to strengthen your abdominals, you can make under leg passes to yourself. Swing the kettlebell around the front of your right leg and through your legs by passing the kettlebell to your left hand behind your left leg. Joshua really enjoys kettlebell workouts and has learned proper technique very quickly. Even Nicki has become a kettlebell aficionado.

Kettlebell workouts may be the answer to those who don't live near a fitness center or can't afford an expensive membership to a local gym. To get going, you should read Pavel's book, *Enter the Kettlebell!* and/or watch the companion DVD, where you'll learn about good beginning exercises and even dare to undertake the Russian kettlebell rite of passage.

For more information on Pavel and Russian kettlebells, visit www.dragondoor.com, where you'll find everything you need to begin your journey to extraordinary fitness.

NATURAL BODY THERAPIES

After my father attended the National College of Naturopathic Medicine, we moved from Portland, Oregon, to New York and later to the Atlanta area so that Dad could attend Life College and study chiropractic medicine.

I was a preschooler at the time, and my parents lived in a neighborhood almost entirely comprised of chiropractic students. Since most of the students were not married, they didn't have any children. In a way, I became an "adjusting dummy" for some of Dad's colleagues in the classroom. They would bribe me with toys if I would let them practice the chiropractic adjustments on me.

So I've probably had more adjustments on the neck than you can shake a stick at. I remain a big believer in chiropractic medicine. I think it's important for people to utilize chiropractic care for proper spinal alignment and nerve energy, not just to relieve back pain and correct spinal issues, but for overall body care. I'm also a fan of massage and other forms of body work.

SKIN AND BODY CARE

When I speak before large groups of women, I tell them straight out that I will not put anything on my skin that I would not eat. That's because the skin is superabsorbent, and a good way to prove that is to rub some crushed garlic on the soles of your feet.

Twenty minutes later, you may be running to the bathroom to brush your teeth because you'll smell garlic on your breath. Similarly, when you rub a tube of lipstick across your lips, you're introducing potentially damaging agents to your bloodstream.

Toxic chemicals are plentiful in our everyday cosmetics and toiletries. Products such as lipstick, lip gloss, hair conditioner, hair coloring, hairspray, shampoo, and soap routinely contain chemical solvents and phthalates, though you could never tell from reading the labels. That's because the long list of ingredients contain multisyllabic words that defy pronunciation, let alone comprehension, by the average consumer. Nowhere on the label will you find an explanation of how these ingredients work, leaving health-conscious women in the dark.

Even the natural and organic brands struggle with being toxin-free, so you need to be very careful. I frequently recommend the internal and external use of organic essential oils. Try rubbing a few drops of myrtle, coriander, hyssop, galbanum, or frankincense onto the palms, then cup your hands over your mouth and nose and inhale. Taking a deep breath will soothe the mind and invigorate the spirit.

An eyedropper or two of these essential oils into a hot bath will give you an opportunity to practice hydrotherapy at the same time. You can also use essential oils in a compress or burn them in a diffuser. These essential oils stimulate the powerful sense of smell, and their pleasant fragrances can have a significant impact on how we feel physically and emotionally.

I recommend incorporating these essential oils found in the Bible on a daily basis. Whether you rub these oils into your skin or add them to your bath, you'll experience a renewed sense of health.

BEYOND ORGANIC HEALTHY LIVING ACCOUNT

In closing this chapter, I want to reiterate that all of us at Beyond Organic believe not only in helping people change their diet, but also in changing their lives. Having a healthy body is important to us, and so is the health of those who come alongside us to share our mission with others.

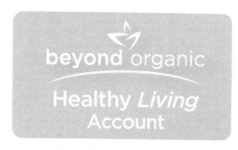

You could be a natural health practitioner such as a chiropractor or acupuncturist, a massage therapist or fitness trainer, a pastor or ministry leader, or perhaps you are a passionate individual who wants to share this message of health and hope with those you know and love.

Those who become leaders in Beyond Organic will have an opportunity to qualify to be Healthy Living Account members. What this means is we will put financial resources in the hands of our leading mission marketers for the sole purpose of enjoying natural health care such as chiropractic and integrative medical care, massage, acupuncture, gym memberships, spa visits, and trips to your local health food store.

When you become a leader in Beyond Organic, you will actually have a Healthy Living membership card and the opportunity to receive hundreds of dollars each month that you can utilize to enhance your health through natural health therapies. This could also mean an opportunity to earn money toward a healthy vacation, buying a far infrared sauna for the home, purchasing your own set of kettlebells or Battling Ropes, or shopping at your favorite health food store.

We are building a network of Healthy Living Account preferred providers that we partner with that will continue to grow nationwide and will give preferred treatment to our Healthy Living Account holders.

FOR MORE INFORMATION ON
THIS AMAZING PROGRAM, VISIT
WWW.LIVEBEYONDORGANIC.COM.

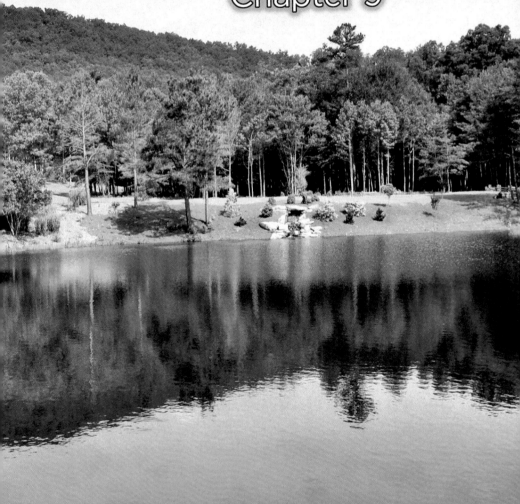

Healthy Mind
Chapter 9

When I arrived in San Diego in the spring of 1996, deathly ill and hoping that my cross-continental journey could turn my health around, Bud Keith—the nutritionist who encouraged me to eat a diet based on biblical principles—took me aside.

"Jordan, while you're here in San Diego, there are two things that you can't do," he said sternly. "You can't say anything negative, and you can't frown."

I nodded, which I figured was better than frowning again. This was going to take some getting used to. There's a Yiddish term to describe what I was like back in those dark days—*ungeblusen*, which means mopey.

You see, for nearly two years, I had worn a perpetual frown. Battling Crohn's disease, symptoms of rheumatoid arthritis, chronic fatigue syndrome, fibromyalgia, and diabetes had taken its toll on both my body and my mind. I had doctors and well-meaning people in my life telling me that my diseases were incurable, that I'd never get well, that I had to just learn to live with my grim circumstances.

But Bud Keith would not tolerate any negativity from me—no complaints, no "woe is me" utterances. He forced me to examine my negative thinking and how that was holding me back. He asked me to memorize and live the verse from Philippians 4:8: " . . . whatever is true, whatever is noble, whatever is right, whatever is pure, whatever is lovely, whatever is admirable—if anything is excellent or praiseworthy—think about such things" (NIV).

Thinking about such things and putting on a happy face wasn't easy at first. Sure, some of my smiles were forced, but they became easier as my health improved. Then it was like the floodgates opened. When I came back even stronger than before, the sun shined in my life.

But I'm going to tell you something: even after my health and life was restored, and I began my mission to transform the health of this nation and world one life at a time, I consistently heard voices telling me what I couldn't do:

- You can't write a book.

- You can't formulate nutritional supplements if you don't have a biology or chemistry background.

- You can't run a multimillion-dollar company with two hundred employees without an MBA.

- You can't buy a ranch because you don't know anything about raising cattle or making dairy products.

Seems like my entire life has been marked by the two-word phrase: *You can't.* I'm even hearing whispers today that starting a company like Beyond Organic in today's tough economic climate is foolhardy at best and a recipe for financial disaster at the worst.

I refuse to think that way—ever since Bud Keith coached me to set aside any negativity fifteen years ago. I made the decision that *I can,* to believe that I was fearfully and wonderfully made, as God's Word says in Psalm 139. To believe what God's Word said even though the mirror told me I was a shriveled up, deformed shadow of myself back in 1996.

I decided not to buy into the doctors' prognoses, which said I was incurable. I refused to listen when support groups told me the best I could hope for was to "manage" my diseases. I wasn't convinced when experts declared that a certain percentage of young people stricken with my illnesses die within a short period of time.

I believed I was going to get well, and I did. Scripture bolstered my confidence in a positive outcome. During my time in San Diego, I stood on God's Word that "I can do all things through Christ who strengthens me" (Philippians 4:13, NKJV).

I REALIZED THE IMPORTANCE OF THINKING AND SPEAKING IN ACCORDANCE WITH GOD'S PROMISES FROM THESE VERSES:

- **"For as he thinketh in his heart, so is he . . ."
  (Proverbs 23:7, KJV)**

- **"For out of the abundance of the heart his mouth speaks."
  (Luke 6:45, NKJV)**

- **"Death and life are in the power of the tongue . . ."
  (Proverbs 18:21, NKJV)**

The idea that what you think and what you say determines who you are has long fascinated me. I found a kindred spirit in this belief in Alex Loyd, N.D., Ph.D., who is the creator of *The Healing Codes.* This biblically based system provides a proactive way to reduce stress in your life, and since stress is the overall number-one cause of doctor visits, this tool may be just what the doctor ordered for many people and perhaps for you.

BELOW IS A SAMPLE SERIES OF STRESS-REDUCING EXERCISES DEVELOPED BY DR. LOYD:

1. Focus on your overall stress level and rate it from 0 to 10, with 10 being highest.

2. Place your hands one on top of the other, with your right palm over your belly button and your left palm over the back of your right hand.

3. Focus on the stress you want to leave your body—physical, emotional, or spiritual.

4. Do Power Breathing for ten seconds. Breathe rapid and powerful "belly breaths" in and out.

5. Forcefully blow out and suck in through your mouth, using your diaphragm so your belly moves out as you breathe in and moves in as you breathe out. If you feel a little lightheaded, breathe the same way, but reduce the intensity.Leave your right hand over your belly button and move your left hand over your heart as you relax for fifty seconds. Say "Stress Out" while you focus on the stress leaving your body. If you like, you can also visualize stress leaving your body as you relax and think or say "Stress Out."

6. Move your left hand back on top of your right hand over your belly button.

7. Focus on physical, emotional, or spiritual peace.

8. Do Power Breathing for ten seconds. Breathe rapid and powerful "belly breaths" in and out. Forcefully blow out and suck in through your mouth, using your diaphragm so your belly moves out as you breathe in and moves in as you breathe out. If you feel a little lightheaded, breathe the same way, but reduce the intensity.

9. Leave your right hand over your belly button and move your left hand over your heart as you relax for fifty seconds. Think or say "Peace" while you focus on peace entering your body. If you like, while you say "Peace," imagine peace flowing into your body from God or visualize a peaceful scene that calms and strengthens you.

10. Re-rate your overall stress level from 0 to 10, as you did in step 1.

11. Re-rate your overall stress level ten minutes later.

12. Do another Healing Codes exercise if your stress level is still at 4 or above.

Dr. Loyd believes that no matter what the issue is—physical or emotional—it all stems from the heart, which, in Scripture, is synonymous with the brain. He explained that it all came together for him when he studied what wise King Solomon had to say in Proverbs 4:23 (NLT): "Above all else, guard your heart, for it affects everything you do."

What Solomon was saying was that heart issues were the source of 100 percent of our problems. Today, science is backing up this biblical wisdom. If you read the more than eleven hundred passages in the Bible that talk about the heart, including what Solomon said about the heart affecting everything you do, and then consider what the research from the University of Texas Southwestern Medical Center says about how our cells record their experiences and have a cellular memory—then you understand that according to the Bible and science, the issues of the heart—or mind—are the source of just about any problem we have in our lives.

Said another way, if we can fix the issues of the heart, then we can fix just about any problem we have.

TURNING OVER A NEW LEAF

While writing this book, I appeared on a TBN "Praise the Lord" program with hosts Matt and Laurie Crouch to talk about Beyond Organic and the "Joseph mandate." One of the other guests on the talk show was Dr. Caroline Leaf, a native of South Africa.

I met Dr. Leaf during my 2006 trip to Johannesburg when I learned about the Maasai tribe and the cultured dairy product that I would later call Amasai. We were both speaking at the annual Rhema Women's Conference, which attracted 8,000 women to Rhema Bible Church in Randburg, a Johannesburg suburb. Rhema is South Africa's largest church with 20,000 members and is a showcase of racial diversity.

Dr. Leaf's message was called, "Who Switched Off My Brain?", which happened to be the title of a book that she had just written. Her main point was that our thoughts chemically affect our behavior, personal diseases, and the healing process. She explained that she had solid neuroscientific research backing up another wise saying from Solomon: that as people think in their hearts, allowing their spirit, mind, will, emotions, and body to absorb those thoughts and images, to that degree they will become in their spirit, soul, and body.

Heavy stuff.

Dr. Leaf had moved to the U.S. since I last saw her five years ago in Johannesburg. Her book *Who Switched Off My Brain?*, which released in this country in 2008, had become a sensation, selling a half-million copies. The book's premise is that since our thoughts ultimately determine our actions and our thoughts, they build a network of positive and negative proteins in the brain. Dr. Leaf called these proteins "black trees" or "green trees."

What happens scientifically in the brain is that our unconscious minds are filled with billions of thoughts, much like a dense forest of trees. The forest is a mixture of black trees (negative thoughts) and green trees (positive thoughts), but hopefully the forest is more green than black.

Brain imaging illustrates that positive thoughts look like beautiful, lush, and healthy green trees, whereas negative thoughts look like ugly, mangled, and dark trees. Dr. Leaf believes toxic thoughts build toxic memories, which upset the chemical feedback loops in your brain, thereby putting your body in a harmful state. Your brain grows heavy with thick memories that release a toxic load, which interferes with how you live life.

She asserts that if you have been verbally or sexually abused as a child, then all the thoughts associated with those experiences will release negative chemicals that travel throughout your body, which can change the shape of the receptors on cells lining your heart, thereby increasing susceptibility to cardiovascular illness. Simply put, **positive experiences and thoughts** induce brain cells to expand while **negative experiences and thoughts** cause brain cells to shrivel and die.

Dr. Leaf was asked on the show what was the most destructive thought you could have.

Her answer: "It's *I can't*."

I nodded my head in agreement. When you say or think *I can't*, that act dashes hope, halts effort, destroys ambition, and jeopardizes the future. The thought that should come to mind in those situations is *I can do all things through Christ who strengthens me.*

Because you can.

In order to have a healthy mind, the theme of this chapter, I want to encourage you—wherever you are in life—to have the attitude, the thoughts, and the actions that say *I can.*

After hearing over and over that I couldn't be healed, couldn't start a health and wellness company, couldn't have a successful publishing career, I made a conscious decision that *I can.* That attitude has served me well, although I will confess that there have been times when I took two steps forward and one back, causing a few too many black trees to grow in my brain. These thoughts bounced around the recesses of my mind, and they weren't healthy:

No one wants to listen to what you have to say, Jordan.

No one will show up to hear you speak.

You're wasting your time. You should go back to being a stock boy at a health food store.

But I made a decision to cut down those black trees and make room for positive thoughts in my life. Now, when dark thoughts come out of nowhere and try to pull me back into the part of the forest where the black trees are the densest, I refuse to go there.

That's easier said than done in this culture. We have a tendency today to "be negative" and constantly talk about all of the bad things that could happen. You hear it in the way some people talk about their poor health, their marriage on the rocks, their children struggling in school, or their nearly empty bank account. What they're really saying is . . . they can't. They can't turn their health around, they can't save their marriage, they can't control their kids, and they can't stay above water financially.

You don't want to go down that road. If you're a Gloomy Gus, someone wearing a permanent frown, you will have to get to work and repeat God's reminder that as you think in your heart, then that's the person you are. Only then can you change *I can't* into *I can.*

As you begin your journey of living beyond organic, I want you to be thinking about what you're going to do with the message I've shared so far. Since you've made it this far in the book, you're either at one of three places:

1. **You're interested in Beyond Organic, but you're on the fence.**

2. **You've decided that you really do want to live beyond organic.**

3. **Not only have you decided to live beyond organic, but you also want to share the Beyond Organic message with those you know and love.**

We, at Beyond Organic, will train you to succeed. We've put together a great education program that starts with **Beyond Organic University**, which is an online training resource designed by a professional educator to allow you to become a health coach and proficient in the principles that you're reading about and the science behind them.

In some cases, you don't have to convince someone to eat and live differently. All you have to do is hand them a copy of this book. We are making copies of *Live Beyond Organic* available so you can give them away as gifts to those who need this message.

We are also producing a magazine, *Beyond Organic Living*, loaded with cutting-edge health and wellness information, fitness tips, and articles designed to train you on sharing this important message effectively. To learn more about *Beyond Organic Living* magazine, go to LiveBeyondOrganic.com today. And last but not least, each week you can join millions of viewers by tuning into our brand-new television program *Living Beyond Organic,* which airs on several cable networks starting in the fall of 2011. Visit www. LiveBeyondOrganic.com for listings of when and where the program is aired in your hometown.

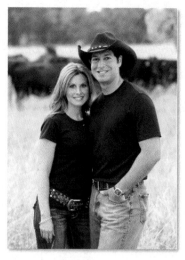

In closing, our goal at Beyond Organic is to help you turn your I can't into I can.

I can be healthy.

I can be successful.

I can fulfill God's calling on my life.

At the end of the day, if you believe God's Word is true, then you're looking at life through a positive lens. I'm not talking about living outside of the realm of reality. But what's the worst that could happen if you have faith and confess God's truth instead of the world's lies? Some refer to the confession of God's Word as the "name it and claim it" doctrine.

I've lived long enough to know that many speak exactly what they *don't* want in their lives into existence.

They talk about how they are going to go broke, that they're destined for bankruptcy. They do lose everything. They named it and claimed it.

They talk about their failing marriage and imminent divorce, and they lose their husband or wife. They named it and claimed it.

They talk about how their diagnosis of cancer means they are going to die, and they die very quickly—days or weeks after the diagnosis. They named it and claimed it.

I believe that out of the overflow of the heart (or mind), the mouth speaks. I also believe that life and death is in the power of the tongue, which is directed by the mind.

Because as you think in your heart, so you are. And today, I declare that you are forgiven, healed, alive, and free in the name of Jesus!

Healthy Spirit

Chapter 10

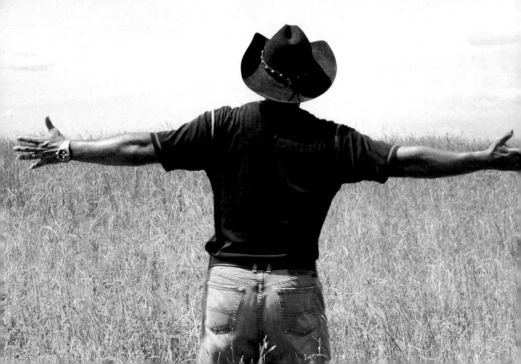

When I was eight years old, my parents let me play my first organized sport—Little League baseball.

I was pretty excited to put on a ballcap and uniform and play "real" baseball for the Atom League White Sox. Our family had settled in Palm Beach Gardens by this time, and it seemed like all the kids in my class had signed up to play. I loved everything about baseball—the freshly mowed field of grass, the baselines lined in chalk, and the challenge of hitting a pitched baseball.

Every time I stepped into the batter box, though, I struggled with the difficulty of hitting any sort of pitch thrown in my direction. I'd swing—and miss . . . and miss . . . and miss. Strike three, and you're out.

And back to the bench I'd go, very frustrated.

My coach *had* to play me two innings, according to Little League rules stating that every ballplayer must get a chance to be in the game. If I had a turn at bat, though, it was a lock that the scorekeeper would write a "K" marking my at-bat as a strikeout. I don't know how many late-inning rallies I ruined with each whiff.

One time, I knelt down in the on-deck circle waiting for my turn to hit. I was in the midst of a terrible slump. When it was my turn to step up to the plate, my coach called me over.

I thought he would tell me something encouraging like "You can do it, Jordan. You're due," or "Just keep your eyes on the ball and make contact." Instead he uttered something that I haven't forgotten to this day. He said in his sternest voice possible, "Jordan, if you strike out one more time, I'm going to do something terrible to you."

I shivered in fear. "Yes, Coach," I mumbled.

I couldn't get the bat off my shoulder and struck out for the fifteenth time in a row. My coach was so disgusted that he couldn't look at me as I hung my head and found a seat at the end of the bench.

I still remember that incident like it happened yesterday. My coach extinguished whatever passion I had for baseball that afternoon. Think about it. Little League baseball was supposed to be fun, especially for carefree eight-year-olds, yet I was miserable and had lost all confidence.

But that was nothing compared to what happened a few years later. I was twelve years old, in the seventh grade, and going through a tough patch at school. Several of my classmates, who were Jewish, went around the halls saying horrible things about me. They also cornered me at my locker and bullied me in front other students. They called me awful names, but the one that hurt the most was, "You're a fake Jew, Jordan." (I'll tell you why they said that in a moment.)

Overnight, I had no friends. No one wanted to hang out or talk with the kid who was a "fake Jew" and a weirdo. I went from spending weekend nights at friends' houses and having lots of buddies to an ostracized kid who had *no* friends. My classmates looked the other way when I walked into the cafeteria, so I ate lunch alone. It was brutal. I even found swastikas drawn on my desk in my homeroom.

The situation deteriorated to the point where I begged my parents to let me transfer to another school, even though that would mean an inconvenient long commute. I can remember telling Mom through tears that she was my best friend, which is profoundly sad for a boy of any age to say.

Just when I thought life couldn't get worse, it did. Shortly after Halloween, I saw something far worse than any Fright Night exhibition. I was walking to the school bus stop one morning when I noticed huge block letters in the street that filled a lane in my neighborhood.

Spray-painted in white letters atop the black pavement was a certain four-letter word followed by my name.

My heart lumped in my throat, and warm tears welled in my eyes. I turned around and trudged in the direction of home, blinking back tears that nonetheless cascaded down my cheeks. I couldn't go to school that day.

Why had my life deteriorated to something out of *Les Misérables*?

The situation had been building to a head for several years, but the main reason I was tormented stemmed from being a Messianic Jew—a Jewish Christian—and sharing my faith with my Jewish friends. You see, I had accepted Jesus as my personal Lord and Savior when I was around eight years old, and I wasn't afraid to evangelize my friends and tell them, "You won't go to heaven unless you have Jesus in your heart." My Jewish friends, however, resented my attempts to proselytize them.

They all knew I was Jewish since I told them so and still observed the Hebraic feasts. Rubin is also a Jewish name. But they also knew I had become a Christian, which is an anathema for any Jew.

As for my spiritual upbringing, I was definitely raised in a Bible-believing home. My parents became Messianic Jews when I was two years old. A Messianic

Jew believes that Jesus is the chosen Messiah who came and will return again. My school friends, however, were told at synagogue that Messianic Jews, known by the same name as the evangelistic ministry Jews for Jesus, were dangerous to their faith and their tradition.

So in typical *Lord of the Flies* tradition, my old friends turned on me. If they weren't yelling out "fake Jew!" in the hallway so that everyone could hear and snicker, they were spitting in my direction when I passed them on the school grounds. And, unfortunately, I found more black swastikas etched on my desk each day.

My parents, of course, noticed that the sparkle had left my eyes and how there were more and more times when I wanted to stay home from school even though I wasn't sick.

One night, they were having a Bible study at out house, and one of their friends heard about my plight. She took a 3x5 note card and wrote two verses from Jesus' Sermon on the Mount that are found in Matthew 6:14-15: "For if you forgive men their trespasses, your heavenly Father will also forgive you. But if you do not forgive men their sins against you, neither will your Father forgive your sins."

"Jordan," my parents' friend said, "I know that some kids at school are saying some really mean things about you, but you need to forgive them like God forgives you. Keep these verses of Scripture with you and read and reread them."

I thanked her for thinking of me. That night in my bedroom, just before I turned out the lights to go asleep, I reread those verses from Matthew that reminded me that I had to forgive my former best friends who had now become my enemies. Then I slipped the note card under my pillow.

Praying for those who tormented me helped. I was not granted the transfer to another school, however, so I moved into high school with very few friends and a desperate desire to fit in. But things spiritually kicked up a notch when my good friend Kenny Duke invited me to the First Baptist Church of West Palm Beach. The youth group at First Baptist was amazing, and I began to grow in my faith.

During my junior year of high school, I went on a choir tour with our youth group and was introduced to a Bible study called *Experiencing God* by Dr. Henry Blackaby, which was a thirteen-week curriculum that helped me learn how to recognize when God was speaking to me. Even though I had been a believer since the second grade, I never truly understood what it meant to have a personal relationship with Jesus until *Experiencing God*.

Experiencing God helped me see the importance of His timing and how to respond obediently. I learned to pray for God-sized things, meaning that I needed to ask God to do things that only He could do. I realized that if I had a need, then God could cause anyone in the world to meet that need.

Everything changed after *Experiencing God*. I went from being the persecuted kid who had no friends and wanted to change schools to waking up every morning wanting to serve God and tell others about Jesus. I went from being an outcast to somebody who didn't care about being popular or fitting in. I took to heart what the Jesus says in Matthew 6:33: "But seek first the kingdom of God and His righteousness, and all these things shall be added onto you."

The Lord sure added those things to me during my senior year of high school. I ended up going from the least popular and least likely to succeed to being awarded "Most Talented" by my fellow students. I was voted onto the Homecoming Court and Prom Court. Palm Beach Gardens High was a huge school with 2,500 students, and we had more than six hundred kids in my class, yet I was one of the four guys on Homecoming Court, along with Ryan Buckner, captain of our wrestling team; Rodney Nubin, our all-district tailback and top player on the football team; and Jesse Vicky, our salutatorian and National Honor Society member.

When I walked out through the tunnel at halftime of the Homecoming football game, I heard the PA announcer recite the words I had written for her:

"Our next member of the Homecoming Court is Jordan Rubin. Jordan believes that the key to one's happiness is a personal relationship with God. Jordan enjoys attending church and spending time studying the Bible. He plans to go into full-time ministry."

After graduating from Palm Beach Gardens High School, I enrolled at Florida State University on an academic scholarship. I made the cheerleading squad,

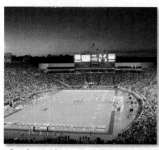

winning a spot as a late walk-on and getting to lead cheers for the No. 1 football team in the nation in front of 72,000 fans at Doak Campbell Stadium. I pledged to a fraternity that had lost its charter but was making a comeback— Pi Kappa Alpha, or the Pikes. Our house was definitely the place to be at Florida State in the Greek system. I became the fraternity chaplain as a *freshman* even though

Doak Campbell Stadium, Florida State University.

the Pikes had mostly fifth-year seniors.

All I really cared about in college was being a witness for my Lord. I found a great church near campus with the second-largest student ministry in the nation, running over 1,000 college students in Sunday worship. I joined a traveling music group that was part of the church's outreach, played intramural football, and somehow found time to get all my schoolwork done—at least most of the time.

I went home after my freshman year and worked as a camp counselor at Lake Swan near Gainesville, located in central Florida. Camp Swan, as it was called, was sponsored every summer by my home church, First Baptist Church.

And then I became deathly ill, which was the start of a two-year health odyssey that resulted in numerous hospitalizations, dozens of doctor visits, and long-shot trips to Mexico and Germany in search of an elusive cure. When I took a cross-country flight to San Diego, I wondered if Bud Keith could do as he promised he would: show me how to regain my health by following God's plan.

I had a miraculous recovery, as I described in the Introduction. Since that time, I realized that forgiveness was a key to my healing. I believed this so strongly that I took the time to write down every negative memory I had that involved someone hurting me, or me hurting someone else. I began with my earliest memory and worked up to the present. This took hours and hours. Each time I came upon a memory that had strong emotions attached to it, I would ask God to heal that memory. If it involved me hurting someone, I asked Him to forgive me.

I recalled the Little League coach who told me that I better not strike out—or else. The kids who spray-painted a vile message to me at the school bus stop. The doctors who told me that my illness was my fault. The relatives and friends who said they would be there for me, but I never heard from them again. Jesus said that if I didn't forgive these people, then He wouldn't forgive me of my sins.

I had sinned, too. I remembered all of the times I hurt others, spoke negatively about them, lied, or cheated. I asked the Lord to forgive me for each and every offense, praying with a contrite heart, seeking His mercy and forgiveness.

Let me tell you: I felt like a huge weight was lifted from my shoulders when I was done. I believe that the memories we store that relate to hurt feelings can act in the body like a cancer. In fact, a friend of mine once said that when you harbor unforgiveness that has turned to bitterness against anyone, it's like drinking poison and expecting it to kill the other person.

This spiritual cleansing was very important to my life and health. Of course, it's an ongoing process. The key is to nip these feelings in the bud before they become stored memories that—as Dr. Caroline Leaf says—"create dark trees in the brain."

Forgiving those that have hurt you is important for your health and well-being because unforgiveness is an emotion that God calls a sin and can cause great bodily harm and even shorten one's life span. When these feelings are allowed to fester, unforgiving hearts turn hard with bitterness. But forgiveness reduces stress-producing anger and improves mental, emotional, and physical health.

In fact, I'll take things a step further: forgiveness is an integral part of healing. I think healing is about faith, followed by confession, combined with action.

If you look at how I was healed, I had faith in God's sovereignty and in the work that He'd already done for me. I believe that *everyone* can be healed. I believe that because nowhere in the Bible does it say that Jesus went through a town and healed some of the people. I believe that everyone who came before Jesus, seeking healing for their diseases, were healed. That's what Scripture says and that's what I believe.

God's desire is for us to be healthy and whole, and if we have faith, if we believe and confess and take action, we can be. I also believe that faith without action is dead, meaning that you can have faith that you're going to be healed, but still live in the same circumstances physically, mentally, emotionally, and spiritually that caused the illness and allowed it to exist, and not get better.

It doesn't matter what happened in the past or what happened to anyone else you know who sought healing but may not have received it. This is your life, so if you're facing a health challenge, then I urge you to spend more time confessing the Word of God by praying *out loud*.

The reason you want to pray out loud for healing is two-fold. First, I believe that life and death is in the power of the tongue. We must speak life into our future, and when what we speak lines up with the word of God, then it is truth.

Second, just as I believe there is a heaven, there's also a hell, meaning there is a devil and his demons. When you pray and confess Scripture out loud, I believe Satan and his demons have to cover their ears as Scripture and the name of Jesus pierces the spirit realm—like a dog whistle that hurts a dog's ears. They can't stand to hear the name of Jesus and His words of truth.

Here's an example of a prayer that I've shared with friends and family members who were facing a cancer diagnosis in their lives. My inspiration for this prayer comes from Bible teacher Charles Capps, author Germaine Copeland (*Prayers That Avail Much*), and wisdom from my father.

If you are facing a health challenge, feel free to adapt this prayer to your situation, but pray this prayer out loud at least three times per day, using this prayer as your medicine. By doing so, you will be confessing with your mouth what you believe in your heart—that you will be healed in the name of Jesus:

> *Every organ and tissue of my body functions in the perfection that God created it to function. I forbid any malfunction in my body in Jesus' name.*
>
> *The same Spirit that raised Jesus from the dead dwells in me, permeating His life through my veins, sending healing throughout my body.*
>
> *The spirit and life of God's Word flows in me cleansing my blood of every disease and impurity.*
>
> *My immune system grows stronger day by day. I speak life to my immune system. I forbid confusion in my immune system.*
>
> *Lymph glands (or insert any part of the body where the cancer is or any other disease affecting your body), you are healed in Jesus' name. I command you to be normal in size and to function normally as my God created you to function. No weapon formed against me shall prosper. Because the Lord is for me, no disease can be against me.*
>
> *Every cell that does not promote life and health in my body is cut off from its life source. My immune system will not allow tumorous growth to live in my body in Jesus' name.*
>
> *That which God has not planted is dissolved and rooted out of my body in the name of Jesus. 1 Peter 2:24 is engrafted into every fiber of my being, and I am alive with the life of God.*
>
> *Jesus bore the curse for me. Therefore, I forbid growths and tumors to inhabit my body. The life of God within me dissolves growths and tumors, and my strength and health is restored.*

Growths and tumors have no right to my body. They are a thing of the past, for I am delivered from the authority of darkness."

The law of the Spirit of Life in Christ Jesus has made me free from the law of sin and death, therefore I will not allow sin, sickness or death to lord it over me.

I will not allow the devil any inroad to attempt to steal, kill, and destroy me. The Bible says that I have already been healed; I am more than a conqueror; an overcomer; I am above only and not beneath; that He wishes above all things that my soul prosper and that I would be in good health. These are not just words, these are God's promises to me. He loves me, and He wants me to be victorious on earth as it is in heaven.

I have set a boundary around my family with a bloodline that is the blood of our Messiah. No weapon formed against me can cross this bloodline that is surrounding me! No defeated demon from the pit of Hell can affect me or harm me.

Even though I walk through the valley of the shadow of death, I will not fear! Satan, you have no authority here and must get out of my life and out of my body because I have been redeemed by the blood of the Lamb. I have been translated from the powers of darkness and translated into God's kingdom!

I am healed and nothing, and I mean nothing, can or will come against me. Only what God has planted in my body will be in my body and remain there. Anything that God has not planted is rooted out of my body, in the name of Jesus. I have had it with the enemy and his attacks. I stand on the Word of God and trust Him fully. Only He can bring me through these circumstances, victoriously. Only Him! No food, medicine, or manmade thing can do what my Savior has already done and will continue to do for me. I will trust in God because He loves me.

I don't have to bow down to the name "cancer." Cancer has to bow down to me because God's spirit indwells me and I have become a joint heir with Jesus as the Righteousness of Christ. He says in His Word that He has given me power to tread on serpents and trample on our enemy. The devil is defeated, and God has given me victory when He shed His blood on the cross.

God's Word is sharper than any two-edged sword and better able to heal than any surgeon's blade. God's promises are true and better able to cure than any physician's medicines. I am the healed of God. It has already been done for me.

Amen!

WHAT REALLY MATTERS

Many an outsider would look at my life and say that I built a great company, Garden of Life, and have now fulfilled my dream in starting Beyond Organic. That I have a successful publishing career, have appeared on hundreds of TV programs, and been interviewed by hundreds of writers, sharing the principles of extraordinary health to millions in this country and around the world.

Many would say that since I've been blessed to earn a lot of money, written a *New York Times* best-seller, been on TV shows like *Good Morning America*, own a nice house, and have a wonderful family, that I must have everything I could ever wish for—especially for someone who came so close to dying at the age of twenty. But I would give up *everything* for the one thing that matters, which is my relationship with Jesus.

I sincerely mean that. If I didn't have a relationship with the God who created me through His Son Jesus, none of what I have "accomplished" in this thing called life would matter. The Word of God says, "What does it profit a man if he gains the whole world and loses his soul?"

The bottom line is this: You can eat beyond organic, get physically fit, and have a sound mind, but if you do not have a personal relationship with Yeshua, Jesus, the son of God, then you're missing out on what truly matters.

I don't want you to miss out on experiencing eternal life on earth as it is in Heaven in relationship with the God that loves you. I want you to experience a healing of the body, soul, and spirit from salvation that comes only through the Son of God who came to this earth and died a horrible death as atonement for our sins.

So my question to you is this: Do you know where you will spend eternity? The Bible teaches us that:

- **Everyone has sinned (Romans 3:23)**

- **The penalty for our sin is death (Romans 6:23)**

- **Jesus the Messiah died for our sins (Romans 5:8)**

- **To be forgiven for our sins, we must believe and confess that Jesus is Lord because salvation only comes through Him who paid the price (Romans 10:8-10)**

I don't believe the fact that you're reading *Live Beyond Organic* is an accident. I believe you are reading this book for a greater purpose than to change your diet. I want to introduce you to the God who created you and His son Jesus and ask that you receive Him as your Lord and Savior and experience forgiveness and fullness of joy.

If you've never received the salvation of God and you're ready to make Jesus Lord of your life, you only need to stretch out your hand to Him. You can do so by praying this prayer with me:

Lord Jesus, I know that I am a sinner. I know that I have made mistakes and done things wrong in my life. And I do know that there needs to be an atonement for my sins. You have paid the price for my sickness and for my sins. I ask you to forgive me for my sins and grant me eternal life with You. I confess You as Lord and Savior and I want to live for you all the days of the rest of my life. In Jesus' name, I pray, amen.

If you prayed this prayer for the first time, I urge you to join a local Bible-believing congregation and begin to fellowship with other believers. Make a commitment to read your Bible and watch as the Word of God comes alive in your life.

I want to leave you with a passage of Scripture that gave me hope during my darkest days. Let it be an encouragement for you as you begin the first day of the rest of your life:

PSALM 40: 1-3 (NKJV), WRITTEN BY DAVID:

I waited patiently for the LORD;
And He inclined to me,
And heard my cry.
He also brought me up out of a horrible pit,
Out of the miry clay,
And set my feet upon a rock,
And established my steps.
He has put a new song in my mouth—
Praise to our God;
Many will see it and fear,
And will trust in the LORD.

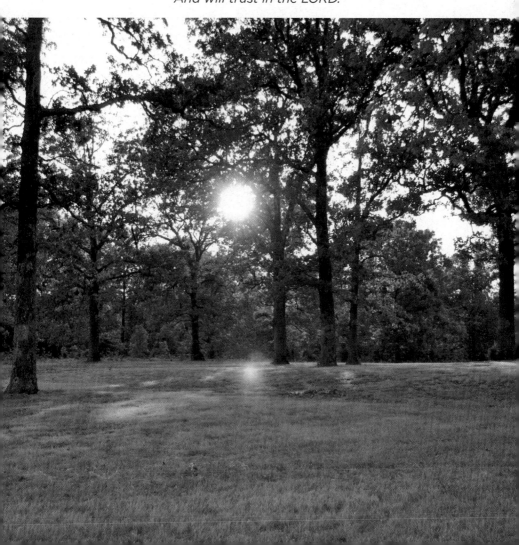

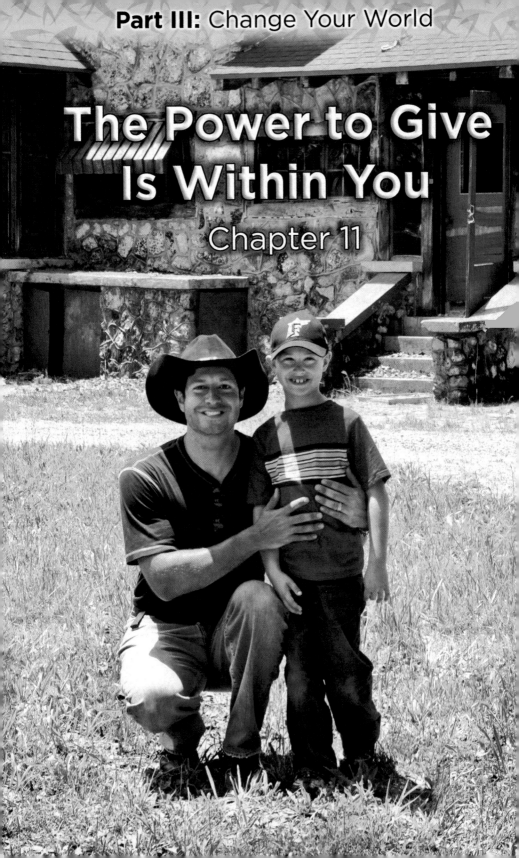

The Power to Give Is Within You

Chapter 11

Looking back, I remember the conversation like it happened yesterday.

I was about to fall asleep late one evening while Nicki was sitting up in bed, flipping through channels. She landed on a program that immediately caught her interest—a documentary about children growing up in a Russian orphanage.

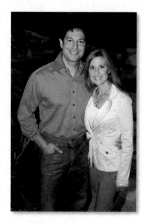

"Jordan, look at this. I think we should adopt someday."

Her casual but out-of-left-field comment got my attention, but since I was tired, I simply responded, "Okay, honey."

When Nicki voiced her desire for adoption that night, we already had a child. I thought we'd have more in the near future. Like millions of parents elsewhere, I believed that we would have multiple children biologically.

Adoption? I wasn't so sure about that. I had heard horror stories, especially about kids from foreign countries, the great expense, and frequent disappointments prospective parents face. I was also aware of something called reactive attachment disorder in adopted children who didn't form healthy bonds with their adoptive parents. Reactive attachment disorder develops because the child's basic needs for comfort, affection, and nurturing weren't met in the orphanages, which proved to be devastating to establishing future relationships with those around them, especially adoptive parents.

There are other issues with foreign adoption. You often have to travel to Russia or China or some foreign country multiple times, where there are language problems and daunting red tape. The authorities there won't tell you if the child has a disability or a deformity. We heard stories about American parents flying to

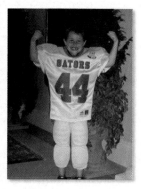

Russia to pick up their child only to be told at the last minute that a long-lost sibling had been "discovered" in another orphanage. There was no way to verify if this eleventh-hour revelation was true or not, but the prospective parents either had to take both children or make the long journey home empty-handed.

My take on adoption was that it was a difficult endeavor that demanded expensive overseas travel, considerable attorney fees, and no guaranteed outcome. There was a strong possibility of heartache and disappointment down the line. And while the financial implications were not a challenge for us, the time commitment certainly was.

"It's very sad what those kids have to go through," I finally said to Nicki that night. While I admired her tender heart, I just didn't see adoption in our future.

A few days later, though, Nicki brought up the topic again. At that point, I realized that she was serious about adopting. I heard her out and kept an open mind.

At one point, I heard Nicki say, "I think we're supposed to adopt." When you hear your wife say something like that, what she really means is this: *We're adopting.*

I said I understood and asked if we could have a little more time to think and pray about it. I began to realize that what the Bible says in James 1:27 about taking care of orphans applies to all of us. When taking that perspective, you realize that God uses us—His children—to be His hands and feet to care for children who have no homes or no hope.

A little later, Nicki and I traveled to Australia in March 2006 when I was invited to speak at the Hillsong Colour Conference in Sydney. This was a big deal to us since we've been worshipping to Hillsong music for years. I was honored to be the first male speaker in the ten-year history of this all-women conference that attracted Christian women from all over the world. Over the course of nine days, I would give two messages a day during the three-day conferences before full houses of energetic and excited women filling the 4,500-seat church auditorium.

What an awesome time, but the cherry on top was the opportunity to lead worship with the Hillsong team and the thrill of singing with Darlene Zschech (pronounced "check"), who penned one of the most popular worship songs in the world, "Shout to the Lord."

Because I was one of the few men in the auditorium, the organizers asked me to serenade the ladies with the Michael Bublé version of "The Way You Look Tonight" during the evening program. At the end of the conference and as a surprise to the ladies, I walked down from the rafters with confetti filtering through the air as I hammed it up singing the words popularized by Frank Sinatra. The spotlight was on me until I reached the stage, where I joined several guys—in tuxes—singing. That was an amazing experience and one I'll never forget.

One of the best parts about the Hillsong conference was meeting fascinating people from all over the world and from the United States. One of those people was Nancy Alcorn, who founded Mercy Ministries, a non-profit Christian organization that cares for young women and girls who've been sexually and physically abused, or who are battling eating disorders and self-mutilation issues.

Nancy told me that she had received a copy of *The Maker's Diet* through Kenneth Copeland Ministries and loved the message. "Your book changed the way I eat and changed my life," she said. Nancy added that she used *The Maker's Diet* principles for healthy living in her Mercy homes in Nashville, St. Louis, and Monroe, Louisiana.

I thanked her, and when I saw Nancy speak and share her heart about how lives were being changed at Mercy Ministries, I was greatly impressed. Before we left Australia, she asked me if I would like to come to Nashville, where the main home and corporate offices for Mercy Ministries were located, and speak to the girls on how to have a proper perspective on food and how it contributes to the health of their bodies.

I replied that I would love to come when time opened up in my schedule. In the meantime, before Nicki and I flew home from Australia, we also met the pastors for Rhema Bible Church in Randburg, South Africa, who invited me to come speak at *their* annual women's conference later in the year. Because of that invite, I learned about the Maasai tribe and their cultured dairy beverage known as *maas*, which would become the inspiration for Beyond Organic's Amasai.

As you can see, the Hillsong Colour Conference impacted Nicki and me in ways that we couldn't see at the time but definitely see today. Little did we know that the hand of God was shaping our future and the future of our family in unimaginable ways.

TRANSITION TIME

I didn't make it to Mercy Ministries until the early part of 2007, when Nicki joined me on the trip. She normally doesn't travel with me because that means arranging for someone to watch Joshua, but she wanted to see Mercy Ministries after meeting Nancy Alcorn in Australia.

Around forty girls resided at the Nashville campus. During a chapel service, I couldn't help but be impressed by how these girls were sold out for Jesus in the midst of their pain. They had been rescued from the trash heap of life and arrived at Mercy Ministries with the "wounds" to prove it. I also noticed scars on the arms and wrists of girls who cut themselves with razors—a way to mask pain by administering pain. Yet there they were, praising the Lord with hands held high as the worship songs played.

As I got to speak with a few of the girls after my presentations, the young women told me that they had lived for years by skipping breakfast and subsisting on fast-food fare—burgers-and-fries and pepperoni pizza—for their nutritional needs. Others practiced binging and purging. A few thought they were getting their "fruit" when they ordered a raspberry-topped sundae.

I soon figured out the message that they needed to hear—how to appreciate the value of food. Frankly, these girls were either scared to eat and deathly afraid of any fats in food, or they didn't know what *was* healthy to eat. I took my time explaining the role of healthy, organic food in our lives and gave them examples of what was healthy and not healthy to eat—and why.

Sometime during our first day, Nicki and I received a tour of the Mercy Ministries facility. Nancy led us down a hallway, and as we passed by a closed door, she casually said, "And this is where our adoption office is."

"You place children for adoption?" I asked.

"Yeah, we have several girls who come in with unplanned pregnancies. We either counsel them to place their children or to keep them."

"That's great," I said. I looked at Nicki, but she didn't say anything.

I knew why Nicki was mute. Yes, she was still interested in adopting and she told me that she believed that one day we would adopt, but she was very firm that God would *bring us* the opportunity. There would be no waiting list, or taking adoption classes, or searching for the right child to adopt. God would bring us the child, she said. Nicki was quite adamant about this.

At the end our tour, though, I asked Nancy if we could get a packet containing information on adoption through Mercy Ministries. Not that we were interested, I said, but we just wanted to know what the process entailed.

Back at our hotel room, however, Nicki was almost irritated with me for asking for the packet, even though I tried to explain that I was just being supportive of her. She reminded me that she believed God was going to bring the child to us and that we would receive a child without applying or doing anything to move the process along.

We took the packet home with us, but it sat on the kitchen counter a few days.

Then Nicki tossed it in the trash. If we were supposed to adopt, then God would bring us a child, she reiterated.

Several months later, I received a voice mail at the end of a Friday afternoon, a little after five o'clock, from a woman named Jana Evans at Mercy Ministries' adoption office. "Jordan, I'd like to talk to you about one of our girls," she said.

I had a feeling what Jana was calling about, but I didn't want to say anything to Nicki until I spoke with Jana.

By the time I called back, Jana had left for the day, so I left her a message. But I was dying to hear more details, so I texted Nancy Alcorn, who is the second fastest human being on a BlackBerry—after me, of course.

Nancy, what's going on? Jana Evans wants to talk to me.

Her response came back in a text: *Jordan, one of our girls who's beautiful, who looks like she could be your sister, wants to give up her child for adoption. Call me.*

I did, and Nancy said an eighteen-year-old pregnant girl who heard me speak at Mercy Ministries thought that Nicki and I would make great parents for the son— she knew she was having a boy—that she would deliver in two months. Nancy added that Kayla wanted the boy to be named Samuel because she was devoting her child to God, just as Hannah in the Bible did with her Samuel.

Nicki, of course, was thrilled to hear about this development, and she felt like the Lord had opened this door to adoption. The following day, we attended the Saturday night church service at Palm Beach Gardens Christ Fellowship. Nicki and I had pretty much decided that we wanted to go ahead with the adoption, and when our pastor preached out of the Book of Samuel that evening, we felt a great confirmation.

We informed Nancy that our answer was *yes.* We immediately began a home study course through a social worker and put together a book for Kayla with

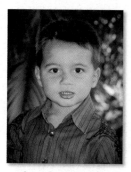

pictures of our family and our home. Samuel was born August 6, 2007, in Nashville's Vanderbilt Hospital, and we had a chance to visit him when he was two days old. Our hearts melted for this precious newborn.

We couldn't take Samuel home with us, however. While Kayla was cooperative, wonderful, and happy about her decision, we still needed the birthfather to sign off on the adoption and complete other paperwork. We were hesitant

Our son, Samuel Tyler Rubin.

to tell Joshua that he would be getting a little brother, but it was hard to hold back the news just as it was hard not to call Samuel our son.

A foster mom named Karri took care of Samuel during this interim time, and she was great. We would visit him every month in Nashville, holding him and spending time with him. When it looked like we were getting close to bringing him home, we bought Samuel a tiny T-shirt with "I'm the Little Brother" printed on the front and an "I'm the Big Brother" T-shirt for Joshua.

Joshua, three years old at the time, was excited to have a little brother. But the adoption process dragged out. We had to hire an attorney who specialized in interstate adoption.

One day our attorney, Earl Mallory, called Nicki while I was in Chicago doing a seminar at Wheaton College.

"Nicki, I just wanted to check up on you," Earl began. "I'm sorry the adoption of Samuel is taking longer than expected, but there's a little girl who will be born in a week. Her prospective adoptive parents have decided not to adopt. She's being born to a birthmother who's a former resident of the Place of Hope children's home."

Place of Hope was founded by Pastor Tom and Donna Mullins of Palm Beach Gardens Christ Fellowship, the church where Nicki and I met and married.

Earl facilitated a lot of their adoptions. In this case, a seventeen-year-old girl was pregnant and was going to have a baby girl in seven days. The prospective adoptive parents dropped out because the birthfather was suspected of having bipolar disorder, which could be genetically passed down to the child.

Nicki listened. "Well, Earl, we believe Samuel is ours, and it's going to work out," she said. "We're getting one baby already, so I don't think we're interested. But I'll call Jordan and see what he says."

Then Nicki reached me while on my way to Wheaton College, just before I was supposed to do my seminar. "Jordan, you won't believe this, but Earl called and there's a girl going to be born in seven days, and he wanted to see if we would be interested in adopting her."

"Of course, we are," I excitedly answered.

"We are?" Nicki asked.

"Sure. We always said if the Lord brings us a child . . ."

So Nicki and I talked things through and agreed that we should check this out.

I called Earl back and said Nicki and I were interested, but we wanted to find out if the prospective adoptive parents were not going to adopt for sure.

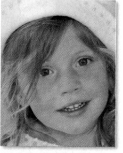

When told that they were out of the picture, Nicki and I decided to go for it. Nine days later, after a series of sleepless and prayerful nights, Alexis Nicole Rubin was born on October 29, 2007, and we brought her home two days later.

Our daughter, Alexis Nicole Rubin.

Joshua was confused, however. He thought he was getting a brother. He obviously didn't understand where kids came from, and now he had a sister when he thought he was getting a brother. He walked around the house saying things like, "Dad, the next brother and sister I get, I want their names to be Princess and Jack."

Both Nicki and I fell in love with Alexis the first time we held her, and she is definitely Daddy's little girl.

But baby Samuel was still out there, and we wanted very much for him to join our family. Finally, in mid-February 2008, the paperwork got resolved, and Nicki and I held him as we experienced an awesome adoption placement ceremony at the Mercy Ministry headquarters in Nashville. With two infants less than three months apart, we had our work cut out for us.

Now there's one part of the story I haven't talked about yet, and it's that before Nicki and were approached to adopt Samuel or Alexis, I had written a new book called *Perfect Weight America* and had agreed to support the book launch by going on a year-long bus tour around America promoting the Perfect Weight America campaign and filming shows for a TV program with the same name.

I couldn't be in two places at once, but I was able to come home one day every week. I took red-eye flights to get home nearly every Saturday night, and on Sundays I would make five gallons of infant formula for my two babies from ingredients like raw goat's or sheep's milk, whey, colostrum, cod liver oil, and extra virgin coconut oil. This would be enough to get both kids through the week until my return the following weekend.

This was not a job; this was a joy. Since neither Samuel or Alexis could be fed breast milk, I was able to provide the nourishment their growing bodies desperately needed. Making homemade infant formula wasn't an easy chore and sometimes took three or four hours, but what father gets to do that for their children?

Since then, I've learned a couple of things about what it means to be an adoptive parent. One, it's almost like a fraternity. When you're outside, you don't even think adoption is possible, but when you do adopt, you can't even imagine why everyone doesn't do it. The other thing that I've realized is that these children are every bit as loved by Nicki and me as our biological son, Joshua.

When I run into people who have heard the story of how Nicki and I adopted two newborns born within three months of each other, they invariably say, "Jordan, you've done such a great thing."

My response: "Are you kidding me?" In my mind, we were presented with this opportunity, and we stepped forward in the faith that this was where the Lord was leading Nicki and me. We were given two beautiful children, and best of all for Nicki, no pregnancy, labor, or delivery!

Now that we've entered the world of adoption, our eyes are open to the plight of the children who *don't* get adopted. What about them? The verse from James 1:27 (NLT) pierces our hearts: "Pure and genuine religion in the sight of God the Father means caring for orphans and widows in their distress and refusing to let the world corrupt you."

Nicki and I talked about this, and we decided that one of the main reasons we are embarking on the Beyond Organic mission is that we want to open children's homes around the world where children would be brought up in health—spiritually and physically. We're looking at starting our first children's home on one of our properties near Birch Tree, Missouri. There are some well-constructed older buildings on the property that haven't been used in a while and need some tender loving care, but we believe that will be the site of our first home. Our goal is to be able to fund this children's home and change the lives of dozens or hundreds or thousands of kids because two is just not enough.

The mandate in James 1:27 is the impetus behind a world-changing program that we are launching at Beyond Organic, and the inspiration comes from a recent family trip to Disney World in Orlando.

As Nicki and I were standing at Will Call with three little kids in tow, I heard one of the "cast members" with a badge yelling to the crowd, "Is anyone here from the 'Give a Day, Get a Disney Day' program?" Apparently, they needed to be in a special line to receive their free admission tickets.

During 2010, Disney instituted a program where if you spent a day volunteering for various charities like Habitat for Humanity or local food banks, you would receive free admission to Disney World, Disneyland, or other Disney theme parks. Disney had a goal of one million volunteers, which was quickly reached.

What if we could do something similar at Beyond Organic? While we were certainly going to change people's diets by providing great food, and we were going to change people's lives by providing educational resources and the Healthy Living Account, I wanted to help people change their world.

That's when I conceived an idea I would call "Give a Meal, Get a Meal." In this program, we partner with ministries and non-profit organizations that care for people who can't care for themselves. We would provide financial resources to improve the health and lives of those in need.

This is the way "Give a Meal, Get a Meal" works. Each time you place an order by phone or online, you will be asked or prompted to give a meal, which we've valued at $10, to one of three ministries of your choice.

In other words, you will be making a $10 donation to that ministry, which we will pass along. Then the next time you place an order with Beyond Organic, you will receive a $10 credit from us toward Beyond Organic foods and beverages. It's a completely sustainable loop. We'll be adding ministries and charities in the future, but in the meantime, we have selected three worthy organizations:

- FEED THE CHILDREN, which distributes food, medicine, clothes and goods to the poor and hungry. Back in the 1980s, Larry Jones was attending a meeting in Haiti. Outside his hotel, a young Haitian boy asked him for a nickel so he could buy a slice of bread. The boy said he hadn't eaten that day, and Larry believed him.

Larry handed the lad a nickel, but as he kept walking to the hotel, he thought about the surplus wheat stored back in silos back in his home state of Oklahoma. When he returned to Oklahoma City, he began asking around for extra wheat, and farmer said they would give it away if someone could haul if off. Then truck drivers who heard his story offered to drive the wheat to Miami, where it could be shipped to Haiti.

More and more surplus wheat was donated, and suddenly Larry was acting as a middleman between food producers and government and charitable organizations. Today Larry oversees a non-profit organization that accepts donations of leftover food, medical supplies, clothes, and toys. Feed the Children's trucks—they have dozens of semis crisscrossing the country—pick up and deliver everything from canned vegetables, meats, food bars, water, coats, and other clothing.

The foodstuffs and goods are delivered to Red Cross chapters, Salvation Army offices, Federal Emergency Management (FEMA) shelters and international hunger relief organizations. Eighty percent of the food is distributed in the United States, the rest internationally.

- URBAN YOUTH IMPACT seeks to love, equip, and empower inner-city youth and their parents to fulfill their God-given purpose. I know about this ministry because it's local to us in West Palm Beach and I know the founder, Bill Hobbs, who's known as Mr. Bill to the kids and teens who participate in summer work programs, camps, and youth ministries.

Urban Youth Impact also offers a Community Health Center, which is the largest free clinic in Palm Beach County, but its flagship project is The Leadership Academy, which serves nearly two hundred after-school students through tutoring, literacy learning, life-skills lessons, and faith-based instruction.

- MERCY MINISTRIES, which I've already talked about at length. This international Christian organization (there are also homes in Vancouver, B.C., Auckland, New Zealand and Bradford, United Kingdom) offers a long-term residential program for young women from the ages of thirteen to twenty-eight who are dealing with eating disorders, sexual abuse, emotional and verbal abuse, self-harm, depression, chemical dependency, physical abuse, and crisis pregnancies.

Nancy Alcorn founded the organization with three core principles: take girls in free of charge; tithe 10 percent of their budget to other ministries; and never accept money with strings attached, such as state or federal funding.

I encourage you to participate in the "Give a Meal, Get a Meal" program every time you purchase healthy foods and beverages with Beyond Organic. Think about the opportunity you have to provide for those in need as God has blessed you.

There's one more chapter—a *long* chapter—in *Live Beyond Organic*: the Beyond Organic Diet Plans. But before you turn the page, I want to pray over you a prayer that I try to pray daily. This prayer comes out of God leading me to study the Scriptures to truly understand His economy, which is firmly based on the Earth's resources.

I encourage you to pray this prayer each and every day and truly understand that by following God's plan for beyond organic agriculture, together we can transform the health of our bodies, our economy, our culture, and even our planet:

MY PRAYER FOR YOU

*Today I pray that like Job, God would surround you with
a hedge of protection and that you would have greater
blessings in the latter part of your life from this day forward.*

*I pray that like Abraham, you would grow
wealthy with cattle, gold, and silver.*

*That like Isaac, you'd plant a field and
reap a hundred-fold harvest.*

*That like Jacob, with wisdom and discernment,
you would grow your flocks and herds.*

*That like Joseph, the dream that God's given
you will be salvation to many.*

*That like Moses, the Lord will reveal himself to
you and show you His glory.*

*That like Bazalel, who helped build the
Tabernacle, that the Lord would anoint you for the
specific task that He's called you to accomplish.*

That like Joshua, God will fill you with the spirit of wisdom.

That like the children of Israel, you'd live in lands that you didn't buy, with barns and houses that you didn't build, drinking from springs and wells that you didn't know existed and eating from vineyards that he didn't plant.

That He'd bless the fruit of your trees, the grass of your fields and the calves of your herds. That He'd bring the spring and autumn rains, and that there would be none sick among you, and none barren.

That like David, God would give you a blueprint of what He would like you to build for him.

That like Solomon, He would give you a wise and understanding heart.

That like Uzziah, there would be good men caring for your cattle in the foothills and that you'd have a love and understanding of the soil.

That like Daniel, God would give you ten times the wisdom, favor, and discernment of all those that don't know him.

And that like Peter, you'd cast your net on the right side of the boat and catch one hundred and fifty-three fish in Jesus' name!

THIS IS MY PRAYER FOR YOU.

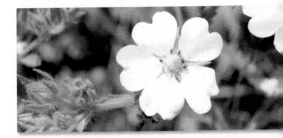

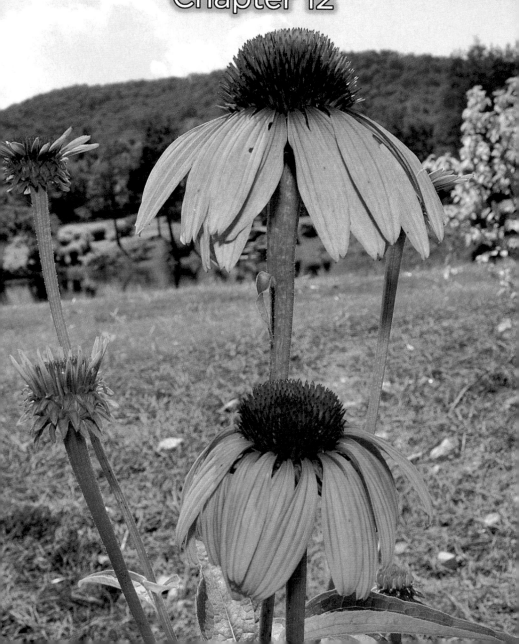

Live Beyond Organic: Your Daily Plan

Chapter 12

THE BEYOND ORGANIC ASSESSMENT

Before beginning your Beyond Organic diet, I'd like you to take the following health assessment. Based on your results, you will be directed to one of three Beyond Organic diet plans.

Regardless of your score on the assessment, you can still follow the Advanced (Live) Plan since it's the most effective diet for providing your body with optimal nutrition.

Once you complete approximately six weeks on your selected plan, re-take the assessment and see if you've graduated to the next plan. If so, begin your new plan for six weeks and then take the assessment once again. But even if you've graduated from the Advanced (Live) Plan, you can always repeat that plan if you feel your body needs a tune up.

But first, you need to start with the assessment questionnaire. Be honest in your answers since the only person you're shortchanging would be yourself.

THE BEYOND ORGANIC ASSESSMENT
FOR SCORING, PLEASE NOTE THAT 1 IS THE WORST AND 4 IS THE BEST.

1. **How many bowel movements do you have per week?**

   ☐ 1-3 = 1 point
   ☐ 4+ = 2 points
   ☐ 4-6 = 3 points
   ☐ 1-3 daily = 4 points

2. **How would you describe your skin?**

   ☐ very dry = 1 point
   ☐ dry = 2 points
   ☐ extremely oily = 3 points
   ☐ balanced = 4 points

3. **How many rounds of antibiotics have you taken in past two years?**

   ☐ 3+ = 1 point
   ☐ 2 = 2 points
   ☐ 1 = 3 points
   ☐ 0 = 4 points

4. **On average, how many servings of cultured dairy (yogurt, kefir, or amasai) do you consume each week?**

   ☐ 0-1 = 1 point
   ☐ 2-3 = 2 points
   ☐ 4-6 = 3 points
   ☐ 7+ = 4 points

5. **You experience gas and bloating:**

   ☐ daily = 1 point
   ☐ frequently = 2 points
   ☐ occasionally = 3 points
   ☐ rarely = 4 points

6. **Describe your gallbladder health:**

   ☐ gallbladder removed = 1 point
   ☐ regular gallstones = 2 points
   ☐ rare gallstones = 3 points
   ☐ never had gallstones = 4 points

7. **Have you been told that you have age-related bone loss?**

   ☐ yes = 1 point
   ☐ no = 4 points

8. **How would you rate the growth of your hair and nails?**

   ☐ poor = 1 point
   ☐ average = 2 points
   ☐ good = 3 points
   ☐ excellent = 4 points

9. **How many servings of organic protein (beef, chicken, fish, eggs, or dairy) do you consume weekly?**

   ☐ 0-2= 1 point
   ☐ 3-5= 2 points
   ☐ 6-9 = 3 points
   ☐ 10+ = 4 points

10. **How often do you consume conventionally raised meat, farm-raised fish, conventional meats, and non-organic dairy products weekly?**

    ☐ 6+ = 1 point
    ☐ 4-5 = 2 points
    ☐ 2-3 = 3 points
    ☐ 0-1 = 4 points

11. **How many glasses of purified water or spring water do you drink per day (not from the tap)?**

    ☐ 0-1 = 1 point
    ☐ 2-4 = 2 points
    ☐ 5-7 = 3 points
    ☐ 8+ = 4 points

12. **Do you regularly drink, bathe, or swim in chlorinated water?**

    ☐ yes = 1 point
    ☐ no, I have a home filtration system = 4 points

13. **Do you ever feel tired or lack of energy?**

    ☐ daily = 1 point
    ☐ often = 2 points
    ☐ sometimes = 3 points
    ☐ rarely = 4 points

14. **How many cups/servings of coffee or energy drinks (or other caffeinated beverages) do you drink per day?**

    ☐ 3+ = 1 point
    ☐ 2 = 2 points
    ☐ 1 = 3 points
    ☐ 0 = 4 points

15. **Do you live or work in a city? If so, how often are you exposed to air pollution?**

    ☐ daily = 1 point
    ☐ frequently = 2 points
    ☐ occasionally = 3 points
    ☐ rarely = 4 points

16. **Are you ever exposed to first- or second-hand smoke?**

    ☐ daily = 1 point
    ☐ frequently = 2 points
    ☐ occasionally = 3 points
    ☐ rarely = 4 points

17. **Do you work with commercial solvents, household cleaners, or paints? How often are you exposed to these items?**

    ☐ daily = 1 point
    ☐ frequently = 2 points
    ☐ occasionally = 3 points
    ☐ rarely = 4 points

18. **How many silver (amalgam) fillings do you have in your teeth?**

    ☐ 5+ = 1 point
    ☐ 3-4 = 2 points
    ☐ 1-2 = 3 points
    ☐ 0 = 4 points

19. **How often do you use conventional personal care products with non-organic ingredients?**

    ☐ daily = 1 point
    ☐ frequently = 2 points
    ☐ occasionally = 3 points
    ☐ rarely = 4 points

20. **Have you had a flu shot or vaccine in the past five years?**

    ☐ yes = 1 point
    ☐ no = 4 points

21. **How many servings of wild-caught fish do you eat per week?**

    ☐ 0 = 1 point
    ☐ 1 = 2 points
    ☐ 2 = 3 points
    ☐ 3+ = 4 points

22. **How would you rate your blood pressure, cholesterol, and triglyceride levels?**

    ☐ below average = 1 point
    ☐ average = 2 points
    ☐ good = 3 points
    ☐ excellent = 4 points

23. **How many servings of vegetables and fruits do you consume each day?**

    ☐ 0 = 1 point
    ☐ 1-3 = 2 points
    ☐ 4-6 = 3 points
    ☐ 7+ = 4 points

24. **How many servings of grains (wheat bread, oatmeal, rice, etc.) do you consume each day?**

    ☐ 7+ = 1 point
    ☐ 5-6 = 2 points
    ☐ 3-4 = 3 points
    ☐ 0-2 = 4 points

25. **How many hours of intense exercise (weight training, interval training, burst training, running, biking, swimming, etc.) do you perform each week?**

☐ 0 = 1 point
☐ 1-2 = 2 points
☐ 3-4 = 3 points
☐ 5+ = 4 points

26. **How many pounds overweight are you?**

☐ 30+ = 1 point
☐ 15-29 = 2 points
☐ 5-14 = 3 points
☐ 0 = 4 points

27. **Do you ever experience joint stiffness or a lack of flexibility?**

☐ constantly = 1 point
☐ frequently = 2 point
☐ occasionally = 3 points
☐ rarely = 4 points

28. **How many times do you miss work or school each year due to not feeling well?**

☐ 6+ = 1 point
☐ 4-5 = 2 points
☐ 2-3 = 3 points
☐ 0-1 = 4 points

29. **Rate your upper respiratory health:**

☐ terrible = 1 point
☐ below average = 2 points
☐ average = 3 points
☐ good = 4 points

30. **How much sunlight do you get each week?**

☐ 0-30 minutes = 1 point
☐ 30-60 minutes = 2 points
☐ 60-120 minutes = 3 points
☐ 2+ hours = 4 points

31. **Are you a vegetarian, someone who doesn't eat beef, poultry, eggs, fish, or dairy?**

☐ yes = 1 point
☐ yes, but I consume dairy = 2 points
☐ yes, but I consume dairy and eggs = 3 points
☐ I'm an omnivore = 4 points

32. **How many times a week do you consume artificial sweeteners like aspartame, sucralose, or saccharin?**

☐ daily = 1 point
☐ 4-6 days a week = 2 points
☐ 1-3 days a week = 3 points
☐ never = 4 points

33. **On average, how many hours do you sleep per night?**

☐ less than 5 = 1 point
☐ 6-7 = 2 points
☐ 7-8 = 3 points
☐ 8+ = 4 points

34. **During the past month, how many days have you felt sad or down?**

☐ 10+ = 1 point
☐ 7-9 = 2 points
☐ 4-6 = 3 points
☐ 0-3 = 4 points

35. How many days a week are you involved in group activities?

☐ 0 = 1 point
☐ 1 = 2 points
☐ 2 = 3 points
☐ 3+ = 4 points

36. How often do you attend a faith-based activity, such as a church service?

☐ never = 1 point
☐ a few times a year = 2 points
☐ every few weeks = 3 points
☐ weekly = 4 points

37. How satisfied are you with your work life?

☐ I hate it = 1 point
☐ it's OK = 2 points
☐ it's good = 3 points
☐ I'm passionate about my work = 4 points

TOTAL SCORE

ADD UP YOUR SCORES, AND DEPENDING ON THE RESULTS, YOU CAN START WITH ONE OF THE FOLLOWING HEALTH PLANS:

- **BELOW 100 POINTS = ADVANCED (LIVE) PLAN**

- **101-119 POINTS = INTERMEDIATE (BEYOND) PLAN**

- **120 POINTS AND ABOVE = LIFETIME (ORGANIC) PLAN**

THE BEYOND ORGANIC DIET

Take a deep breath.

The following chapter—by far the longest one in *Live Beyond Organic*—introduces and outlines the Beyond Organic Diet plans. While each of the three diet plans offers only the highest quality foods and nutrients, the Advanced (Live) Plan is the most restrictive. Each successive plan becomes easier with a wider offering of food choices.

The Advanced (Live) Plan is for those who are in real need of a health transformation. This plan restricts the consumption of disaccharide carbohydrates and removes common allergens. The Intermediate (Beyond) plan is for those who are in reasonably good health but want to improve.

The Maintenance (Organic) plan is a healthy eating plan that you and your family can follow for the rest of your lives. This eating plan will give you and your loved ones the nutrients and beneficial compounds you need to thrive.

The results of your Beyond Organic assessment score determine the plan you will start with. I recommend you redo your assessment every six weeks to determine if your score has increased, which will indicate that you can move on to the next plan.

THE BEYOND ORGANIC
ADVANCED (LIVE) PLAN

The Beyond Organic Diet Advanced (Live) plan is the most rigorous because you must be very careful about the carbohydrates, fats, and proteins that you eat.

By definition, carbohydrates are the sugars and starches contained in plant foods, and while they are a necessary part of a well-rounded diet, our modern-day diet revolves around sweetened or sugared foods such as breakfast cereals, blueberry muffins, cookies, ice cream, and flavored coffees.

The predominant form of carbohydrates contained in grains, fluid dairy products, sugar, potatoes, and corn are known as disaccharides, as I outlined in Chapter 5. A disaccharide is a "double sugar" that is composed of two molecules of single molecules (monosaccharides) linked to each other. When you consume too much refined white sugar, white flour, and other disaccharide-rich foods, you're feeding the "bad" microorganisms and upsetting the balance of the intestinal flora—prompting digestive problems to strike.

While following the Advanced (Live) Plan, you should avoid eating sugar unnecessarily and cut back on your starches considerably. I know that avoiding sugar and its sweet relatives—high fructose corn syrup, sucrose, molasses, and maple syrup—is easier said than done, but all those sweets can turn your health sour!

The carbohydrates you want to consume are low glycemic, high nutrient, low sugar, and high in monosaccharides. These would be mostly high-fiber fruits, especially berries, vegetables, nuts, seeds, and some legumes.

Eating unrefined carbohydrate-containing foods introduces nutrient-, antioxidant-, and fiber-rich foods into your body. Fiber is the indigestible remnants of plant cells found in vegetables, fruits, whole grains, nuts, seeds, and beans. Fiber-rich foods take longer to break down and are partially indigestible, which means that as these foods work their way through the digestive tract, they absorb water and increase the elimination of waste in the large intestine.

GOOD SOURCES OF FIBER ARE:

- Berries

- Fruits with edible skins (apples, pears, and grapes)

- Citrus fruits

- Whole non-gluten grains (quinoa, millet, amaranth, and buckwheat) that are introduced in the Maintenance (Organic) plan

- Green peas

- Carrots

- Cucumbers

- Zucchini

- Tomatoes

Green leafy vegetables such as spinach and micro greens are also fiber-rich. Eating foods high in fiber and low in starches will immediately improve your digestion as you begin to "starve off" the potentially harmful microorganisms in your gut.

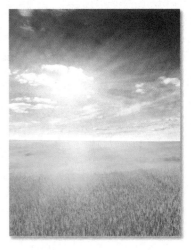

You'll see in the approved foods lists that white sugar, artificial sweeteners, and preservatives are forbidden. If you're currently consuming high amounts of carbohydrates and/or artificial sweeteners on a regular basis, reducing the amounts may cause temporary withdrawal-type symptoms such as headaches, dry mouth, carbohydrate cravings, less energy, mood swings, or even changes in your bowel habits. These "detox" reactions are indications that the program is working as the body works to cleanse toxins from the system. When you have the "blahs," increase water intake and rest.

This plan restricts disaccharide-heavy carbohydrate foods such as pastas and breads but makes up for it in the variety of delicious, filling foods you can enjoy. You are likely to see weight loss during this initial four-week period due to the reduction in high-carbohydrate foods.

During the Advanced (Live) Plan, you will also be avoiding unhealthy fats and proteins that have deleterious effects on the body. This includes the avoidance of many dairy products containing a protein known as beta casein A1, which causes dairy intolerances in many individuals. In addition, stay away from any alcohol— wine, beer, or spirits.

When following the Advanced (Live) Plan, consume only those dairy products specified in the recommended food list. The types of fats you consume are extremely important and can have a great influence on your overall health.

You also need to pay attention to the amount of pure water you're drinking. The goal is a half-ounce of water for every pound you weigh, so someone weighing 150 pounds should drink 75 ounces of water daily, which is a little more than a half-gallon.

Consuming highly pure, natural spring water is an ideal way to enhance the delivery of nutrients and facilitate the removal of waste.

DISCLAIMERS REGARDING RAW DAIRY, RAW EGGS, RAW FISH, AND RAW JUICE

THE FOLLOWING ARE GOVERNMENT-ISSUED WARNINGS FOR THE CONSUMPTION OF RAW OR UNDERCOOKED FOODS AND BEVERAGES.

- Raw milk products may contain disease-causing microorganisms. Persons at highest risk for of disease from these organisms include newborns and infants, the elderly, pregnant women, those taking corticosteroids, antibiotics and antacids, and those having chronic illnesses and other conditions that weaken their immunity.

- Consuming raw or undercooked eggs may increase your risk of food-borne illness.

- Consuming raw or undercooked seafood may increase your risk of food-borne illness.

- Juice that has not been pasteurized may contain bacteria that can increase the risk of food-borne illness. People most at risk are children, the elderly and persons with a weakened immune system.

I am the founder of Beyond Organic and Garden of Life, and, where applicable, I am recommending these companies' products. Regarding other companies that I recommend, I do so because I consume their products and find them to be of good nutritional quality and taste. Beyond Organic and Garden of Life cannot be held responsible for the quality or claims of these products. Please do your research and consult with your healthcare practitioner prior to starting any new diet or supplement program.

THE ADVANCED (LIVE) PLAN FOODS AND BEVERAGES

MEAT (GREENFED, WILD, PASTURE-RAISED, OR GRASS-FED)

⌁ beef	⌁ veal	⌁ lamb
⌁ buffalo	⌁ venison	⌁ elk
⌁ goat bone soup/stock	⌁ liver and heart (must be GreenFed)	

⌁ GreenFed beef sausage (no pork casing—natural and nitrite/nitrate free)

⌁ GreenFed beef hot dogs (no pork casing—natural and nitrite/nitrate free)

✗ alligator	✗ pork	✗ ham
✗ bacon	✗ sausage (pork)	✗ ostrich
✗ imitation meat product (soy)	✗ frog	✗ turtle
✗ veggie burgers	✗ emu	
✗ grain-fed beef (conventional or organic)		

FISH (WILD FRESHWATER/OCEAN-CAUGHT FISH; MAKE SURE IT HAS FINS AND SCALES)

⌁ salmon (sockeye is best)	⌁ halibut	⌁ tuna
⌁ cod	⌁ grouper	⌁ haddock
⌁ mahi mahi	⌁ pompano	⌁ wahoo
⌁ trout	⌁ orange roughy	⌁ sea bass
⌁ snapper	⌁ mackerel	⌁ herring
⌁ sole	⌁ whitefish	⌁ fish bone
⌁ soup/stock	⌁ tuna (canned in spring water)	⌁ scrod
⌁ salmon (canned in spring water)		
⌁ sardines (canned in water or olive oil only)		

✗ farm-raised fish of any kind	✗ fried, breaded fish	✗ catfish
✗ eel	✗ squid	✗ shark
✗ tilapia (which is typically farm-raised)		

✗ avoid all shellfish, including crab, clams, oyster, mussels, lobster, shrimp, scallops, and crawfish

POULTRY (PASTURE-RAISED)

✅ chicken   ✅ Cornish game hen   ✅ Guinea fowl

✅ turkey   ✅ duck   ✅ bone soup/stock

✅ natural chicken or turkey hot dogs (no pork casing—organic and nitrite/nitrate free)

✅ chicken or turkey bacon (no pork casing—organic and nitrite/nitrate free) natural deli meats, including chicken and turkey

✅ liver and heart (must be GreenFed)

✅ chicken or turkey sausage (no pork casing—natural and nitrite/nitrate free, but use sparingly in Advanced (Live) Plan)

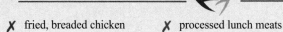

✗ fried, breaded chicken   ✗ processed lunch meats

EGGS (PASTURE-RAISED)

✅ chicken eggs (whole with yolk)   ✅ duck eggs (whole with yolk)

✗ imitation eggs (such as Egg Beaters)

DAIRY (GREENFED, BETA CASEIN A1-FREE, TRUE WHOLE MILK)

✅ Amasai sheep's milk yogurt (plain)   ✅ goat's milk yogurt (plain)

✅ raw cow's, sheep's or goat's milk cheeses

✅ raw, homemade almond milk

✅ whole milk plain goat's milk kefir

✗ rice milk

✗ soy milk

✗ goat's milk dairy (grain-based diet)

✗ cow's milk dairy (non-GreenFed, not true whole milk)

✗ any regular milk, ice cream, or processed cheese food

✗ flavored, low-fat, or fat-free cheese, yogurt, and kefir

✗ dry milk (many processed foods contain this ingredient)

FATS AND OILS (ORGANIC)

- flaxseed oil (not for cooking)
- hempseed oil (not for cooking)
- pasture-raised cow's milk butter
- extra-virgin coconut oil (best for cooking)
- extra-virgin olive oil (not best for cooking)
- coconut milk/cream (canned or fresh)

- pasture-raised butter oil (ghee)
- avocado
- pasture-raised goat's milk butter
- red palm oil

✗ sesame oil	✗ peanut oil	✗ grapeseed oil
✗ lard	✗ margarine	✗ shortening
✗ soy oil	✗ safflower oil	✗ canola oil
✗ sunflower oil	✗ corn oil	✗ cottonseed oil
✗ any partially hydrogenated oil		

VEGETABLES (ORGANIC OR HYDROPONICALLY GROWN, FRESH OR FROZEN)

broccoli	asparagus	beets
cauliflower	Brussels sprouts	cabbage
carrots	celery	cucumber
eggplant	pumpkin	garlic
onion	okra	mushrooms
peas	peppers	string beans
tomatoes	lettuce (all varieties)	spinach
squash (winter or summer)	micro veggies (hydroponically grown)	

- artichokes (French, not Jerusalem)
- leafy greens (kale, collard, broccoli rabe, mustard greens, etc.)
- sprouts (broccoli, sunflower, pea shoots, radish, etc.)
- sea vegetables (kelp, dulse, nori, kombu, hijiki, etc.)
- raw, fermented vegetables (lacto-fermented only, no vinegar)

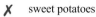

✗ corn	✗ sweet potatoes	✗ white potatoes

BEANS AND LEGUMES (ORGANIC AND SOAKED OR FERMENTED ARE BEST)

- lentils
- small amounts of fermented soybean paste (miso) as a broth

✗ soy beans	✗ tofu	✗ black beans
✗ kidney beans	✗ navy beans	✗ white beans
✗ garbanzo beans	✗ lima beans	✗ pinto beans
✗ red beans	✗ split beans	✗ broad beans
✗ black-eyed peas	✗ tempeh (fermented soy bean loaf)	

NUTS, SEEDS AND THEIR BUTTERS (ORGANIC, RAW, OR SOAKED ARE BEST; CHEW WELL)

almonds	pumpkin seeds	hempseed
flaxseed	sunflower seeds	almond butter
hempseed butter	sunflower butter	pecans
hazelnuts	macadamia nuts	walnuts
Brazil nuts	chia seeds	
tahini, sesame butter	pumpkin seed butter	

| ✗ honey-roasted nuts | ✗ peanuts |
| ✗ peanut butter | ✗ cashews |

CONDIMENTS, SPICES, SEASONINGS, COOKING INGREDIENTS, AND SALAD DRESSINGS (ORGANIC)

ketchup (organic)	hot sauce (preservative-free)
salsa (fresh or canned, organic)	guacamole (fresh)
tomato sauce (no added sugar)	apple cider vinegar
soy sauce (wheat-free, tamari)	mustard
Herbamare seasoning	omega-3 mayonnaise
umeboshi paste	Coconut Aminos
balsamic vinegar	red wine vinegar
capers	wasabi (preservative and color free)

- Bragg brand salad dressings   herbs and spices (no added stabilizers)
- whole mineral sea salt (Celtic, Real Salt, Himalayan salt)
- pickled ginger (preservative and color free)
- cooking wine (organic red and white de-alcoholized after cooking)
- homemade salad dressings and marinades using Advanced (Live) Plan-recommended ingredients
- organic flavoring extracts (alcohol-based, no sugar added, vanilla, almond, etc.)

X all spices that contain added sugar   X commercial ketchup with sugar
X commercial barbecue sauce with sugar   X white vinegar

FRUITS (ORGANIC FRESH OR FROZEN, BUT NO MORE THAN TWO SERVINGS PER DAY AND ALWAYS EATEN WITH HEALTHY FATS)

- blueberries   strawberries   blackberries
- raspberries   aronia berries   grapefruit
- lemon   lime   olives
- green apple   cranberries (fresh or frozen, not dried)

X pomegranate	X apples (with skin)	X melons
X apricots (not dried)	X peaches	X grapes
X orange	X pears	X papaya
X kiwi	X nectarines	X pineapple
X plums	X fresh figs	X cherries
X bananas	X mangoes	X dried fruit
X canned fruit		

BEVERAGES

- botanically infused pure spring water with low total dissolved solids
- cultured beverages (SueroViv, kombucha, and kvass)
- coconut water (must be raw and not packaged)
- herbal teas (organic)—unsweetened or with a small amount of raw, unheated honey
- raw vegetable juice (mostly green with beet or carrot juice—maximum 50 percent of total)

X alcoholic beverages of any kind   X fruit juices   X sodas
X pre-ground commercial coffee   X chlorinated tap water
X natural sparkling water, no carbonation added (such as Gerolsteiner)
X certified organic coffee—buy whole beans, freeze them, and grind fresh when desired; flavor only with organic cream and a small amount of honey

SWEETENERS

✒ **honey in small amounts**
✒ **coconut sap sugar (in small amounts)**

✗ Agave nectar   ✗ Stevia   ✗ Lo Han Guo

✗ maple syrup   ✗ fructose or corn syrup

✗ all artificial sweeteners, including aspartame, sucralose, and acesulfame K

✗ sugar alcohol, including sorbitol, malitol, and xylitol
   (in small quantities or in mints and gum)

✗ sugar (all-natural cane sugar and organic brown sugar, including organic sugars)

SNACKS/MISCELLANEOUS

✒ **goat's milk protein powder**
✒ **sprouted raw protein powder**

✗ soy protein powder   ✗ rice protein powder
✗ milk or whey protein powder from cow's milk

GRAINS AND STARCHY CARBOHYDRATES

✗ bread   ✗ pasta

✗ cereal   ✗ rice

✗ oatmeal   ✗ pastries

✗ baked goods   ✗ corn tortillas

✗ popcorn   ✗ avoid all grains and starchy foods

✗ arrowroot powder (as a substitute for cornstarch)

THE ADVANCED (LIVE) PLAN
SAMPLE 3-DAY DIET

DAY 1

Upon waking
Reign Awaken (16 ounces)

BREAKFAST

Beyond Organic Living Smoothie—mix in a blender with the following ingredients:

1 cup plain Amasai (Amasai is best, or substitute cultured diary such as yogurt or kefir—goat or sheep's milk preferably)

1 tablespoon organic flaxseed oil

1 tablespoon organic raw honey

1 cup of organic berries (fresh or frozen)

2 pasture-raised eggs (see disclaimer on pg 198)

dash of vanilla extract (optional)

MID MORNING

Reign Fruit Infusion (16 ounces)

LUNCH

Beyond Organic Green Salad with micro cruciferous veggies, mixed greens, tomatoes, avocado, carrots, cucumbers, celery, red cabbage, red peppers, red onions, and sprouts with three hard-boiled pasture-raised eggs.

Beyond Organic Salad Dressing: mix extra-virgin olive oil, apple cider vinegar or lemon juice, Celtic sea salt, herbs, and spices, or you may mix 1 tablespoon of extra-virgin olive oil with 1 tablespoon of a healthy store-bought dressing.

One green apple with skin

Drink 8 ounces of SueroViv or other live cultured beverage.

MID AFTERNOON

Reign Veggie Infusion (16 ounces)

DINNER

Baked, poached, or grilled wild-caught salmon

Steamed or stir-fried veggies

Beyond Organic Green Salad

Beyond Organic Salad Dressing

Drink 8 ounces of SueroViv or other live cultured beverage.

BEYOND ORGANIC SNACK

Eat 2 ounces of GreenFed raw cheese and 2-4 ounces of raw almonds.

Drink 8-16 ounces of Reign Supreme Pure Mountain Spring water.

BEFORE BED

Consume 8 ounces of plain Amasai (Amasai is best, or substitute cultured dairy such as yogurt or kefir—goat or sheep's milk preferably).

THE ADVANCED (LIVE) PLAN SAMPLE 3-DAY DIET

DAY 2

UPON WAKING

Reign Awaken (16 ounces)

BREAKFAST

Two or three eggs any style, cooked in one tablespoon of extra-virgin coconut oil

Stir-fried onions, mushrooms, and peppers

Drink 8 ounces of SueroViv or other live cultured beverage.

MID MORNING

Reign Fruit Infusion (16 ounces)

LUNCH

Beyond Organic Green Salad with three ounces of high omega-3 tuna.

Beyond Organic Salad Dressing (see page 205 for recipe)

Drink 8 ounces of SueroViv or other live cultured beverage.

MID AFTERNOON

Reign Veggie Infusion (16 ounces)

DINNER

GreenFed cheeseburgers

cooked vegetables (carrots, onions, peas, etc.)

Beyond Organic Green Salad

Beyond Organic Salad Dressing (see page 205 for recipe)

Drink 8 ounces of SueroViv or other live cultured beverage.

BEYOND ORGANIC SNACK

Eat 8 ounces of plain amasai and a half-cup of raspberries.

Drink 8-16 ounces of Reign Supreme mountain spring water.

BEFORE BED

Drink 8 ounces of plain Amasai.

DAY 3

UPON WAKING

Reign Awaken (16 ounces)

BREAKFAST

Beyond Organic Living Smoothie (see page 205 for recipe)

MID MORNING

Reign Fruit Infusion (16 ounces)

LUNCH

Beyond Organic Green Salad and three ounces of wild salmon

Beyond Organic Salad Dressing (see page 205 for recipe)

Drink 8 ounces of SueroViv or other live cultured beverage.

MID AFTERNOON

Reign Veggie Infusion (16 ounces)

DINNER

Beyond Chicken Soup (see the Appendix for the recipe)

Beyond Organic Green Salad

Beyond Organic Salad Dressing (see page 205 for recipe)

Drink 8 ounces of SueroViv or other live cultured beverage.

BEYOND ORGANIC SNACK

Eat 1-2 ounces of GreenFed raw cheese and blueberries.

Drink 8-16 ounces of Reign Supreme mountain spring water.

BEFORE BED

Drink 8 ounces of plain Amasai.

THE BEYOND ORGANIC INTERMEDIATE (BEYOND) PLAN

The Intermediate (Beyond) Plan allows for a greater variety of foods, which are listed below, but grains and high-lactose, beta-casein A1-containing dairy products are still restricted.

MEAT (GREENFED, WILD, PASTURE-RAISED, OR GRASS-FED)

- beef
- buffalo
- oat
- veal
- venison
- bone soup/stock
- lamb
- elk
- beef (GreenFed) sausage (no pork casing—natural and nitrite/nitrate free)
- liver and heart (must be GreenFed)
- beef (GreenFed) hot dogs (no pork casing—natural and nitrite/nitrate free)

- ✗ pork
- ✗ bacon
- ✗ imitation meat product (soy)
- ✗ veggie burgers
- ✗ frog
- ✗ alligator
- ✗ ham
- ✗ sausage (pork)
- ✗ ostrich
- ✗ emu
- ✗ turtle
- ✗ grain-fed beef (conventional or organic)

FISH (WILD FRESHWATER/OCEAN-CAUGHT FISH; MAKE SURE IT HAS FINS AND SCALES)

- salmon (sockeye is best)
- halibut
- cod
- grouper
- mahi mahi
- wahoo
- orange roughy
- snapper
- herring
- whitefish
- tuna (canned in spring water)

- fish bone soup/stock
- tuna
- scrod
- haddock
- pompano
- trout
- sea bass
- mackerel
- sole
- salmon (canned in spring water)
- sardines (canned in water or olive oil only)

- ✗ fried, breaded fish
- ✗ eel
- ✗ shark
- ✗ catfish
- ✗ squid
- ✗ tilapia (which is typically farm-raised)
- ✗ avoid all shellfish, including crab, clams, oyster, mussels, lobster, shrimp, scallops, and crawfish

POULTRY (PASTURE-RAISED)

- chicken
- Guinea fowl
- duck
- Cornish game hen
- turkey
- bone soup/stock
- liver and heart (must be GreenFed)
- natural deli meats, including chicken and turkey
- chicken or turkey bacon (no pork casing—organic and nitrite/nitrate free)
- natural chicken or turkey hot dogs
  (no pork casing—organic and nitrite/nitrate free)
- chicken or turkey sausage (no pork casing—natural and nitrite/nitrate free, and use sparingly in Advanced (Live) Plan)

- ✗ fried, breaded chicken
- ✗ avoid processed lunch meats

EGGS (PASTURE-RAISED)

✓ chicken eggs (whole with yolk)   ✓ duck eggs (whole with yolk)

✗ imitation eggs (such as Egg Beaters)

DAIRY (GREENFED, BETA CASEIN A1-FREE, TRUE WHOLE MILK

✓ Amasai   ✓ sheep's milk yogurt (plain)

✓ goat's milk yogurt (plain)   ✓ whole milk plain goat's milk kefir

✓ raw, homemade almond milk

✓ GreenFed, raw cow's, sheep or goat milk cheeses

✗ cow's milk dairy (non GreenFed, not true whole milk)

✗ goat's milk dairy (grain-based diet)

✗ soy milk

✗ rice milk

✗ avoid milk, ice cream, processed cheese food

✗ flavored, low-fat, or fat-free cheese, yogurt, and kefir

✗ dry milk (many processed foods contain this ingredient)

FATS AND OILS (ORGANIC)

✓ flaxseed oil (not for cooking)   ✓ pasture-raised butter oil (ghee)

✓ hempseed oil (not for cooking)   ✓ avocado

✓ pasture-raised cow's milk butter   ✓ pasture-raised goat's milk butter

✓ coconut milk/cream (canned or fresh)   ✓ red palm oil

✓ sesame oil (cold pressed)   ✓ peanut oil (cold pressed)

✓ extra-virgin coconut oil (best for cooking)

✓ extra-virgin olive oil (not best for cooking)

✗ grapeseed oil   ✗ lard

✗ margarine   ✗ shortening

✗ soy oil   ✗ safflower oil

✗ canola oil   ✗ sunflower oil

✗ corn oil   ✗ cottonseed oil

✗ any partially hydrogenated oil

VEGETABLES (ORGANIC OR HYDROPONIC, FRESH OR FROZEN)

- broccoli
- beets
- Brussels sprouts
- carrots
- cucumber
- pumpkin
- onion
- mushrooms
- peppers
- tomatoes
- spinach
- squash (winter or summer)
- asparagus
- cauliflower
- cabbage
- celery
- eggplant
- garlic
- okra
- peas
- string beans
- lettuce (all varieties)
- sweet potatoes
- micro greens (hydroponically grown)
- artichokes (French, not Jerusalem)
- leafy greens (kale, collard, broccoli rabe, mustard greens, etc.)
- sprouts (broccoli, sunflower, pea shoots, radish, etc.)
- sea vegetables (kelp, dulse, nori, kombu, hijiki, etc.)
- raw, fermented vegetables (lacto-fermented only, no vinegar)

✗ corn ✗ white potatoes

BEANS AND LEGUMES (ORGANIC AND SOAKED OR FREMENTED ARE BEST)

- lentils
- kidney bean
- white beans
- lima beans
- red beans
- broad beans
- black beans
- navy beans
- garbanzo beans
- pinto beans
- split beans
- black-eyed peas
- tempeh (fermented soy bean loaf)
- small amounts of fermented soybean paste (miso) as a broth

✗ soy beans ✗ tofu

NUTS, SEEDS AND THEIR BUTTERS (E.G. ALMOND BUTTER), ORGANIC, RAW, OR SOAKED ARE BEST; CHEW WELL

- almonds
- hempseed
- sunflower seeds
- hempseed butter
- tahini, sesame butter
- macadamia nuts
- pecans
- Brazil nuts
- cashews
- pumpkin seeds
- flaxseed
- almond butter
- sunflower butter
- pumpkin seed butter
- hazelnuts
- walnuts
- chia seeds

✗ honey-roasted nuts ✗ peanuts ✗ peanut butter

CONDIMENTS, SPICES, SEASONINGS, COOKING INGREDIENTS, AND SALAD DRESSINGS (ORGANIC)

- ketchup (organic)
- salsa (fresh or canned, organic)
- tomato sauce (no added sugar)
- soy sauce (wheat free), tamari
- Herbamare seasoning
- umeboshi paste
- Coconut Aminos
- red wine vinegar
- hot sauce (preservative-free)
- guacamole (fresh)
- apple cider vinegar
- mustard
- omega-3 mayonnaise
- Bragg brand salad dressings
- balsamic vinegar
- capers
- herbs and spices (no added stabilizers)
- pickled ginger (preservative and color free)
- wasabi (preservative and color free)
- whole mineral sea salt (Celtic, Real Salt, Himalayan salt)
- cooking wine (organic red and white de-alcoholized after cooking)
- homemade salad dressings and marinades using Advanced Live Plan-recommended ingredients
- organic flavoring extracts (alcohol-based, no sugar added, vanilla, almond, etc.)

✗ all spices that contain added sugar ✗ commercial ketchup with sugar
✗ commercial barbecue sauce with sugar ✗ white vinegar

FRUITS
(ORGANIC FRESH OR FROZEN, NO MORE THAN TWO SERVINGS PER DAY AND ALWAYS EATEN WITH HEALTHY FATS)

blueberries	strawberries	blackberries
raspberries	aronia berries	grapefruit
lemon	lime	olives
green apple	pomegranate	apples (with skin)
melons	apricots (not dried)	peaches
grapes	orange	pears
papaya	kiwi	nectarines
pineapple	plums	fresh figs
cherries	cranberries (fresh or frozen not dried)	

✗ bananas	✗ mangoes
✗ dried fruit	✗ canned fruit

BEVERAGES

- pure, spring water with low total dissolved solids
- botanically infused pure spring water
- cultured beverages (SueroViv, kombucha, and kvass)
- purified water
- coconut water (must be raw and not packaged)
- herbal teas (preferably organic)—unsweetened or with a small amount of honey
- raw vegetable juice (mostly green with beet or carrot
- juice—maximum 50 percent of total)
- natural sparkling water, no carbonation added (such as Gerolsteiner)
- certified organic coffee—buy whole beans, freeze them, and grind fresh when desired; flavor only with organic cream and a small amount of honey

---

✗ alcoholic beverages of any kind	✗ fruit juices
✗ pre-ground commercial coffee	✗ chlorinated tap water
✗ sodas	

SWEETENERS

- honey in small amounts
- Lo Han Guo
- coconut sap sugar/nectar
- sugar (organic cane sugar, evaporated cane juice, and organic brown sugar)
- sugar alcohol, including sorbitol and malitol, xylitol (in small quantities or in mints and gum)

- Stevia
- maple syrup
- agave nectar (in very small quantities)

✗ fructose or corn syrup
✗ all artificial sweeteners, including aspartame, sucralose, and acesulfame K

SNACKS/MISCELLANEOUS

- goat's milk protein powder
- raw, sprouted protein powder

✗ soy protein powder
✗ milk or whey protein powder from cow's milk
✗ rice protein powder

GRAINS AND STARCHY CARBOHYDRATES

✗ bread
✗ cereal
✗ oatmeal
✗ baked goods
✗ popcorn
✗ arrowroot powder (as a substitute for cornstarch)

✗ pasta
✗ rice
✗ pastries
✗ corn tortillas
✗ avoid all grains and starchy foods

THE INTERMEDIATE (BEYOND) PLAN SAMPLE 3-DAY DIET

DAY 1

UPON WAKING

Reign Awaken (16 ounces)

BREAKFAST

Beyond Organic Living Smoothie—mix in a blender with the following ingredients:

1 cup plain Amasai (Amasai is best, or substitute cultured diary such as yogurt or kefir—goat or sheep's milk preferably)

1 tablespoon organic flaxseed oil

1 tablespoon organic raw honey

1 cup of organic berries (fresh or frozen)

2 pasture-raised eggs (see disclaimer on pg 198)

dash of vanilla extract (optional)

MID MORNING

Reign Fruit Infusion (16 ounces)

LUNCH

Beyond Organic Green Salad with micro cruciferous veggies, mixed greens, tomatoes, avocado, carrots, cucumbers, celery, red cabbage, red peppers, red onions, and sprouts with three hard-boiled pasture-raised eggs.

Beyond Organic Salad Dressing: mix extra-virgin olive oil, apple cider vinegar or lemon juice, Celtic sea salt, herbs, and spices, or you may mix 1 tablespoon of extra-virgin olive oil with 1 tablespoon of a healthy store-bought dressing.

One green apple with skin

Drink 8 ounces of SueroViv or other live cultured beverage.

MID AFTERNOON

Reign Veggie Infusion (16 ounces)

DINNER

Baked, poached, or grilled wild-caught salmon

Steamed or stir-fried veggies

Beyond Organic Green Salad

Beyond Organic Salad Dressing

Drink 8 ounces of SueroViv or other live cultured beverage.

BEYOND ORGANIC SNACK

Eat 2 ounces of GreenFed raw cheese and 2-4 ounces of raw almonds.

Drink 8-16 ounces of Reign Supreme Pure Mountain Spring water.

BEFORE BED

Consume 8 ounces of plain Amasai (Amasai is best, or substitute cultured diary such as yogurt or kefir—goat or sheep's milk preferably).

DAY 2

UPON WAKING

Reign Awaken (16 ounces)

BREAKFAST

Two or three eggs any style, cooked in one tablespoon of extra-virgin coconut oil

Stir-fried onions, mushrooms, and peppers

One orange

Drink 8 ounces of SueroViv, Amasai, or other live cultured beverage.

MID MORNING

Reign Fruit Infusion (16 ounces)

LUNCH

Beyond Organic Green Salad with three ounces of canned high omega-3 tuna

Beyond Organic Salad Dressing (see page 214 for recipe)

One apple

Drink 8 ounces of SueroViv or other live cultured beverage.

MID AFTERNOON

Reign Veggie Infusion (16 ounces)

DINNER

Nicki's GreenFed Meatloaf (see the Appendix for the recipe)

Sweet potato with butter

Beyond Organic Green Salad

Beyond Organic Salad Dressing (see page 214 for recipe)

Drink 8 ounces of SueroViv or other live cultured beverage.

BEYOND ORGANIC SNACK

Amasai (plain or flavored)

GreenFed raw cheese (1 ounce) and a peach

Drink 8-16 ounces of Reign Supreme mountain spring water.

BEFORE BED

Drink 8 ounces of Amasai (plain or flavored).

DAY 3

UPON WAKING

Reign Awaken (16 ounces)

BREAKFAST

Drink 12 ounces of Amasai or Beyond Organic Living Smoothie (see page 214 for recipe)

MID MORNING

Reign Fruit Infusion (16 ounces)

LUNCH

Beyond Organic Green Salad with three ounces of wild salmon (baked or canned)

Beyond Organic Salad Dressing (see page 214 for recipe)

One half cup of fresh pineapple

Drink 8 ounces of SueroViv or other live cultured beverage.

MID AFTERNOON

Reign Veggie Infusion (16 ounces)

DINNER

Roasted pasture-raised chicken

Roasted veggies (peas, carrots, onions)

Beyond Organic Green Salad

Beyond Organic Salad Dressing (see page 214 for recipe)

Drink 8 ounces of SueroViv or other live cultured beverage.

BEYOND ORGANIC SNACK

GreenFed raw cheese (2 ounces) and a half-cup of blueberries

Amasai (plain or flavored)

Reign Supreme mountain spring water (8-16 ounces)

BEFORE BED

Drink 8 ounces of Amasai (plain or flavored).

NEED RECIPES?

You'll find healthy and delicious recipes in the Appendix, "Beyond Organic Recipes." For additional recipes, please visit **LiveBeyondOrganic.com**

THE BEYOND ORGANIC LIFETIME (ORGANIC) PLAN

The Lifetime (Organic) Plan is the ultimate diet for health and wellness for the entire family. Based on the principles of maximum nutrition and minimal toxicity, your diet will consist of meals balanced with healthy proteins and fats while eliminating refined, processed foods.

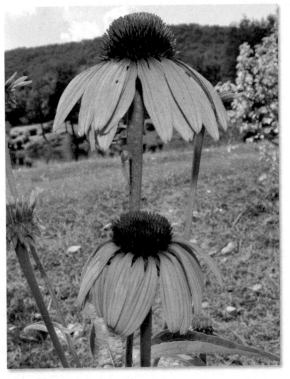

THE LIFETIME (ORGANIC) PLAN FOODS AND BEVERAGES

MEAT
(GREENFED, WILD, PASTURE-RAISED, OR GRASS-FED

- beef
- lamb
- venison
- goat
- liver and heart (must be GreenFed)
- beef (GreenFed) sausage (no pork casing—natural and nitrite/nitrate free)
- beef (GreenFed) hot dogs (no pork casing—natural and nitrite/nitrate free

- veal
- buffalo
- elk
- bone soup/stock

- ✗ grain-fed beef (conventional or organic)
- ✗ ham
- ✗ sausage (pork)
- ✗ ostrich
- ✗ emu
- ✗ turtle

- ✗ pork
- ✗ bacon
- ✗ imitation meat product (soy)
- ✗ veggie burgers
- ✗ frog
- ✗ alligator

FISH
WILD FRESHWATER/OCEAN-CAUGHT FISH; MAKE SURE IT HAS FINS AND SCALES

- salmon (sockeye is best)
- tuna
- scrod
- haddock
- pompano
- trout
- sea bass
- mackerel
- sole
- fish bone soup/stock
- salmon (canned in spring water)

- halibut
- cod
- grouper
- mahi mahi
- wahoo
- orange roughy
- snapper
- herring
- whitefish
- tuna (canned in spring water)
- sardines (canned in water or olive oil only)

- ✗ tilapia (which is often farm-raised)
- ✗ catfish
- ✗ squid
- ✗ avoid all shellfish, including crab, clams, oyster, mussels, lobster, shrimp, scallops, and crawfish

- ✗ fried, breaded fish
- ✗ eel
- ✗ shark

219

POULTRY (PASTURE-RAISED)

- chicken
- Cornish game hen
- Guinea fowl
- turkey
- duck
- bone soup/stock
- chicken or turkey bacon (no pork casing—organic and nitrite/nitrate free)
- natural deli meats, including chicken and turkey
- chicken or turkey sausage (no pork casing—natural and nitrite/nitrate free)
- liver and heart (must be pasture-raised)
- natural chicken or turkey hot dogs (no pork casing—organic and nitrite/nitrate free)

✗ fried, breaded chicken   ✗ avoid processed lunch meats

EGGS (PASTURE-RAISED)

- chicken eggs (whole with yolk)
- duck eggs (whole with yolk)

✗ imitation eggs (such as Egg Beaters)

DAIRY
(GREENFED, BETA CASEIN A1 FREE, TRUE WHOLE MILK)

- Amasai
- sheep's milk yogurt (plain)
- goat's milk yogurt (plain)
- raw, homemade almond milk
- whole milk plain goat's milk kefir
- GreenFed, raw cow's, sheep or goat milk cheeses

✗ soy milk

✗ rice milk

✗ cow's milk dairy (non GreenFed, not true whole milk)

✗ goat's milk dairy (grain-based diet)

✗ avoid milk, ice cream, processed cheese food

✗ flavored, low-fat, or fat-free cheese, yogurt, and kefir

✗ dry milk (many processed foods contain this ingredient)

FATS AND OILS (ORGANIC)

- flaxseed oil (not for cooking)
- hempseed oil (not for cooking)
- pasture-raised cow's milk butter
- coconut milk/cream (canned or fresh)
- sesame oil (cold pressed)
- extra-virgin coconut oil (best for cooking)
- extra-virgin olive oil (not best for cooking)

- pasture-raised butter oil (ghee)
- avocado
- pasture-raised goat's milk butter
- red palm oil
- peanut oil (cold pressed)

- ✗ grapeseed oil
- ✗ margarine
- ✗ soy oil
- ✗ canola oil
- ✗ corn oil
- ✗ any partially hydrogenated oil

- ✗ lard
- ✗ shortening
- ✗ safflower oil
- ✗ sunflower oil
- ✗ cottonseed oil

VEGETABLES (ORGANIC OR HYDROPONIC, FRESH OR FROZEN)

- micro greens (hydroponically grown)
- broccoli
- sweet potatoes
- cauliflower
- cabbage
- celery
- eggplant
- garlic
- okra
- peas
- string beans
- lettuce (all varieties)

- squash (winter or summer)
- asparagus
- beets
- Brussels sprouts
- carrots
- cucumber
- pumpkin
- onion
- mushrooms
- peppers
- tomatoes
- spinach

- artichokes (French, not Jerusalem)
- leafy greens (kale, collard, broccoli rabe, mustard greens, etc.)
- sprouts (broccoli, sunflower, pea shoots, radish, etc.)
- sea vegetables (kelp, dulse, nori, kombu, hijiki, etc.)
- raw, fermented vegetables (lacto-fermented only, no vinegar)

✗ corn

✗ white potatoes

BEANS AND LEGUMES
(ORGANIC AND SOAKED OR FERMENTED
ARE BEST)

- lentils
- kidney bean
- white beans
- lima beans
- red beans
- broad beans
- tempeh (fermented soy bean loaf)
- small amounts of fermented soybean paste (miso) as a broth

- black beans
- navy beans
- garbanzo beans
- pinto beans
- split beans
- black-eyed peas

✗ soy beans   ✗ tofu

NUTS, SEEDS AND THEIR BUTTERS
(E.G. ALMOND BUTTER), ORGANIC, RAW OR
SOAKED ARE BEST; CHEW WELL

- almonds
- hempseed
- sunflower seeds
- hempseed butter
- tahini, sesame butter
- macadamia nuts
- pecans
- Brazil nuts
- cashews
- peanut butter

- pumpkin seeds
- flaxseed
- almond butter
- sunflower butter
- pumpkin seed butter
- hazelnuts
- walnuts
- chia seeds
- peanuts

✗ honey-roasted nuts

CONDIMENTS, SPICES, SEASONINGS, COOKING INGREDIENTS, AND SALAD DRESSINGS (ORGANIC)

- ketchup (organic)
- salsa (fresh or canned, organic)
- tomato sauce (no added sugar)
- soy sauce (wheat free), tamari
- capers
- omega-3 mayonnaise
- Bragg brand salad dressings
- balsamic vinegar
- herbs and spices (no added stabilizers)
- pickled ginger (preservative and color free)
- whole mineral sea salt (Celtic, Real Salt, Himalayan salt)
- cooking wine (organic red and white de-alcoholized after cooking)
- homemade salad dressings and marinades using Advanced (Live) Plan-recommended ingredients
- organic flavoring extracts (alcohol-based, no sugar added, vanilla, almond, etc.)

- hot sauce (preservative-free)
- guacamole (fresh)
- apple cider vinegar
- mustard
- Herbamare seasoning
- umeboshi paste
- Coconut Aminos
- red wine vinegar
- wasabi (preservative and color free)

- ✗ all spices that contain added sugar
- ✗ commercial barbecue sauce with sugar
- ✗ commercial ketchup with sugar
- ✗ white vinegar

FRUITS
(ORGANIC FRESH OR FROZEN, NO MORE THAN TWO SERVINGS PER DAY AND ALWAYS EATEN WITH HEALTHY FATS)

- blueberries
- raspberries
- lemon
- green apple
- melons
- grapes
- papaya
- pineapple
- cherries
- canned fruit
- cranberries (fresh or frozen not dried)

- strawberries
- aronia berries
- lime
- pomegranate
- apricots (not dried)
- orange
- kiwi
- plums
- bananas
- dried fruit (sulfite-free)

- blackberries
- grapefruit
- olives
- apples (with skin)
- peaches
- pears
- nectarines
- fresh figs
- mangoes

BEVERAGES

- ☙ purified water
- ☙ coconut water
- ☙ pure, spring water with low total dissolved solids
- ☙ botanically infused pure spring water
- ☙ cultured beverages (SueroViv, kombucha, and kvass)
- ☙ natural sparkling water, no carbonation added (such as Gerolsteiner)
- ☙ herbal teas (preferably organic)—unsweetened or with a small amount of honey
- ☙ raw vegetable juice (mostly green with beet or carrot juice—maximum 50 percent of total)
- ☙ certified organic coffee—buy whole beans, freeze them, and grind fresh when desired; flavor only with organic cream and a small amount of honey

- ✗ alcoholic beverages of any kind
- ✗ pre-ground commercial coffee
- ✗ sodas
- ✗ fruit juices
- ✗ chlorinated tap water

SWEETENERS

- ☙ honey in small amounts
- ☙ Lo Han Guo
- ☙ agave nectar
- ☙ Stevia
- ☙ maple syrup
- ☙ sugar (organic cane sugar, evaporated cane juice, and organic brown sugar)
- ☙ sugar alcohol, including sorbitol and malitol, xylitol (in small quantities or in mints and gum)

- ✗ fructose or corn syrup
- ✗ all artificial sweeteners, including aspartame, sucralose, and acesulfame K

SNACKS AND MISCELLANEOUS

- ☙ goat's milk protein powder

- ✗ soy protein powder
- ✗ rice protein powder
- ✗ milk or whey protein powder from cow's milk

GRAINS AND STARCHY CARBOHYDRATES
(ORGANIC, SOAKED ARE BEST)

- quinoa
- buckwheat
- brown rice
- sprouted, Ezekiel-type bread
- corn grits (organic only)
- whole-grain yeast-free bread
- spelt
- barley

- amaranth
- millet
- sprouted cereal
- sprouted Essence bread
- corn tortillas (organic only)
- kamut
- oats
- rye

Grains such as wheat, kamut, spelt, oats, barley, and rye contain gluten but may be consumed in yeast-free whole grain breads

- ✗ pastries
- ✗ white rice
- ✗ instant oatmeal
- ✗ bread (except sprouted or sourdough)
- ✗ pastas (except whole-grain kamut or spelt)

- ✗ baked goods
- ✗ dried cereal

SNACKS/MISCELLANEOUS

- healthy trail mix
- cocoa powder
- healthy popcorn
- macaroons (made with simple ingredients and naturally sweetened)

- organic chocolate spreads
- carob powder
- cacao, naturally sweetened

- ✗ soy protein powder
- ✗ rice protein powder
- ✗ milk or whey protein powder (byproduct of cheese manufacturing, denatured)

THE BEYOND ORGANIC DIET LIFETIME (ORGANIC) PLAN SAMPLE 3-DAY DIET

DAY 1

UPON WAKING
Reign Awaken (16 ounces)

BREAKFAST
12 ounces of flavored Amasai or Beyond Organic Living Smoothie (see page 214 for recipe)

MID MORNING
Reign Fruit Infusion (16 ounces)

LUNCH
Beyond Organic Green Salad and three ounces of canned high omega-3 tuna (see page 214 for recipe)
Beyond Organic Salad Dressing (see page 214 for recipe)
Grapes
Drink 8 ounces of SueroViv or other live cultured beverage.

MID AFTERNOON
Reign Veggie Infusion (16 ounces)

DINNER
Halibut (see the Appendix for the recipe)
Steamed quinoa (see the Appendix for the recipe)
Stir-fried veggies (see the Appendix for the recipe)
Beyond Organic Green Salad (see page 214 for recipe)
Beyond Organic Salad Dressing (see page 214 for recipe)
Drink 8 ounces of SueroViv or other live cultured beverage.

BEYOND ORGANIC SNACK
GreenFed raw cheese and raw almonds (2 ounces of each)
Beyond Organic Chocolate bar
Drink 8-16 ounces of Reign Supreme Pure Mountain Spring water.

BEFORE BED
Consume 8 ounces of Amasai (plain or flavored).

DAY 2

UPON WAKING
Reign Awaken (16 ounces)

BREAKFAST
Two or three eggs any style, cooked in one tablespoon of extra-virgin coconut oil

Stir-fried onions, mushrooms, and peppers. One orange

Drink 8 ounces of SueroViv, Amasai, or other live cultured beverage.

MID MORNING
Reign Fruit Infusion (16 ounces)

LUNCH
Organic roasted or smoked chicken sandwich on sprouted or yeast-free sourdough whole grain bread with GreenFed really raw cheese

One apple

Drink 8 ounces of SueroViv or other live cultured beverage.

MID AFTERNOON
Reign Veggie Infusion (16 ounces)

DINNER
Filet of GreenFed Beef
(see the Appendix for the recipe)

Beyond Organic Green Salad
(see page 214 for recipe)

Beyond Organic Salad Dressing
(see page 214 for recipe)

Drink 8 ounces of SueroViv or other live cultured beverage.

BEYOND ORGANIC SNACKS
8 ounces of Amasai (plain or flavored)

Beyond Organic chocolate bar

Drink 8-16 ounces of Reign Supreme Mountain Spring Water.

BEFORE BED
Drink 8 ounces of Amasai (plain or flavored).

DAY 3

UPON WAKING
Reign Awaken (16 ounces)

Breakfast

Drink 12 ounces of Amasai or Beyond Organic Living Smoothie (see page 214 for recipe)

MID MORNING
Reign Fruit Infusion (16 ounces)

LUNCH
Beyond Organic Green Salad with three ounces of wild salmon (baked or canned)

Beyond Organic Salad Dressing
(see page 214 for recipe)

One half-cup of fresh pineapple

Drink 8 ounces of SueroViv or other live cultured beverage.

MID AFTERNOON
Reign Veggie Infusion (16 ounces)

DINNER
GreenFed Beef Fajitas
(see the Appendix for the recipe)

Beyond Organic Green Salad
(see page 214 for recipe)

Beyond Organic Salad Dressing
(see page 214 for recipe)

Drink 8 ounces of SueroViv or other live cultured beverage.

BEYOND ORGANIC SNACK
GreenFed raw cheese (2 ounces) and a half-cup of blueberries

8 ounces of Amasai (plain or flavored)

Beyond Organic Chocolate Bar

Drink 8-16 ounces of Reign Supreme Mountain Spring Water

BEFORE BED
Drink 8 ounces of Amasai (plain or flavored).

SHOPPING TIPS FOR THE BEYOND ORGANIC DIET

When it comes to following the Beyond Organic Diet, changing the way you shop for foods will change the way you eat.

The great news is that with the Beyond Organic online virtual farmers market, you will be able to purchase some of the world's healthiest foods and beverages from our farms delivered directly to your family. For the foods and beverages that Beyond Organic doesn't offer, you will want to purchase these from health food stores and natural markets as well as progressive grocery stores and, of course, local farmers markets or even better, local farms.

I wouldn't blame you, though, if you walked into your local health food store and felt totally confused. You may have no idea where to begin, or you don't know how to read the food labels. You may not even be sure that everything in the store is truly healthy for you—and you'd be right about that. Don't worry. I have some advice for you.

First, I highly suggest you ask the staff members at your local health food store for advice and assistance. They are almost always informed, friendly, and eager to help out.

Our bodies were not designed to operate at optimum levels on all the junk food, fast food, prepackaged food, or any of the genetically modified, antibiotic-laden, and growth hormone-laden foods that most Americans eat today. Yes, organic products do cost more, but organic foods give you a higher percentage of nutrients, no residual pesticides, no antibiotics, no growth hormones, no foods made from genetically modified crops, no potential long-term health effects, and no negative environmental effects. Any extra money you do spend is well worth it. Don't you want to feel better?

If you can't afford or find organic produce, however, the next best thing to organic is to apply a veggie wash to your conventionally grown vegetables and fruits. Keep in mind that it's much better to consume fruits and vegetables than not to, even if they are not organic. That said, many regular grocery stores are now carrying certified organic produce.

CONSUMING HEALTHY FRUITS AND VEGETABLES

Certified organic fruits and vegetables have an incredible amount of nutrients— vitamins, minerals, live enzymes, antioxidants, and many other healthy compounds. Depending on what season it is, there are different fruits and vegetables available, but every fruit and vegetable has something unique to offer. Let's take a closer look at some of the healthiest foods on the planet:

Berries such as strawberries, blueberries, blackberries, and raspberries are all high in antioxidants and some of the most important fruits you can consume. Antioxidants are nutrients found naturally in the body and in plants such as fruits and vegetables—especially berries.

As cells function normally, they produce damaged molecules called free radicals. Free radicals are highly unstable and steal components from other cells, including DNA, thereby spreading the damage. This damage continues in a chain reaction, and entire cells soon become damaged and die off. This process can be beneficial because it helps the body destroy cells that have outlived their usefulness and kills germs and parasites. When left unchecked, this process can destroy or damage healthy cells. Eating high-antioxidant foods, though, can help the body produce healthy cells.

Of course, buying your berries fresh is best, but frozen berries are a great source of antioxidants year round.

CHECK OUT THESE AMAZING FOOD BENEFITS:

BLUEBERRIES are prized as a high source of antioxidants, with great anti-aging benefits.

CRANBERRIES, usually consumed seasonally, are another great source of antioxidants. They are excellent for urinary tract health and come to a harvest peak in November; thus their association with Thanksgiving.

RASPBERRIES contain ellagic acid, which is an antioxidant with immune-boosting properties and excellent benefits for female health. They are also high in pectin, which makes them an excellent thickener in homemade jellies and jams.

PINEAPPLE has something called bromelain, an enzyme that aids indigestion and causes fruit salads to get soggy after only a short period of time. Eat pineapple fresh, not canned.

So for your fruits, focus on strawberries, raspberries, blueberries, blackberries, cherries, lemons, limes, and grapefruit.

If you eat dried fruits, avoid the kind with sulfate or sulfite preservatives. Sulfites, or sulfur-based preservatives, are artificial chemicals added to hundreds of foods to stop spoilage, but these chemicals can be toxic to the human body. Some studies have shown sulfur additives may contribute to chronic inflammatory diseases such as ulcerative colitis, Crohn's disease, as well as irritable bowel syndrome. So choose your pineapple and all other dried fruits sulfite- and preservative-free.

AVOCADOS, a much-maligned food, is a fruit, not a vegetable. Avocados contain high-quality fats as well as vitamin E and are a great source of fiber and other minerals. Avocados are 75 percent water and contain good fats, similar to olive oil.

LETTUCE comes in several varieties and is high in fiber, but it's difficult to know which ones to choose. Americans are used to consuming iceberg lettuce, but today there are many great brands of mixed salad blends. These mixed blends contain things like organic baby lettuces, including green oak leaf, organic baby spinach, red and green chard, and arugula. They're popular, they're pre-washed, and they're easy for people who don't have a lot of time on their hands. These greens contain virtually every mineral and trace element and large amounts of beta-carotene, which fits into the nutritional category of carotenoids, a class of very important antioxidants that give fruit and vegetables their bright colors.

CABBAGE is excellent for the digestive tract, particularly when cooked or juiced. It contains something called vitamin U, which is the anti-ulcer vitamin. Cabbage is also extremely effective in its cultured or fermented form as sauerkraut, making it very bio-available.

MUSHROOMS are high in nutrients, particularly the mineral selenium, which work with vitamin E as an antioxidant and bind with toxins in the body, rendering them harmless. Mushrooms are over 90 percent water and are high in biotin, one of the B-complex vitamins.

Mushrooms are one of those foods that should be eaten organically because of where they are grown. Mushrooms pick up many nutrients from the soil and the trees they are grown on. If they are grown in a non-organic environment, however, they are often high in heavy metals, so you want to be careful about eating non-organic mushrooms. Despite what you hear, eating mushrooms does not contribute to yeast overgrowth in the body. Some people who are yeast sensitive, however, have cross-sensitivities to mushrooms.

PEPPERS are rich in antioxidants, which clean up and prevent cell damage. Green peppers may be more difficult to digest than other colored peppers, so if you have complicated digestive problems, you should eat yellow, orange, or red peppers. The different colors are rich in different nutrients as well. Red peppers are substantially higher in vitamins C and A than green peppers.

SWEET POTATOES are vegetables with one of the highest sources of beta-carotene. Studies have linked the high intake of foods rich in beta-carotene to a reduced risk of cancer, particularly lung cancer. Sweet potatoes also contain vitamin C, calcium, potassium, carbohydrates, and fiber.

EGGS contain all the known nutrients except for vitamin C. They are good sources of the fat-soluble vitamins A and D as well as certain carotenoids that guard against free radical damage to the body. They also contain lutein, which has been shown to prevent age-related macular degeneration, the leading cause of blindness in America. But please note that when it comes to healthy kinds of eggs, not just any old egg will do.

What kind of eggs should you look for in your health food store? Organic pasture-raised, high omega-3 eggs. They are nature's perfect food. When possible, try to buy eggs from farms where the chickens are allowed to roam free and eat their natural diet. Eggs produced from chickens in their natural environment contain a healthy balance of omega-3 to omega-6 fatty acids and DHA, which is good for the brain and eyes. High omega-3/DHA or organic eggs have six times the vitamin E and nine times the omega-3 fatty acids as regular store-purchased eggs.

You have heard that you should watch how many eggs you eat because they are high in cholesterol. The myths about cholesterol are completely unfounded. Eggs can be a healthy addition to anyone's diet and actually help reduce the risk of both heart disease and cancer. They can be consumed in a variety of ways: fried, hard-boiled, soft-boiled, and poached. Eggs can be used in baking and can even be added to the smoothie recipes found in the Beyond Organic Eating Plan.

CONSUMING HEALTHY POULTRY AND FISH

I recommend organic, pasture-raised chicken, turkey, and duck. When purchasing poultry, look for chicken and turkey that has been raised on a soy-free diet. Poultry is healthiest when consumed in a soup or stock, and the dark meat has more nutrients than the white meat.

For seafood, eat only fish with fins and scales caught in the ocean or freshwater, not farm-raised fish. Salmon, halibut, tuna, cod, sea bass, and sardines are highly recommended, but don't eat shellfish and crustaceans because they contain abundant toxins from their water-bound scavenging habits. In fact, scientists gauge the contaminant levels of our oceans, bays, and rivers by measuring the biological toxin levels in the flesh of crabs, oysters, clams, and lobsters.

WILD SALMON, with sockeye being one of the best varieties, is loaded with healthy protein, omega-3 fatty acids, vitamin D, and the antioxidant astaxanthin, which has been extensively studied and shown to benefit the entire body with its powerful antioxidant effects.

Believe it or not, you can find very healthy seafood in a can. The big key is whether the can is marked "wild caught" rather than "farm raised." You want to choose the former. The good news is that when you are looking for salmon, sardines, and even herring, canned is almost always going to be wild.

HIGH-QUALITY SARDINES are one of the world's greatest foods, although many people hold their nose just thinking about them. Whole, canned sardines are an extremely rich source of omega-3 fats and contain as much calcium as a glass of milk. Make sure to obtain sardines that contain edible soft bones and organs of the fish, which make it a total package.

I also recommend WILD-CAUGHT CANNED TUNA, but it would be wise to restrict canned tuna to one or two cans a week based upon the possible contamination of heavy metals and PCBs. Research shows chunk light tuna contains less mercury than other types because the natural oils contained in fish are detoxifiers of heavy metals.

So, when consuming tuna, try to eat chunk light. You can also look for high omega-3 tuna, which is a more premium product coming from younger, fattier fish. Look for tuna canned in spring water with a high amount of fat (6-8 grams) per serving. Tuna higher in fats are usually lower in toxins such as heavy metals. The advantage of buying tuna in a health food store is that the product doesn't contain additives or preservatives. The fewer ingredients, the better.

Omega-3 fatty acids—the fats we lack the most in our diet—are critical in negating the effects of the overabundance of omega-6 acids and hydrogenated fats found in the standard American diet. The ratio of omega-3 to omega-6 fatty acids can be balanced by consuming more omega-3 foods such as ocean-caught fish with fins and scales (salmon, tuna, and sardines) and eggs high in high in omega-3 fats.

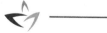

CONSUMING HEALTHY GRAINS

When on the Lifetime (Organic) Plan, you can include grains like quinoa, buckwheat, and brown rice, as well as cereal and breads made with sprouted grains. Feel free to enjoy whole organic grain products in your diet as long as they have been properly prepared through soaking, sprouting, or fermenting.

When choosing bread, look for the term "sprouted" on the label. Brands such as Ezekiel and Essence are extremely high in fiber and can be very nutritious. You can tell a good whole-grain sourdough bread when the label lists a handful of ingredients such as whole grain spelt, water, and sea salt and has the designation as a "whole-grain yeast-free bread." When you buy bread made from sprouted organic grains or whole grain sourdough bread, you can be assured that you're getting the highest-quality products.

Most breads you find in the grocery store have been treated with pesticides and other sprays that inhibit mold. White bread is totally devoid of any nutritional properties and should never be eaten—never. In fact, a diet high in white bread, white rice, and white potatoes puts women at much higher risk of pancreatic cancer, especially if they are overweight and don't get adequate exercise, according to a National Cancer Institute report from 2002.

Whole-grain sourdough and sprouted breads and cereals are healthy grains. Before the advent of modern food processing technology, it was common for our ancient ancestors to soak their grains overnight and then allow them to dry in the open air until they sprouted. Many times they allowed their grains to go through an ancient leavening process that resulted in whole-grain sourdough bread.

Be aware that white rice is just like white bread, meaning that it is a high-glycemic carbohydrate that is absorbed quickly into the bloodstream and can raise insulin levels rapidly. As a result, white rice causes a spike of blood sugar and a surge of insulin. Instead, try whole-grain brown rice, quinoa, amaranth, buckwheat, or oats soaked overnight. Instant oatmeal is processed and refined and is much less healthy than slowly cooked whole oats. Puffed or flaked wheat, oats, and rice have been processed by high heat and pressure. They also shoot your insulin levels way up.

Some of the largest sources of mineral-depleting nutrients are contained in the sugary breakfast cereals lining the shelves of America's grocery stores. Studies show these cereals can have even more detrimental effects on blood sugar than refined sugar and white flour.

As a healthier alternative, I recommend hot cereals made from soaked or sprouted whole grains during the Lifetime (Organic) Plan. They are not processed and do not have preservatives, artificial flavors, added colors, added synthetic vitamins, hidden sugars, or artificial sweeteners.

CONSUMING HEALTHY OILS, SPICES, CONDIMENTS, AND SALT

When it comes to **oils**, I suggest cooking and baking with saturated fats, which are stable, healthy fats. The two best fats to cook with are **extra-virgin coconut oil** and **organic butter** from pasture-raised animals. These fats can withstand high heat without oxidizing.

Coconut oil promotes a healthy microbial balance and supports healthy digestion and immune system function. High-quality extra-virgin coconut oil produced through natural fermentation should have the aroma of a fresh coconut.

Margarine is a man-made fat produced by using bleaching agents, deodorization, and high heat, destroying nearly all of its nutrients. Margarine contains harmful hydrogenated oils. These hydrogenated oils contain trans fatty acids and are the real culprits behind many of our nation's health problems.

OLIVE OIL is extremely healthy, but olive oil should be used only on food and never heated. Look for certified organic extra-virgin olive oil in a dark bottle since light coming into clear bottles can decrease some of the important health properties of the oil as well as its freshness. Extra-virgin olive oil is produced from the first cold pressing of the olives, and that's where you'll get the most antioxidants and other nutrients. Choose a colorful oil with a rich aroma. Stay away from the hydrogenated vegetable oils and polyunsaturated oils, especially when cooked, as well as soy, sunflower, canola, or safflower oils.

When choosing cooking oil, your first choice should be extra-virgin coconut oil or organic butter. Since Extra-virgin olive oil is not as stable under heat as coconut oil or butter, it is best used in salad dressings. Polyunsaturated, hydrogenated oils are unstable fats that should not be used as cooking oils. These include canola oil, sunflower oil, corn oil, safflower oil, soybean oil, and cottonseed oil.

Read the labels of the food you buy because oils are frequently key ingredients in packaged or canned foods. Many contain artificially processed fats and oils that are hydrogenated and partially hydrogenated trans-fatty acids. The processing they undergo makes them more stable, enabling them to sit on a shelf for weeks or even years at a time, but this artificial processing also makes them a foreign and indigestible substance in our bodies, which is It's tough on the digestive system and can harm your health.

The best spices are **organic spices** because they don't contain caking agents and other preservatives that you may find in non-organic spices. Flavored spices are combination seasonings with a variety of organic herbs and spices. Some other favorite seasonings include unrefined sea salt. You can use them in cooking and add them to your favorite foods.

Cultured veggies and spicy kimchi are **condiments** *par excellence*. Be brave and give them a try. This would also be a good time to clear your refrigerator and pantry of any commercial ketchup, mustard, mayonnaise, pickled relish, or other common condiments. Organic versions of these popular condiments are readily available these days, even in supermarkets. They come without refined sugar and unhealthy preservatives.

Regular table salt is highly refined with chemical and high temperature processes. These processes remove many of the valuable minerals, use harmful and potentially toxic additives, and employ bleaching agents to make the salt pristine white. **Unrefined sea salt**, however, still has all the important minerals, and is actually slightly gray or pink in color. Celtic Sea Salt and RealSalt are recommended brands.

CONSUMING HEALTHY SWEETENERS

We've all seen the pink, blue, and yellow packets on restaurant tables. Stay away from those artificial sweeteners! Aspartame, saccharin, sucralose, and their sweet cousins are made from chemicals that have sparked debate for decades. Though the Food and Drug Administration has approved the use of artificial sweeteners in drinks and food, these chemical additives may prove to be detrimental to your health in the long term. The fear is that these highly addictive artificial sweeteners can cross the blood-brain barrier, causing neurological problems.

The best sweetener to use is **raw, unheated honey**, which is a rich storehouse of naturally occurring enzymes. Some other acceptable sweeteners are **organic cane sugar**, **organic maple syrup**, and **coconut sap sugar**.

CONSUMING HEALTHY NUTS AND SEEDS

The good news is that **snacks** have a place in the Beyond Organic Diet. The bad news is that when blood sugar levels fall, many reach for a candy bar or soda for a quick "pick me up." These commercially produced snack foods are loaded with sugar, preservatives, and artificial ingredients that can rob you of your good health.

Some of the most convenient and healthiest snacks are **nuts and seeds**, which are great sources of fiber, healthy fats, and nutrients. If properly prepared, they are extremely nutritious. "Properly prepared" means raw, soaked, or dry-roasted nuts and seeds not roasted in vegetable oil. Just make sure they are organic. Try almonds, walnuts, pecans, pumpkin seeds, and sunflower seeds, or make your own healthy trail mix. The most nutritious seeds are flaxseeds and chia and hemp seeds, all loaded with omega-3 fatty acids and fiber.

Raw nut butters, made from almonds, cashews, and sunflower seeds, are something worth checking out. They're special because when they're raw—not roasted or heated—they're easy to digest and still have their vitamins, minerals, and enzymes. Nut butters can be used as a veggie dip or spread onto sprouted bread or fresh fruit.

It is worthy to note that the phytates found on the covering of grains and seeds "grab" minerals in the intestinal tract and block their absorption. The sprouting process effectively removes these phytates from the outer covering of the natural grain. Germination initiates a chemical transformation in the seed grains that neutralizes the phytates, causing them to come alive, making all of the nutrition within the seed available for digestion.

NEED RECIPES?

You'll find healthy and delicious recipes in the Appendix, "Beyond Organic Recipes." For additional recipes, please visit **LiveBeyondOrganic.com**

DINING OUT TIPS

I'D LIKE TO OFFER YOU SOME TIPS WHEN YOU DINE OUT:

1. Opt for water as your beverage of choice, preferably filtered or bottled (not chlorinated). Avoid alcohol, coffee, tea, juice, and soda.

2. Don't reach for the bread or chips at the table. This includes dinner rolls, bread sticks, sliced bread, muffins, and tortilla chips.

3. Avoid appetizers as much as possible. Eat your soup (grain-, flour-, and dairy-free) or salad before eating your entrée.

4. When ordering soup, make sure no sugar is added. Avoid the use of toppings such as crackers, bacon, cream cheese, or cheese.

5. Choose the house salad over the Caesar salad or other salads with numerous ingredients and toppings. The plainer the salad, the better.

6. Salad dressing is real simple: balsamic vinegar and/or olive oil. Other dressings are full of hydrogenated oils and sugars. It is safer to just order the balsamic vinaigrette as the waiter may not know exactly what is in the other dressings. Also, avoid the croutons.

7. Ask your server how the food is prepared. To avoid some hidden traps in your meal, inquire about the butter, margarine, cream, or oil that may be used in preparing that item. Have your meal cooked in olive oil or butter. Look for the words grilled, poached, baked, roasted, or broiled on the menu.

8. Request that your food be prepared without MSG or sugar.

9. Avoid entrees with a lot of ingredients. Avoid foods that have the following descriptions: fried, buttery, creamy, rich, au gratin, scalloped, béarnaise, Newburg, BBQ, sweet and sour, teriyaki, or breaded.

10. For your main entrée, use the following pecking order when choosing a protein:
    - wild fish
    - wild game (venison or bison)
    - lamb (most lamb is raised well in Australia or New Zealand and fairly well in the States)
    - beef (best if organic or pasture-raised)
    - farm-raised fish (not the healthiest food by any stretch, but still an okay option for dining out)
    - chicken (by far the worst of the biblically clean, conventionally raised animals due to the way factory-farmed poultry is treated and processed)

11. Don't be afraid to make special requests. Most restaurants are willing to accommodate your dietary needs when possible. Order steamed vegetables instead of mashed potatoes, French fries, or coleslaw.

12. There is no need to dress your food up with salt. Most foods already have salt added to them while being cooked.

13. Breakfast can be real simple if you focus on eggs as your main dish. Mix it up a little by requesting diced tomatoes, peppers, and onions—but no ham, please.

14. If you are eating a light dinner, try a salad with grilled wild fish, topped with olive oil and balsamic vinegar for the dressing.

NEED RECIPES?

You'll find healthy and delicious recipes in the Appendix, "Beyond Organic Recipes." For additional recipes, please visit **LiveBeyondOrganic.com.**

BEYOND ORGANIC RECIPES

Living Beyond Organic has never been easier. In this section you will find delicious and nutritious recipes for Beyond Organic breakfasts, lunches, dinners, snacks, beverages, and desserts that your entire family will enjoy. These recipes contain foods and beverages loaded with vitamins, minerals, probiotics, enzymes, proteins, carbohydrate and fats. When preparing these recipes, it is best to use organic ingredients whenever possible.

RED MEAT DISHES

GREENFED BEEF FAJITAS
INGREDIENTS

2 pounds GreenFed beef cut into strips, about   to   inch thick

6 tablespoons extra-virgin coconut oil

    cup lemon or lime juice

4 garlic cloves, peeled and mashed

    teaspoon chili powder

1 red pepper, seeded and cut into strips

1 yellow pepper, seeded and cut into strips

2 medium onions, thinly sliced

extra-virgin coconut oil

12 sprouted whole wheat tortillas

melted butter

amasai for topping

avocado for topping

DIRECTIONS

Make a mixture of oil, lemon or lime juice and spices and mix well with the beef. Marinate for several hours. Remove with a slotted spoon to paper towels and pat dry. Using a heavy skillet, saut the meat, a batch at a time, in coconut oil, transferring to a heated platter and keeping warm in the oven. Meanwhile, mix vegetables in marinade. Saut vegetables in batches in coconut oil and layer over beef. Heat tortillas briefly in a stainless steel pan and brush with melted butter. Serve beef mixture with tortillas and topping.

Serves 4-6.

FI... GREENFED BEEF

ING...TS

GreenFed beef filets
sea salt
black pepper
extra virgin olive oil
chopped herbs (rosemary, thyme, etc.)
2 cups port wine
balsamic vinegar
2 teaspoons of honey
3 chopped shallots
2 chopped garlic cloves
asparagus
porcini mushrooms
soy sauce
GreenFed cheddar blue cheese

DIRECTIONS

Season each filet with salt and black pepper and rub some extra virgin olive oil mixed with chopped herbs, such as rosemary and thyme. Grill or pan sear to desired temperature and taste.

Put 2 cups of port wine in a sauce pan with a good splash of balsamic vinegar, a couple teaspoons of honey, 3 chopped shallots, and 2 cloves chopped garlic. Reduce by ¾ or until slightly thickening. Strain through sieve if you like. Parboil asparagus in a generous amount of boiling water for 1-2 minutes. Shock in a bowl of ice water. Drain.

Season with salt and pepper, extra virgin olive oil, and a little chopped garlic. Chop mushrooms in half and place in roasting pan with some extra virgin olive oil, chopped garlic, salt and pepper, dash of soy sauce, and roast in 400-degree oven for 7-8 minutes or until browning and soft. Place cheddar blue cheese in a double broiler with a few tablespoons of cream and warm until melted. Put cooked filets on plates and stack some asparagus next to them. Place some porcini mushrooms on top of the steak, put a spoonful of cheddar blue cheese over steaks, and drizzle on the port wine sauce.

The yield is 1 serving per beef filet.

Recipe courtesy of Mike and Margie Perrin of 11 Maple Street, a restaurant in Jensen Beach, Florida

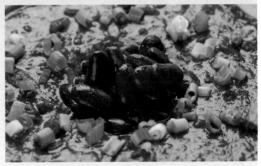

GREENFED BEEF CHILI

INGREDIENTS

1½ pounds ground GreenFed beef
48 ounces tomato juice
1 onion, chopped
3 cans kidney beans, drained
1 can Italian-style diced tomatoes
chili powder
salt and pepper to taste

DIRECTIONS

Brown beef in a skillet. In a large pot, bring tomato juice, chopped onion, drained kidney beans, and diced tomatoes to a boil and then turn down to simmer. Add browned meat after it has been drained. Add chili pepper, salt and pepper to taste. Cook on low for 30 minutes. Serves 8.

RED MEAT DISHES

GREENFED BEEF STUFFED ACORN SQUASH

INGREDIENTS

½ cup GreenFed ground beef, cooked

½ cup quinoa, cooked

1 acorn squash, baked

½ cup onion, chopped

1 tablespoon extra virgin organic coconut oil

¼ cup currants

¼ cup sunflower seeds

1-2 garlic cloves, pressed

1 teaspoon dried basil

½ -1 teaspoon sea salt

½ teaspoon cumin

½ teaspoon paprika

DIRECTIONS

Bake the acorn squash at 400 degrees for 45 minutes, or until tender. The easiest way to cut the squash in half is to bake it for about 20 minutes whole. Remove from the oven and scoop out the seeds and return to the oven to bake until completely cooked through. If you add a little water to the baking pan, it will speed the baking process.

While the squash is baking, cook the ground beef and quinoa in separate pans. Sauté onion in coconut oil until translucent. When cooked, scoop the beef and quinoa into a bowl and add onion, currants, sunflower seeds, garlic, basil, the salt, cumin, and paprika. Stir until well combined. Scoop half the mixture into each half of the acorn squash.

Serves 2.

Adapted from The Juice Lady's Living Foods Revolution *by Cherie Calbom*

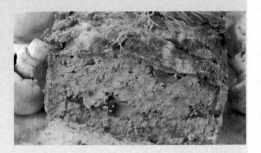

NICKI'S GREENFED MEATLOAF

INGREDIENTS

1½ pounds GreenFed ground beef

1 pasture-raised egg, beaten

½ teaspoon Dijon mustard

½ cup ketchup

1 finely chopped onion

½ finely chopped red pepper (or green)

¼-½ cup organic whipping cream

1½ teaspoon salt

½ cup oats

1 cup buttered sprouted whole grain toast

1½ tablespoons organic cane sugar

TOPPING INGREDIENTS

½ ketchup

3 tablespoons organic cane sugar

2 teaspoons stone ground mustard

½ teaspoon chili powder

DIRECTIONS

Mix ingredients and bake in loaf pan 1½ hours at 350 degrees. Spoon mixed topping ingredients over loaf the last 10 minutes.

Yield is 4-6 servings.

Recipe courtesy of Nicki Rubin

RED MEAT DISHES

SPINACH AND BEEF LASAGNA WITH GREENFED CHEESE

INGREDIENTS

1 pound ground GreenFed beef

12 spelt whole grain lasagna noodles

3 cups pasta sauce (or tomato sauce)

3½ cup ricotta cheese

1 teaspoon olive oil

4 ounces crumbled GreenFed cheddar cheese

2 eggs, beaten

1 tablespoon chopped fresh basil (or 1 teaspoon dried)

½ cup grated parmesan cheese

1 cup shredded GreenFed havarti cheese

salt and pepper or Herbamare seasoning

4 cups raw baby spinach (or regular chopped spinach)

DIRECTIONS

Preheat oven to 400 degrees. Place lasagna noodles in a large shallow dish and cover with boiling water for 15-20 minutes to soften. Cook beef in a large skillet for 10 minutes or until brown, stirring occasionally. Drain fat and return to skillet. Reduce to low heat and add in pasta sauce. Simmer for 5 minutes. In a bowl, mix ricotta, GreenFed cheddar cheese, eggs, basil, parmesan, and salt and pepper or use Herbamare to taste.

Spread 1 cup of sauce on bottom of 9x13-inch baking dish. Place 1/3 of softened noodles on top of sauce. Add Đ spinach, pressing down to make a flat layer. Spread Đ ricotta mixture as the next layer. Top with meat mixture, and then another 1/3 of noodles. Add remaining spinach as a layer, and then the remaining ricotta mixture as a layer. Top with remaining noodles and last cup of sauce. Bake 45 minutes to 1 hour on the middle rack at 400 degrees. Sprinkle GreenFed havarti cheese over sauce during the last 10 minutes of baking. May be prepared and refrigerated up to 24 hours or frozen.

Serves 8.

GREENFED SHEPHERD'S PIE

INGREDIENTS

1 pound GreenFed beef (or other red meat)

1 tablespoon olive oil

1 medium onion, diced

1 cup sliced mushrooms

2/3 cup hummus

3 tablespoons butter

1 squash, julienne

1 zucchini, julienne

2 sweet potatoes

DIRECTIONS

Heat oven to 350 degrees. Place sweet potatoes in oven and cook for 35 minutes. Sauté onion in olive oil for 2-3 minutes over medium heat. Add beef and mushrooms, cooking until done. Stir in hummus and set aside. Sauté squash and zucchini in 1 tablespoon of butter until just tender.

Take sweet potatoes, peel away skin, and mash with 2 tablespoons butter. Grease a 9 x 9 casserole dish with butter. Spread the beef mixture evenly in pan. Cover with vegetable mix. Spread mashed sweet potatoes over top. Cover and cook in 350-degree oven for 20 minutes. Uncover and let cook for 5 minutes.

Serves 4.

Recipe courtesy of Jason Longman

RED MEAT DISHES

HEALTHY POWERBURGERS WITH RAW KETCHUP

INGREDIENTS

1 pound GreenFed ground beef

½ cup chopped veggies such as yellow onions, green onions, zucchini, and yellow squash

2 tablespoons chopped parsley

DIRECTIONS

Sauté the vegetables over medium heat until tender, about 8-10 minutes. In a medium bowl, combine the sautéed vegetables with the ground beef and parsley. Work the mixture with your hands until well combined. Form into four patties and grill until done. Serve on whole grain buns, or as an open-face burger on lettuce leaves, or between two lettuce leaves.

Serves 2-4.

Adapted from The Coconut Diet *by Cherie Calbom*

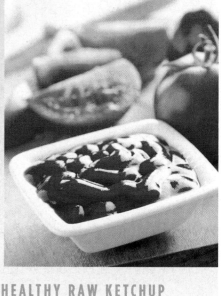

HEALTHY RAW KETCHUP

INGREDIENTS

1 cup chopped tomato

1 cup sun-dried tomatoes, soaked for 30 minutes, drained, and chopped

1 tablespoon fresh garlic, minced

10 fresh basil leaves

3 dates, pitted

¼ cup extra virgin olive oil

1 tablespoon unpasteurized soy sauce or 1 teaspoon sea salt

1- 2 tablespoons apple cider or coconut vinegar

DIRECTIONS

Blend all ingredients together until it forms a paste. Makes about 2½ cups.

From The Juice Lady's Living Foods Revolution *by Cherie Calbom*

FISH DISHES

SEARED TUNA WITH BROWN RICE CAKES AND WAKAME SALAD

INGREDIENTS

4 6-ounce pieces tuna steaks

½ cup sake

½ cup soy sauce

1 teaspoon ginger, grated

2 tablespoons cilantro, chopped

4 tablespoons clarified butter (ghee)

1 medium onion, diced

1 clove garlic, chopped

1 jalapeño, seeded and chopped

1 cup shiitake mushrooms, chopped

3 cups brown rice, cooked

½ cup vegetable or fish stock

4 tablespoons butter

1 ounce dried wakame

DIRECTIONS

Mix together the sake, soy sauce, ginger, and cilantro and marinate tuna steaks for 1-2 hours. Place tuna steaks in a hot pan with 2 tablespoons of clarified butter. Sear to desired doneness. In a 12-inch skillet over medium heat, melt 2 tablespoons of butter. Add onions and garlic and sauté for 4-5 minutes. Add jalapeno and mushrooms and cook for another 6-8 minutes. Take 1 cup of cooked brown rice and place in food processor and pulse until coarsely ground. Put the ground rice and whole rice in a bowl, season with salt and pepper, and add sautéed vegetables. Mix well. Form rice into cakes.

Heat 12-inch skillet over medium-high heat and add remaining 2 tablespoons of clarified butter. Sear rice cakes for about 2 minutes per side. In a medium saucepan, warm 1/2 cup fish or vegetable stock. Add 2 tablespoons of cold unsalted butter and melt. Remove from heat and add wakame. To serve, place wakame (with sauce) on the plate, top with rice cake and then tuna steak.

Serves 4.

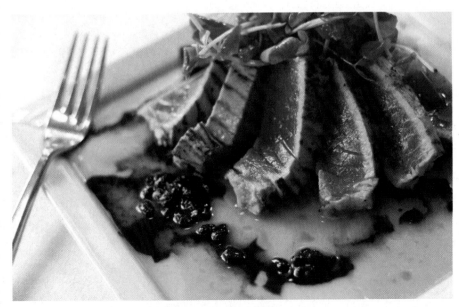

FISH DISHES

HALIBUT DIJON
INGREDIENTS

1½ pounds halibut, cut into four steaks

¼ cup fresh lemon juice

1 cup plain Amasai

½ cup finely chopped onion

1 tablespoon Dijon mustard

¼ teaspoon red pepper flakes

Sea salt and pepper to taste

DIRECTIONS

Make 3 diagonal cuts on each fish steak 2 inches long and ½-inch deep. Place fish in shallow bowl and pour lemon juice over the fish, making sure it seeps into the fish. Let the fish stand in the lemon juice at room temperature for 30 minutes.

Preheat broiler. In a shallow bowl, stir together Amasai, onion, Dijon mustard, and red pepper flakes.

Salt and pepper the halibut steaks, as desired.

Scoop the mustard-mustard mixture on a plate and dip each halibut steak in the mixture, coating both sides. Arrange halibut on broiler tray and broil 5 minutes, then flip the steaks. Apply the rest of the amasai mixture to the top of the steaks and return to the broiler for another 4-5 minutes, or until the fish is opaque in the center.

Serves 4.

Adapted from The Coconut Diet *by Cherie Calbom*

HERB-BAKED WILD SALMON
INGREDIENTS

4 6-ounce pieces of salmon

1 tablespoon Trocomare or other mixed spice blend seasoning

1 teaspoon tarragon (dry)

1 teaspoon coriander crushed seeds

juice of 2 lemons

2 tablespoons of pasture-raised butter

DIRECTIONS

Marinate fish in herbs, spices, and lemon juice for 1-2 hours. Sear in hot butter, 2 minutes on each side. Finish in oven 5 minutes at 385° F.

Serves 4.

Recipe courtesy of Sheila Barcelo of Eden's Wellness Lifestyle in Lakeland, Florida

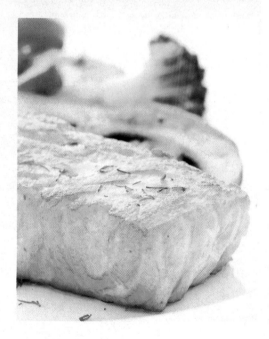

FISH DISHES

WILD SALMON BURGERS WITH GINGER-LEMON SAUCE
INGREDIENTS

16 ounces pre-cooked or canned wild salmon sockeye, drained and flaked

2 pasture-raised eggs

¼ cup chopped fresh parsley

2 tablespoons finely chopped onion

¼ cup cooked quinoa

2 tablespoons lemon juice

½ teaspoon dried basil

1 pinch red pepper flakes or cayenne pepper

1 tablespoon extra virgin coconut oil

GINGER-LEMON SAUCE
INGREDIENTS

2 tablespoons mayonnaise

1 tablespoon lemon juice

¼ teaspoon fresh ginger juice or 1/8 teaspoon ginger powder

1 pinch dried basil

DIRECTIONS

In a medium bowl, mix together the salmon, eggs, parsley, onion, 2 tablespoons of lemon juice, ½ teaspoon of basil, and red pepper flakes. Form into 6 firmly packed patties, about ½ inch thick. Heat the oil in a large skillet over medium heat. When the oil is hot, add the patties and cook for 4 minutes per side, or until nicely browned. In a small bowl, mix together the mayonnaise, 1 tablespoon of lemon juice and a pinch of basil. Use as a sauce for your patties.
Serves 2-4.

BLACKENED SEA BASS
INGREDIENTS

6-ounce pieces of fish, cover completely with blackening spice mix

1 tablespoon extra virgin coconut oil

2 tablespoons cumin seed, ground

2 teaspoons coriander seed, ground

1 tablespoon dulse flakes

3 tablespoons tamari

1 teaspoon organic cane sugar

1 tablespoon capers

DIRECTIONS

Heat cumin seed, coriander seed, and dulse for 1 minute in small fry pan with coconut oil. Add tamari, organic sugar, and capers. Blend well. Marinate fish for minimum 3 hours. Heat under broiler on high. Cook fish 2 minutes on each side.

Serves 4.

Recipe courtesy of Sheila Barcelo of Eden's Wellness Lifestyle in Lakeland, Florida

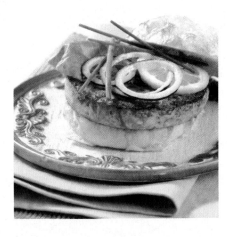

POULTRY DISHES

CHICKEN PICCATA WITH DIJON HIZIKI DRESSING

INGREDIENTS

5 6-ounce marinated boneless chicken breasts

4 ounces clarified butter oil (ghee)

1 ounce amaranth flour

1 lemon

1 serving garlicky green beans (see recipe on page 263)

4 ounces Italian zucchini

4 ounces Dijon Hiziki (see below)

2 ounces cultured vegetables

1/8 teaspoon Herbamare or mixed spice blend

DIRECTIONS

In a large sauté pan, melt the clarified butter. Coat the chicken breast in amaranth flour. Sautee chicken 1½ minutes to sear on both sides. While searing, add the juice from ½ lemon. Continue to sauté until nearly completed cooking, turning occasionally to lightly brown. Add the juice from ½ lemon and finish cooking in the oven. Remove the cooked chicken piccata from the oven and slice diagonally into 5 even strips. Season the sauce to taste with a pinch of sea salt. While the chicken is cooking, prepare the garlicky green beans. In a large sauté pan with olive oil, sauté garlic, oil and sea salt 1 minute. Add green beans and sauté.

Serves 1.

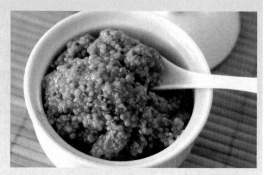

DIJON HIZIKI DRESSING

INGREDIENTS

2 ounces hiziki boshu

⅛ cup extra virgin coconut oil

1 quart diced yellow onions

¼ cup Dijon mustard

⅛ gallon water

½ tablespoon sea salt

1½ quarts chopped white cabbage

¼ quart red peppers

DIRECTIONS

Soak hiziki in a large pan of filtered water, then transfer to a fresh pan and soak again. Transfer to a colander and rinse. In a pot, heat the oil and sauté the onions on low heat.

Stir in mustard. Dissolve the salt into the water. Add the hiziki to the cooked onions. Then add the salt water solution and bring up to heat. Reduce to simmer and cover.

Check back in 10 minutes.

Fold washed and small diced cabbage into the above mixture and continue to simmer. After liquid has cooked down, fold in peppers, remove from heat and let cool. Store, cover and refrigerate. Shelf life 3 days.

Yield: 1 quart.

Recipe courtesy of R. Thomas Deluxe Grill in Atlanta, Georgia

POULTRY DISHES

SWEET AND SOUR CHICKEN

INGREDIENTS

1 pound boneless cubed chicken

1 tablespoon extra virgin coconut oil

½ red bell pepper cut into thin strips

½ green bell pepper cut into thin strips

1 tablespoon cornstarch

¼ cup soy sauce

1 cup pineapple cut into small chunks

¼ cup pineapple juice

3 tablespoon vinegar

3 tablespoons organic cane sugar

½ teaspoon ground ginger

½ teaspoon garlic powder

1½ cup brown rice

DIRECTIONS

Prepare brown rice as directed on package. Heat coconut oil in a large skillet and stir-fry chicken until well browned. Add peppers and cook another 2 minutes. Mix cornstarch and soy sauce. Pour into skillet. Add pineapple and juice, vinegar, organic cane sugar, ginger, and garlic powder. Bring to a full boil. Serve chicken over brown rice.

Serve 4.

HERBED STIR-FRIED CHICKEN AND MIXED VEGGIES

INGREDIENTS

2 pounds chicken, cut into thin strips

½ cup fennel, thinly sliced

1 cup red and green bell peppers, thinly sliced

1 tablespoon red chilies, diced

½ cup carrots, thinly sliced

2 tablespoons mint leaves, roughly chopped

2 tablespoons sweet basil, roughly chopped

½ cup coconut oil

1 tablespoon tamari

¼ cup Mirin sauce

4 cloves garlic, finely chopped

2 teaspoons coriander seeds, crushed

1 teaspoon cumin, ground

DIRECTIONS

Season chicken with coriander seeds, tamari, and cumin. Marinate for 3 hours. Stir-fry carrots in coconut oil for 3 minutes. Add fennel, stir-fry for 2 minutes, then add all peppers and garlic, stir-fry for 1 minute.

Combine chicken and veggies; return to heat and add Mirin sauce. Heat for 3 minutes; remove from heat. Add mint and basil leaves. Combine well and serve.

Serves 4.

Recipe courtesy of Sheila Barcelo of Eden's Wellness Lifestyle in Lakeland, Florida

POULTRY DISHES

GREENFED CHEESE-STUFFED FREE-RANGE CHICKEN BREAST

INGREDIENTS

2 pasture-raised chicken breasts

GreenFed havarti cheese

chopped thyme

chopped marjoram

basil pesto (see below)

rhubarb

unsalted pasture-raised butter

balsamic vinegar

honey

black beans

salt

black pepper

chopped garlic

extra virgin olive oil

pine nuts

chopped basil

watercress

red onions

DIRECTIONS

Cut a pocket in the side of each chicken breast and stuff with fresh goat cheese, mixed with some chopped thyme and marjoram. Rub inside and out with basil pesto (recipe follows). Dust each chicken breast with flour and pan sear both sides until nicely browned. Check middle to see if still pink, then finish roasting in oven. Wash and cut rhubarb stalks (1 per person, peel if stringy) on the diagonal into half-inch pieces. Put in roasting pan, drizzle with unsalted butter until well coated. Add ½ cup or so of balsamic vinegar, salt and pepper, and drizzle honey over all. Roast in a 375-degree oven until pieces feel soft and the butter and balsamic begin to caramelize. Do not stir or pieces will dissolve. Taste, and if still very tart, drizzle on a little more honey.

Soak black beans overnight. Drain. Cook black beans in a generous amount of water until tender. Drain and season with salt and pepper, a little chopped garlic and extra virgin olive oil. To make pesto, grind a good pinch of kosher salt and 2 cloves of garlic in a mortar. Add some toasted pine nuts (or substitute almonds, walnuts, etc.) and a little extra virgin olive oil. Grind up good.

Roughly chop some basil, add to mortar, grind up a little, and finish with more olive oil. Carefully spoon some rhubarb on each plate and top with chicken breast (sliced if you like). Toss watercress lightly with black beans, sliced red onions, splash of balsamic vinegar, and extra virgin olive oil. Place salad on chicken and drizzle a little pesto around the plate.

Serves 1-2 persons.

Recipe courtesy of Mike and Margie Perrin of 11 Maple Street, a restaurant in Jensen Beach, Florida

POULTRY DISHES

CHICKEN WITH SUN-DRIED TOMATOES AND SPINACH

INGREDIENTS

2 skinless, boneless chicken breasts

2 tablespoons butter

1 tablespoon extra virgin olive

½ cup white wine

½ cup chicken broth

1 lemon

½ cup sliced sun-dried tomatoes

1 cup fresh spinach

2 tablespoons capers

salt and pepper

DIRECTIONS

Cut both chicken breasts into halves. Pound out to ¼-inch thick. Season both sides with salt and pepper. Heat a large saucepan over medium high heat. Melt 1 tablespoon of butter and add olive oil. Sauté chicken breasts evenly on both sides until done, about 3 minutes per side.

Remove chicken and set aside, keeping warm. Add sun-dried tomatoes and capers and let cook for 1 minute. Add white wine, chicken broth, and juice from one lemon. Reduce by half, then add spinach, cooking until just wilted.

Serves 1 or 2.

Recipe courtesy of Jason Longman

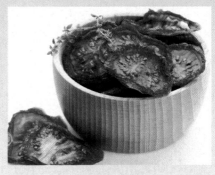

THAI EXPRESS BOWL WITH CHICKEN

INGREDIENTS

3 ounces chicken, cooked and pulled

2 ounces extra virgin olive oil

2 ounces broccoli

2 ounces red cabbage

2 ounces carrots

2 ounces green onions

2 ounces red onions

4 ounces peanut butter sauce

1 cup steamed quinoa

1 teaspoon cilantro

DIRECTIONS

In a large sauté pan, heat the olive oil. Add the vegetables, chicken (slice ¼ inch thick) and sauté until hot. Add peanut butter sauce and toss well only to warm the sauce. In a large bowl, steam the quinoa. Add the above sauté to the hot bowl of quinoa and garnish with cilantro.

Serves 1.

Recipe courtesy of R. Thomas Deluxe Grill in Atlanta, Georgia

POULTRY DISHES

CHICKEN CURRY

INGREDIENTS

6-8 organic, pasture-raised chicken thighs

1½ cups plain Amasai

3 tablespoons fresh lemon juice

3-4 tablespoons extra virgin coconut oil

2 cups chopped onion

1-2 green hot peppers, finely chopped (optional)

1 tablespoon freshly minced garlic*

2 teaspoons coriander

1½ teaspoons turmeric

sea salt to taste (optional)

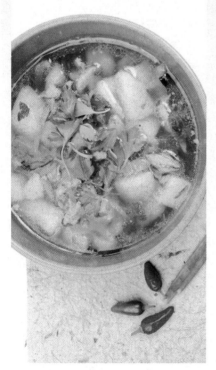

DIRECTIONS

A medley of steamed vegetables and a wild and brown rice bed for the chicken and sauce makes a nice accompaniment and is useful for soaking up this lovely curry sauce. Heat a heavy pan, add the oil and onion, and sauté gently until they are soft and transparent. Don't rush this part. It is very important that the onions be really softened and cooked to a slightly golden color. Only then will they be ready for the spices. This could take as much as 15-20 minutes.

If you like just a little touch of spiciness, seed the peppers (remove the seeds) and chop them up finely. If you like lots of spiciness, then leave the peppers whole with the seeds intact. Now add the minced garlic and spices and sauté for another 3 minutes, stirring constantly. Pushing the onions aside, add the chicken pieces to the pan and cook to a slightly golden color. Turn them around and cover them with the onion spice mixture. Stir in the amasai, then simmer for at least 45 minutes until the chicken is tender. By cooking this dish slowly for a lengthy period, you ensure that the meat will absorb all the lovely flavors of the spices and the amasai. Add the lemon juice and it's ready to serve. If the lemon is very large and juicy, use only half. You may not need any salt in this dish, but if you are a salt aficionado, add a pinch.

Serve hot over a brown and wild rice bed.

Note: Always use fresh garlic, never garlic salt or garlic powder; it will ruin the taste of the dish! A dollop of plain Amasai will be cooling, especially if the "hot" version is used. (A dollop is a large tablespoon or two.) This is an excellent antidote for spiciness and blends very well with any curry flavor.

Serves 3-4.

Adapted from The Coconut Diet *by Cherie Calbom*

POULTRY DISHES

ASIAN CHICKEN LETTUCE WRAPS
INGREDIENTS

1 pound cooked chicken, cut in bite-size pieces

12-16 Boston Bibb or butter lettuce leaves

1 tablespoon extra virgin coconut oil

1 large onion, chopped

2 cloves fresh garlic, minced

1 tablespoon soy sauce

1 tablespoon raw honey

2 teaspoons minced ginger

1 tablespoon rice wine vinegar

pinch of Asian chile pepper sauce or red pepper flakes (optional)

8-ounce can of water chestnuts, drained and finely chopped

1 bunch green onions, chopped

2 teaspoons Asian (dark) sesame oil

DIRECTIONS

Rinse whole lettuce leaves and pat dry, being careful not tear them. Set aside.

In a medium skillet over medium heat with sesame oil, cook the onion, stirring frequently. Add the garlic, soy sauce, honey, ginger, vinegar, and chile pepper sauce to the onions, and stir. Stir in chopped water chestnuts, green onions, sesame oil, and cooked chicken; continue cooking until the onions just begin to wilt, about 2 minutes. Arrange lettuce leaves around the outer edge of a large serving platter, and pile meat mixture in the center. To serve, allow each person to spoon a portion into a lettuce leaf. Wrap the lettuce around the chicken mixture like a burrito, and enjoy!

Serves 4.

Recipe courtesy of Cherie Calbom

EGG DISHES

BASIC OMELET

An omelet is a great way to start the morning and empty out your fridge of leftovers. Below you will find the basic recipe and some fun variations. To get the most nutrition out of your omelet, make sure you choose pasture-raised eggs high in omega-3 fatty acids.

INGREDIENTS

4 fresh eggs, at room temperature

3 tablespoons extra virgin coconut oil or butter

pinch of sea salt

DIRECTIONS

Crack eggs into a bowl. Add water and sea salt, and blend with a wire whisk. (Do not over-whisk or the omelet will be tough). Melt coconut oil or butter in a well-seasoned cast iron skillet or frying pan. When foam subsides, add egg mixture. Tip pan to allow egg to cover the entire pan.

Cook several minutes over medium heat until underside is lightly browned. Lift up one side with a spatula and fold omelet in half. Reduce heat and cook another 30 seconds or so—this will allow the egg on the inside to cook.

Slide omelet onto a heated platter and serve.

EGG DISHES

OMELET VARIATIONS TO SUIT YOUR TASTE

- **Mexican Omelet:** Add salsa, avocado, sour cream, and jack cheese to omelet just before folding.

- **Onion, Pepper, and Goat Cheese Omelet:** Sauté 1 small onion, thinly sliced, and 1/2 red pepper, cut into julienne strips, in a little extra virgin/coconut oil or butter until tender. Strew this evenly over the egg mixture as it begins to cook, along with 2 ounces of goat's milk, cheddar, or feta cheese.

- **Garden Herb Omelet:** Scatter 1 tablespoon parsley, finely chopped, 1 tablespoon chives, finely chopped, and 1 tablespoon thyme or other garden herb, finely chopped, over omelet as it begins to cook.

- **Mushroom Swiss Omelet:** Sauté 1/2-pound fresh mushrooms, washed, well-dried, and thinly-sliced, in extra–virgin coconut oil or butter and olive oil. Scatter mushrooms and grated Swiss cheese over the omelet as it begins to cook.

CHICKEN KING OMELET
INGREDIENTS

3 ounces cooked chicken

3 pasture-raised eggs

2 ounces GreenFed raw cheddar cheese

2 tablespoons extra virgin olive oil

2 ounces mushrooms

2 ounces zucchini

½ ounce sunflower sprouts

1 slice of sprouted whole grain bread

DIRECTIONS

In a sauté pan, sauté the vegetables and the chicken. Mix the eggs and cook in separate pan. Place cheese in the center of the eggs. Add the cooked vegetables and the chicken. Fold in the top and bottom edges of the omelet. Fold and roll the sides of the omelet in. Place omelet on a plate with toasted 9-grain bread and garnish with leftover vegetables and sunflower sprouts. Add piece of toasted bread.

Serves 1.

Recipe courtesy of R. Thomas Deluxe Grill in Atlanta, Georgia

EGG DISHES

SAUSAGE QUEEN OMELET

INGREDIENTS

3 pasture-raised eggs
½ ounce red onion
½ ounce red pepper
2 ounces GreenFed sausage or hot dogs
½ ounce GreenFed raw cheddar cheese
1 ounce shiitake mushroom gravy (See Shiitake Mushroom Gravy recipe on page 254.)
2 ounces roasted rosemary potatoes
1 serving of veggies
½ ounce sprouts
1 slice of sprouted whole grain bread

DIRECTIONS

Cook together all of the onions, peppers, and hot sausage or hot dog (reserve 1 piece of sausage or hot dog for garnish on top of the omelet). Cook the omelet eggs. Add the above veggie mix, mushroom gravy, and cheese to the omelet. Fold omelet to the size of the spatula. Place on plate, garnish with sausage and sprouts on top. Add piece of toasted bread.
Serves 1.
Recipe courtesy of R. Thomas Deluxe Grill in Atlanta, Georgia

BLENDER HOLLANDAISE SAUCE

INGREDIENTS

3 large pasture-raised egg yokes
dash of cayenne pepper
2 tablespoons fresh lemon juice
4 ounces butter from pastured cows, melted and bubbling hot

DIRECTIONS

In a blender, combine egg yolks, lemon juice, and cayenne pepper and blend on high for about 3 seconds. Remove lid, and with the motor running, slowly pour in hot butter in a steady stream over the egg mixture. When butter is poured in, blend for 5 seconds. Taste and adjust seasoning as desired. Serve immediately, or keep the Hollandaise sauce warm by standing the blender in a bowl of warm water.
Makes 12 servings.
Recipe adapted from The Coconut Diet *by Cherie Calbom*

EGGS BENEDICT

INGREDIENTS

8 large pasture-raised eggs
1 tablespoon pasture-raised butter
8 sprouted whole grain English muffins, split
1 tablespoon finely chopped fresh chives or finely chopped fresh flat-leaf parsley leaves

DIRECTIONS

Pour enough water into 2 large skillets to reach a depth of about 3 inches. Bring both skillets to a gentle simmer over medium heat. Crack an egg into a cup and carefully slide it into the hot poaching liquid. Quickly repeat with all the eggs. Poach the eggs, turning them occasionally with a spoon, until the whites are firm, or to the desired degree of doneness, about 3 to 5 minutes.

Using a slotted spoon, remove the eggs and place on top of the buttered English muffins. Or, use an egg poacher pan. To serve, toast the English muffin halves and divide them among 4 warmed plates. Butter each half and set an egg on top. Spoon the hollandaise sauce over the eggs and garnish with the chives. Serve immediately.
Serves 4 (2 Eggs Benedict each).

GRAIN AND STARCH DISHES

EASY WHOLE GRAIN WAFFLES
INGREDIENTS

1⅓ cups whole grain flour (spelt or kamut)

¾ teaspoon sea salt

2 teaspoons non–aluminum baking powder

2 tablespoons unheated honey

1 cup water

2 tablespoons plain Amasai

4 tablespoons extra virgin coconut oil

2 eggs, separated

DIRECTIONS

Soak the flour in water with 2 tablespoons of yogurt for at least 7 hours. Separate the eggs. Beat the yolks and add the amasai and butter. Combine salt, honey, and flour and add this to the first mixture. Beat the egg whites until they form stiff peaks, and then fold them into the mix. Mix in the baking powder quickly. Cook in your waffle iron.

Serves 6.

SHIITAKE MUSHROOM GRAVY
INGREDIENTS

1½ ounces dried Shiitake mushrooms

¼ cup extra virgin coconut oil

¾ cup yellow onions

¼ cup garlic in extra virgin olive oil

1 cup amaranth flour

⅝ gallon hot water

1 tablespoon Herbamare or sea salt

SMASHED POTATOES WITH SHIITAKE GRAVY
INGREDIENTS

1½ oz. extra virgin coconut oil

⅛ cup garlic in extra virgin olive oil

½ quart diced celery

1 ounce sea salt

½ gallon hot water

½ gallon red potatoes

¼ tablespoon Herbamare or sea salt

DIRECTIONS

In a large pot, sauté first 3 ingredients until tender. Add in diced potatoes, salt, and water. Bring to a boil and simmer until potatoes become soft. Strain off and drain for 3-4 minutes in a colander. With hand blender, puree all ingredients. Re-season with Herbamare and refrigerate.

Yield: 1 quart

DIRECTIONS

In a thick bottom sauté pot, sauté diced onions with coconut oil until onions are fairly brown. Add in garlic in oil and sauté for a bit longer. Pour in flour and stir frequently until flour is golden brown. Add in water, Herbamare, and mushrooms (with stems trimmed and small diced). Bring to a boil, slow down the heat, and slow simmer, stirring well and often, being sure to reach the bottom of the pot until the gravy is thickened to desired thickness. Allow to cool and refrigerate.

Yield: 2 quarts.

Recipe courtesy of R. Thomas Deluxe Grill in Atlanta, Georgia

GRAIN AND STARCH DISHES

HOBO POTATOES

INGREDIENTS

6-8 medium potatoes

1 large onion

1 stick pasture-raised butter

salt and pepper or Herbamare

DIRECTIONS

Fold heavy duty aluminum foil to make cooking area. (Please note that I do not advocate using aluminum foil regularly.) Slice potatoes and onion thinly in order to make layers. A food processor makes this easy. Layer small pieces of butter, potatoes, onions and salt and pepper. Cover with another sheet of aluminum foil. Attach top and bottom sheets of foils to make a tent over the potatoes. Grill over medium heat for 45 minutes or until tender. Or bake in the oven at 400 degrees for 45 minutes.

Yield: 6 servings

EASY OATMEAL

INGREDIENTS

1 cup of rolled oats

2 cups of water

1 teaspoon Amasai

1 tablespoon extra virgin coconut oil or butter

honey to taste

DIRECTIONS

Soak the oats overnight in 1 cup of water with 1 teaspoon of amasai added. In the morning, add remaining water. Bring to a boil, then simmer for 1–2 minutes. Soaked oatmeal cooks very fast. Add the oil or butter and honey.

Serves 2.

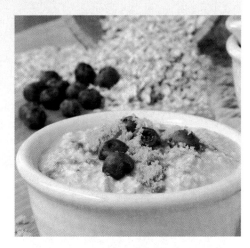

EASY FRENCH TOAST

INGREDIENTS

2 eggs, slightly beaten

1 cup Amasai (milk and honey flavor)

½ teaspoon sea salt

8 slices sprouted or sourdough whole grain bread

DIRECTIONS

Combine eggs, Amasai, honey, and salt in a mixing bowl. Dip each slice of bread quickly into the mixture and brown in extra virgin coconut oil. Serve with butter and unheated honey, maple syrup, or fresh fruit.

Serves 4.

GRAIN AND STARCH DISHES

BLUEBERRY MUFFINS

INGREDIENTS

1 cup blueberries, fresh or frozen

1¼ cups whole wheat, spelt, kamut or buckwheat flour

¾ cup water mixed with 1 tablespoon of Amasai

1 egg, lightly beaten

¼ teaspoon sea salt

½ cup extra-virgin coconut oil

⅓ cup honey

2 teaspoons baking powder

1 teaspoon vanilla

DIRECTIONS

Mix flour with water and Amasai and let stand overnight. Mix in remaining ingredients. Pour into well-buttered muffin tin about three quarters full. Place 5-7 blueberries on each muffin. Berries will fall partway into the muffins. Preheat oven to 400 degrees F. Bake for 18 minutes.
Yield: 12 muffins

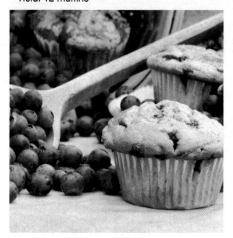

GREEN CORNBREAD

INGREDIENTS

1 cup cornmeal

1 egg

4 stalks celery

3 leaves kale

½ bunch parsley

½ cup barley flour (substitute buckwheat or brown rice flour for gluten-free version*)

1 tablespoon aluminum-free baking powder

½ teaspoon sea salt

1 cup sweet organic corn kernels, cut off the cob

¼ cup almond oil

DIRECTIONS

Juice the celery, kale, and parsley, and reserve ¾+1 tablespoon cup of juice. In a medium bowl, combine the cornmeal, barley flour, baking powder, and salt. Add the corn kernels and mix well. Add the dry ingredients to the green juice and mix until just combined. Turn the batter into an 8 x 8 inch baking dish or a 9-inch cast iron skillet. Bake the cornbread until a toothpick inserted into the center of the bread comes out clean, about 25 minutes. Let the bread cool in the pan for 10 minutes before serving. Serve with organic butter from pastured cows. Makes one 8-inch square loaf or one 9-inch round.

Note: Barley flour has a small amount of gluten; if you are gluten intolerant, you can substitute buckwheat or brown rice flour. Also, only buy organic corn because corn is one of the biggest GMO (genetically modified) crops.

Adapted from Cooking for Life by Cherie Calbom and Vicki Chelf

GRAIN AND STARCH DISHES

PROBIOTIC PANCAKES
INGREDIENTS

1 cup buckwheat, kamut, spelt, or whole wheat flour

½ teaspoon cinnamon

¼ teaspoon sea salt

1⅓ cup Amasai
(milk and honey flavor)

2 tablespoons extra virgin coconut oil

1 egg (pasture-raised)

½ cup blueberries (optional)

½ cup chopped walnuts (optional)

extra-virgin coconut oil for griddle

2 teaspoons aluminum-free baking powder

½ teaspoon baking soda

DIRECTIONS

In a small bowl, mix together dry ingredients and set aside. Whisk together Amasai, oil, and egg. Add dry ingredients and mix until just moistened. Add more Amasai to make batter to your liking. Stir in blueberries and/or walnuts, as desired. Cook on oiled skillet or griddle. Use about ¼ cup batter per pancake. Cook until pancake surface starts to bubble and a few have burst, about 1-2 minutes.

Flip and cook 1-2 minutes more. Top with Amasai and fresh fruit and a small bit of maple syrup or honey and butter.

Serves 4.

Recipe courtesy of Cherie Calbom

QUINOA PILAF
INGREDIENTS

2 cups quinoa

2 tablespoons extra virgin coconut oil

1 medium yellow onion, finely chopped

½ red bell pepper, finely chopped

1 garlic clove, minced

¼ cup currants

¼ cup chopped almonds

4 cups water

⅛ teaspoon pepper

¼ cup chopped fresh basil or 1 tablespoon dried basil

2 tablespoons chopped fresh chives (or green onions including the greens)

sea salt and pepper to taste

DIRECTIONS

Place quinoa in a large sieve and rinse it until the water runs clear. Heat 2 tablespoons of coconut oil on medium high heat in a 3-4 quart pot. Add the onion, bell pepper, garlic, and currants and cook, stirring occasionally until the onions are translucent, but not browned. Add the drained quinoa and cook, stirring occasionally for a couple more minutes. You can let some of the quinoa get a little toasted.

Add 4 cups of water and one teaspoon of salt. Bring to a boil and reduce the heat to low so that the quinoa and water are simmering while the pot is partially covered (enough to let out some steam). Simmer for 20 minutes, or until the quinoa is tender and the water has been absorbed.

Remove from heat and put into a large serving bowl. Stir in the almonds, and fluff up with a fork. Stir in basil, chives, and add salt and pepper to taste.

Serves 2-4.

Recipe courtesy of Cherie Calbom

DESSERTS

DELICIOUS RAW APPLE PIE

INGREDIENTS

10 Medjool dates, pitted
¼ cup honey
2 cups ground almonds (raw, no salt)
1 teaspoon almond extract

DIRECTIONS

Put almonds in food processor. When finely ground, add remaining ingredients until mixture is sticky and can form a ball. Do not overprocess. Oil 9-inch glass pie plate with coconut oil and wipe with paper towel. Press crust mixture evenly in pie plate.
Put in freezer while you make caramel sauce.

CARAMEL SAUCE

INGREDIENTS

15 Medjool dates, pitted
3/4 cup raw butter
¼ cup honey
1 teaspoon vanilla
1 tablespoon cinnamon

DIRECTIONS

Put dates, butter, honey, and vanilla in food processor until mixture is smooth and creamy like caramel. This can take a few minutes. Put in bowl and stir in cinnamon. Set aside while you cut your apples.

Apple Filling Ingredients
6 Honey Crisp or Pink Lady apples

DIRECTIONS

Core peel and slice 6 Honey Crisp or Pink Lady apples. Thin slices are important. As you slice the apples, add them to the caramel mixture. Set aside.

QUICK SPROUTED APPLE CRISP

INGREDIENTS

4 medium baking apples
1 ounce purified water
⅔ cup Ezekiel 4:9 sprouted cereal
1 tablespoon butter
2 tablespoons honey, separated

DIRECTIONS

Preheat oven to 375 degrees. Peel, core, and chop the apples. Place apples in medium–sized pot with water and butter. Cover and cook on medium heat for 15 minutes or until apples can be mashed with a fork to the consistency of apple sauce. Stir in 1 tablespoon of honey. Pour mixture into a medium–sized baking dish. Pour cereal evenly over apple mixture and press down with a fork. Drizzle with remaining 1 tablespoon of honey. Bake for 15 minutes. Remove from heat, let cool, and serve.
Serves 4.

CRUMBLE TOPPING INGREDIENTS

³/₄ cup walnuts
¹/₈ cup honey
2 tablespoons cinnamon

DIRECTIONS

In a food processor, rough chop the walnuts. Take out and put in bowl, add honey, and mix well so all walnut crumbs are coated with honey. Add cinnamon and mix well. Set aside. Then get crust out of freezer. Add apple caramel mixture, then top with crumble topping. Refrigerate overnight or at least 6 hours before serving. Gluten-free, sugar-free, and sodium-free.
Recipe courtesy of Renee Ainlay of Living Coconut

DESSERTS

VANILLA ICE CREAM (AMASAI)

INGREDIENTS

8 ounces Amasai (milk and honey flavor)

1 raw egg yolk (optional)

½ teaspoon organic vanilla extract

dash of sea salt

DIRECTIONS

Combine all ingredients in a blender and pour into a bowl or porcelain baking dish. Cover and place in the freezer for 2-3 hours.

Serves 2.

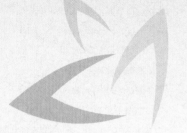

BLACKERRY COBBLER

INGREDIENTS

2½ cups frozen blackberries

1 cup whole spelt or kamut flour

½ cup honey

$1/3$ cup organic cane sugar

2 teaspoons baking powder

1 cup Amasai (milk and honey flavor)

DIRECTIONS

Preheat oven to 375 degrees. Melt ½ stick butter in 8x8 dish. Mix dry ingredients and pour on top of melted butter. Pour 2 ½ cups berries on top of mixture. Bake at 375 degrees for 35-40 minutes.

Serves 2-4.

VARIATIONS:

Blueberry, Blackberry & Cherry, Blueberry & Peach

VANILLA ICE CREAM (AMASAI) PIE

INGREDIENTS FOR CRUST

2 cups pecans or walnuts

1 cup pitted dates, soaked in water for 5 minutes and drained

¼ cup ground flaxseeds

½ teaspoon sea salt

½ ounce pure vanilla extract

INGREDIENTS FOR VANILLA ICE CREAM (AMASAI)

Triple the ice cream recipe above.

DIRECTIONS

To prepare the crust, place pecans in a food processor and process or pulse until finely chopped. Add the dates, flaxseeds, salt, and vanilla and process until mixture forms a ball. Turn out into an 8-inch springform pan and press the mixture into a crust. Chill for about an hour until the crust sets. While the crust sets, prepare the ice cream recipe (be sure to triple the ingredients.)

When the crust has set, pour the ice cream mixture over the crust and place in the freezer for 2-3 hours or until completely frozen. Before serving, top with fresh berries.

Serves 6.

Recipe courtesy of Cherie Calbom and Jordan Rubin

DESSERTS

CREAMY HIGH ENZYME DESSERT
INGREDIENTS

4 ounces Amasai (plain)

1 tablespoon raw, unheated honey

2 tablespoons ground flaxseed or chia seed

½ cup fresh or frozen organic berries

DIRECTIONS

Mix Amasai, honey, and flaxseed or chia seed and top with berries.

BANANA BREAD
INGREDIENTS

5 ripe bananas, mashed

2 eggs, beaten

2 cups whole spelt or kamut flour

1 teaspoon baking powder

½ cup extra virgin coconut oil

½ cup honey

½ cup organic cane sugar

½ teaspoon salt

3 tablespoons Amasai (milk and honey flavor)

½ teaspoon vanilla

½ cup chopped walnuts

DIRECTIONS

Preheat oven to 350 degrees. In a large bowl, beat coconut oil and organic cane. Add eggs and mashed bananas. Add dry ingredients. Add cream and vanilla. Stir in walnuts. Pour in greased 9x13 loaf pan. Bake for 1 hour at 350 degrees.

PAUL'S RAW COCONUT FRUIT PIE
INGREDIENTS FOR THE CRUST

2 cups chopped walnuts

2 cups chopped pecans

½ cup freshly squeezed orange juice

7 pitted Medjool dates

1 ripe banana, thinly sliced

1 ripe mango, peeled, pitted and thinly sliced

INGREDIENTS FOR THE FILLING:

3½ cups young coconut meat (about 4 young coconuts)

1 cup young coconut juice/water (from 1 young coconut)

1 ripe banana (optional)

6 pitted Medjool dates

1 tablespoon ground chia seed

shredded coconut and raisins or pine nuts

DIRECTIONS

To prepare the crust, place walnuts, pecans, orange juice, and dates in a food processor and process until the mixture has the consistency of pastry dough. Press the mixture into an 8-inch glass pie plate to form the crust. Makes 8 servings.

To prepare the filling, place coconut meat, coconut juice/water, optional banana, dates, and ground chia seed in a blender and process until completely smooth. Pour into the pie crust. Garnish the edges of the pie with shredded coconut and raisins or pine nuts.

Recipe courtesy of Paul Nison, author of Raw Food: Formula for Health

SNACKS AND SMALL PLATES

EZ PIZZAS
INGREDIENTS

2 slices sprouted whole grain bread or
1 sprouted whole grain English muffin
pasta sauce
GreenFed cheddar or havarti cheese
green onions, thinly sliced (optional)
sea salt or Herbamare seasoning

DIRECTIONS

Toast bread or English muffins. Place bread on baking sheet.
Spoon pasta sauce over bread. Place onions over pasta sauce.
Cut slices of cheese and place over onions. Sprinkle with
sea salt or Herbamare and cook in oven for 5 minutes or until
cheese melts.

ZESTY POPCORN
INGREDIENTS

$1/3$ cup popcorn
3 tablespoons extra virgin
coconut oil
2 tablespoons garlic-chili flax
2 tablespoons melted butter
Herbamare or sea salt to taste

DIRECTIONS

Melt coconut oil in pan over
medium heat. Pour popcorn into
pan. Cover pan with lid. While
popping melt butter. Cook until
popped. Pour into large bowl. Pour
melted butter and garlic chili flax
and seasoning and mix thoroughly.

BEVERAGES

CULTURED VEGETABLE JUICE
INGREDIENTS

3 red beets
1 carrot
2-4 tablespoons fermented whey
or 1 packet cultured vegetable starter
1 ounce grated ginger
1 teaspoon fine Celtic sea salt
purified water

DIRECTIONS

Peel and chop beets and carrot; combine with peeled
and grated ginger. Place in a 1-2 quart glass container
with a seal. Cover with water and add whey and salt.
Stir well and cover. Leave at room temperature for 2-3
days, then transfer to the refrigerator. Serves 1-2
Recipe courtesy of Jordan Rubin

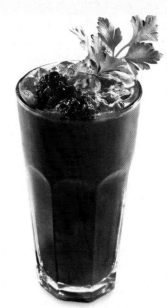

SOUP

CHICKEN SOUP (AND STOCK)
INGREDIENTS

1 whole chicken (free range, pastured, or organic chicken)

3-4 quarts cold filtered water

1 tablespoon raw apple cider vinegar

4 medium-sized onions, coarsely chopped

8 carrots, peeled and coarsely chopped

6 celery stalks, coarsely chopped

2-4 zucchini (medium)

4-6 tablespoons of extra virgin coconut oil

1 bunch parsley

5 garlic cloves

4 inches grated ginger

2-4 tablespoons whole mineral sea salt

DIRECTIONS

If you are using a whole chicken, remove fat glands and the gizzards from the cavity. By all means, use chicken feet if you can find them: they are full of gelatin. (Jewish folklore considers the addition of chicken feet the secret to successful broth.) Place chicken or chicken pieces in a large stainless steel pot with the water, vinegar, and all vegetables except parsley. Bring to a boil and remove scum that rises to the top. Cover and cook for 12 to 24 hours. The longer you cook the stock, the richer and more flavorful the stock will be. About five minutes before finishing the stock, add parsley. This will impart additional mineral ions to the broth. Remove from heat and take out the chicken.

Let cool and remove chicken meat from the carcass. Reserve for other uses such as chicken salads, enchiladas, sandwiches, or curries. (The skin and smaller bones, which will be very soft, may be given to your dog or cat.) Strain the stock into a large bowl and reserve in your refrigerator for use as a base for other soups.

Yield: 6-10 servings.

COCONUT MILK SOUP
INGREDIENTS

1 pound chicken or fish, cut into small cubes

1½ quarts homemade fish or chicken stock

1½ cups coconut milk and cream

3 jalapeño chilies, diced or ½ teaspoon cayenne pepper, dried

1 tablespoon grated fresh ginger

2 tablespoons fish sauce (optional)

2-4 tablespoons lime juice

chopped cilantro for garnish

DIRECTIONS

Simmer all ingredients until meat is cooked through. Garnish with cilantro.

Yield: 6-8 servings.

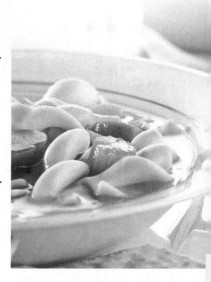

SOUP

TOMATO BASIL SOUP

INGREDIENTS

1 medium onion, halved and sliced

1 tablespoon olive oil

2 large cans of diced tomatoes

4 cups chicken broth

1 clove garlic, minced

½ cup fresh basil, chopped

2 teaspoons balsamic vinegar

½ cup heavy cream (optional)

DIRECTIONS

In a heavy bottomed pan, sauté onions and garlic in oil over medium high heat until soft, being careful not to burn garlic. Add tomatoes, basil, chicken broth, and salt and pepper. Bring to a boil, then reduce heat and simmer for 20 minutes. In a blender, puree the mixture and then strain back into a clean pot. Heat soup and add balsamic vinegar and heavy cream (optional).

Yield: 2 servings.

Recipe courtesy of Jason Longman

RAW ENERGY SOUP

INGREDIENTS

1 cup fresh carrot juice (5-7 medium-sized carrots, or approximately 1 pound, yields about 1 cup)

1 lemon

1-inch chunk ginger root

1 avocado, peeled and seed removed

½ teaspoon ground cumin

½ zucchini, grated (optional)

¼ cup fresh corn cut from the cob (optional)

DIRECTIONS

Juice the carrots, lemon, and ginger. Pour the juice in a blender. Add the avocado and cumin and blend until smooth. Pour into 2 bowls and top with grated zucchini and fresh corn kernels, as desired. Serve chilled. Serves 2.

Adapted from The Juice Lady's Turbo Diet *by Cherie Calbom*

VEGGIES

GARLICKY GREEN BEANS

INGREDIENTS

4 ounces fresh green beans

1 ounce extra virgin olive oil

$\frac{1}{8}$ ounce Herbamare or sea salt

1 teaspoon garlic and extra virgin olive oil

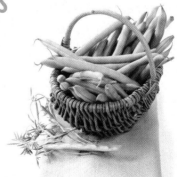

DIRECTIONS

In a large sauté pan, combine olive oil and garlic. Sauté. Add green beans and sauté. Add Herbamare and sea salt to taste.

Yield: 1 serving.

Recipe courtesy of R. Thomas Deluxe Grill in Atlanta, Georgia

VEGGIES

KALE SAUTÉ
INGREDIENTS

1½ pounds young kale, stems and leaves coarsely chopped

3 tablespoons extra virgin olive oil or coconut oil

2 cloves garlic, finely sliced

½ cup vegetable stock or water

sea salt and pepper

2 tablespoons red wine vinegar or balsamic vinegar

DIRECTIONS

Heat oil in a large saucepan over medium-high heat. Add the garlic and cook until soft, but not colored. Raise heat to high, add the stock or water and kale and toss to combine. Cover and cook for 5 minutes. Remove cover and continue to cook, stirring until all the liquid has evaporated. Season with salt and pepper to taste and add vinegar.

Serves 2-4.

ITALIAN ZUCCHINI
INGREDIENTS

1 tablespoon extra virgin olive oil

¼ cup red onion

¼ cup oregano

1 teaspoon garlic in oil

pinch of Herbamare sea salt

⅛ gallon chopped zucchini

DIRECTIONS

In a hot braising pan, heat oil. Stir in onions, garlic, and oregano. Then sauté the veggies for 3 minutes. Add in zucchini and Herbamare and simmer to sweat the zucchini. Pull off and cool immediately. Do not overcook the veggies. Allow to cool and refrigerate.

Yield: 1 quart.

Recipe courtesy of R. Thomas Deluxe Grill in Atlanta, Georgia

SAUTÉED VEGGIES
INGREDIENTS

1 tablespoon extra virgin coconut oil

½ cup onion, thinly sliced

1 cup mix green and red bell peppers

½ cup thinly sliced carrots

1 teaspoon Herbamare or sea salt to season veggies

DIRECTIONS

Sauté veggies in coconut oil, allow cooling.

Serves 1-2.

Recipe courtesy of Mike and Margie Perrin of 11 Maple Street, a restaurant in Jensen Beach, Florida

CREAMED STYLE SPINACH
INGREDIENTS

3 cups spinach, rough chopped

1 cup GreenFed havarti cheese

½ cup Amasai (plain)

2 tablespoons capers

DIRECTIONS

Combine and heat just enough to wilt spinach.

Serves 1-2.

Recipe courtesy of Sheila Barcelo of Eden's Wellness Lifestyle in Lakeland, Florida

VEGGIES

CINNAMON SWEET POTATOES

INGREDIENTS

5 pounds sweet potatoes (yams)

¼ cup extra virgin coconut oil

¼ tablespoon Herbamare and sea salt

¹⁄₁₆ teaspoon cinnamon spice concentrate

¹⁄₁₆ teaspoon ginger spice concentrate

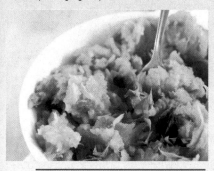

DIRECTIONS

Peel and chop sweet potatoes into 1-inch triangle shapes approximately. Melt coconut oil. In a large bowl, mix sweet potatoes with coconut oil and add Herbamare or sea salt to taste. Divide the mixture evenly to 3 large sheet pans. With 350-degree oven, roast sweet potatoes for 15 minutes. Pull out and stir. Repeat approximately every 10 minutes until the sweet potatoes are soft and brown. Remove sweet potatoes back to the bowl. Add in cinnamon and ginger extracts and gently mix the sweet potatoes by hand. Transfer to large container, label, and refrigerate. Yield: 1 quart.

Recipe courtesy of R. Thomas Deluxe Grill in Atlanta, Georgia

SALADS

CHICKEN SALAD

INGREDIENTS

6 ounces of cooked chopped chicken

1 tablespoon of omega-3 mayonnaise

1 tablespoon flaxseed oil or garlic-chili flax

chopped onions

chopped peppers

chopped celery

DIRECTIONS

Combine all ingredients and serve over lettuce or on toasted sprouted bread.
Yield: 1-2 servings

GREEN SALAD WITH MISO-TAMARI DRESSING

INGREDIENTS

4-6 cups torn red or green leaf lettuce, or a combination of both

1½ cups trimmed and halved snow peas (about 6 ounces)

2 medium carrots, shredded

2 tablespoons sesame oil (cold-pressed)

1 tablespoon red or yellow miso

1 tablespoon apple cider or coconut vinegar

1 tablespoon soy sauce

1 teaspoon finely grated fresh ginger

DIRECTIONS

Whisk oil, miso, vinegar, tamari or soy sauce, and ginger in a large bowl until well combined. Add lettuce, snow peas and carrots; toss to coat.
Serves 4.
Recipe courtesy of Cherie Calbom

beyond organic

APPENDIX

SALADS

CHICKEN SUPREME SALAD

INGREDIENTS

3 ounces cooked and pulled chicken

1 cup chopped romaine lettuce

1 cup mixed field greens

1 fluid ounce extra virgin olive oil

2 ounces fresh green onions

2 ounces carrots

2 ounces red peppers

2 ounces apple

3 tablespoons balsamic honey Dijon dressing

2 ounces pecans

2 ounces GreenFed raw cheddar cheese

¼ ounce sunflower sprouts

1½ sliced oranges

DIRECTIONS

In a large sauté pan with the oil, sauté all vegetables, the apples, and chicken (sliced ¼-inch thick) for 2-3 minutes. Add the dressing and continue to sauté one minute, tossing well. In a large salad bowl, place the romaine lettuce first, then the mixed field greens on top of the romaine lettuce.

Do not mix. Add the sautéed vegetables and chicken to the top of the lettuce.

Add cheese and pecans to the top of the vegetables. Place 1½ slices of orange cut in half on the side of the bowl.

Add sprouts.

Yield: 1 serving.

Recipe courtesy of R. Thomas Deluxe Grill in Atlanta, Georgia

BLENDED RAW SALAD

INGREDIENTS

1 cup spinach or lettuce leaves

1 cup sunflower sprouts (optional)

1 ripe avocado, peeled and pitted

1 ripe tomato, coarsely chopped

½ rep bell pepper, cored, seeded, and cut into 4 or 5 pieces (optional)

½ medium-size cucumber, cut into 3 or 4 pieces

1 stalk celery, cut into 3 or 4 pieces

juice of ½ lemon

1 teaspoon flaxseed oil or cold-pressed extra-virgin olive oil (optional)

DIRECTIONS

Combine all ingredients in a food processor or blender and process until smooth. For better digestion, try blending your salads instead of chewing them.

Makes 2-3 servings.

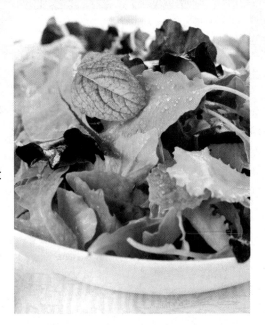

SALADS

EASY ORIENTAL SALMON SALAD
INGREDIENTS

2 salmon filets

5 cups mixed salad greens

1 cup fresh bean sprouts

1 cup fresh snow pea pods, trimmed

½ green bell pepper, thinly sliced

½ red bell pepper, thinly sliced

1 small or medium cucumber, thinly sliced

1 cup sliced green onions

3 tablespoons soy sauce

2 teaspoons grated fresh ginger

2 teaspoons sesame seeds, toasted

Oriental Salad Dressing (see recipe to the right)

Spicy Peanut Sauce (see recipe below and right)

DIRECTIONS

Combine soy sauce and ginger in a shallow baking dish. Add salmon. Cover and marinate in refrigerator up to 4 hours. Remove salmon from marinade and discard remaining marinade. Cook fish until lightly browned. Combine mixed salad greens and next 6 ingredients. Pour a half-cup Oriental Salad Dressing over salad and toss. Arrange cooked salmon and pour more salad dressing on top. Serve with Spicy Peanut Sauce.

Serves 4.

ORIENTAL SALAD DRESSING
INGREDIENTS

4 tablespoons rice vinegar

2 tablespoons soy sauce

2 teaspoons grated ginger

2 teaspoons toasted sesame oil

2 teaspoons finely chopped green onion or chives

2 cloves garlic, peeled and mashed

1 teaspoon raw honey

⅔ cup extra-virgin olive oil

2 teaspoons unrefined flax seed oil

DIRECTIONS

Place all ingredients in a jar and shake vigorously. Yield: one cup.

SPICY PEANUT SAUCE
INGREDIENTS

½ cup peanut butter

⅓ cup coconut milk

2 tablespoons soy sauce

1 tablespoon grated fresh ginger

1 tablespoon sesame oil

¼ teaspoon dried crushed red pepper

¼ cup chicken broth

DIRECTIONS

Combine all ingredients in a bowl and mix well. Yields 1 and ⅓ cups.

SALADS

PAUL'S POWERFUL RAW SALAD

INGREDIENTS

fresh spinach leaves
(as much as you like)

1 ripe avocado, peeled, pitted, and chopped

½ medium-size cucumber, chopped

½ red bell pepper, cored, seeded, and chopped (optional)

½ stalk celery, chopped

juice of 1 lemon

1-2 tablespoons ground flaxseeds

DIRECTIONS

Place spinach, avocado and cucumber, optional bell pepper, and celery in large bowl. Toss gently to combine. Sprinkle with lemon juice and flaxseeds. This salad is called "powerful" because every ingredient is a powerhouse of nutrients.

Makes 1 serving.

Recipe courtesy of Paul Nison, author of Raw Food: Formula for Health

RAINBOW SLAW

INGREDIENTS

¾ cup mayonnaise

⅛ cup yellow mustard

½ teaspoon cayenne pepper

¼ cup raw honey

½ teaspoon celery seed

2 tablespoons apple cider or coconut vinegar

sea salt and freshly ground black pepper

½ green cabbage

½ red cabbage

2 medium carrots, peeled

½ red onion

1 large unpeeled Granny Smith apple

DIRECTIONS

In a medium bowl, whisk together the mayonnaise, mustard, cayenne, honey, celery seed, apple cider vinegar, and salt and black pepper, to taste, until thoroughly combined. Chill until ready to use. Using a large holed grater attachment for a food processor, grate the cabbage, carrots, red onion, and apple. Remove to a large serving bowl and toss with the reserved dressing. Cover with plastic wrap and refrigerate for at least 2 hours.

Recipe courtesy of Cherie Calbom.

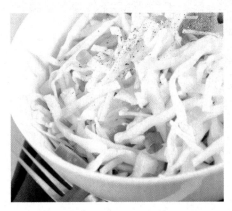

SMOOTHIES

PIÑA COLADA SMOOTHIE
INGREDIENTS

10 ounces of Amasai (plain)

1-2 organic eggs*
(optional; see note on page 198)

1 tablespoon extra virgin coconut oil

1 tablespoon flaxseed oil or hemp seed oil

1-2 tablespoons unheated honey

1 cup fresh or frozen pineapple

1 fresh or frozen banana

½ teaspoon vanilla extract

During my healing process, I consumed this smoothie one to two times per day with raw eggs. Contrary to popular belief, eggs from healthy free-range, pastured chickens are often free of dangerous germs. If the egg has an odor, obviously it should not be eaten. Since germs on the shell cause most of the salmonella infections, for added protection it is best to wash the eggs in the shell with a mild alcohol or hydrogen peroxide solution or a fruit and vegetable wash.

For those who can't stand the thought of consuming raw eggs in their smoothies, you can enjoy healthy smoothies without them, but you should know that the best-tasting ice creams are made with egg yolks.

DIRECTIONS

Combine the ingredients in a high-speed blender.

Yield: 2 8-ounce servings.

BANANA PEACH SMOOTHIE
INGREDIENTS

10 ounces Amasai (plain)

1-2 organic eggs (optional; see note on page 198)

1 tablespoon of extra virgin coconut oil

1 tablespoon flaxseed oil or hemp seed oil

1-2 tablespoons unheated honey

½-1 cup fresh or frozen peaches

1 fresh or frozen banana

½ teaspoon vanilla extract (optional)

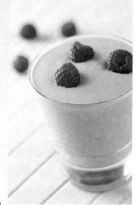

BERRY SMOOTHIE
INGREDIENTS

10 ounces of Amasai (plain)

1-2 organic eggs (optional; see note on page 198)

1 tablespoon flaxseed oil or hemp seed oil

1-2 tablespoons of raw honey

½-1 cup of fresh or frozen berries (blueberries, strawberries, raspberries, blackberries)

vanilla extract (optional)

DIRECTIONS

Combine all ingredients in a high-speed blender and blend until desired texture.

Serves 2.

SMOOTHIES

MOCHACCINO SMOOTHIE
INGREDIENTS

10 ounces Amasai (plain)

1–2 organic eggs (optional, see note on pg 198)

1 tablespoon extra virgin coconut oil

1 tablespoon flaxseed or hemp seed oil

1–2 tablespoons unheated honey

2 tablespoons cocoa or carob powder

1 tablespoon organic whole coffee beans

1–2 fresh or frozen bananas

1/2 teaspoon vanilla extract

DIRECTIONS

Combine the ingredients in a high–speed blender.
Serves 2.

CREAMSICLE SMOOTHIE
INGREDIENTS

8 ounces of Amasai (plain)

4 ounces freshly squeezed orange juice

1–2 organic eggs (optional, see note on pg 198)

1 tablespoon flaxseed oil or hemp seed oil

1–2 tablespoons unheated honey

1–2 fresh or frozen bananas

1/4 teaspoon vanilla extract

DIRECTIONS

Combine the following ingredients in a high–speed blender.
Serves 2.

CHERIE'S HAPPY MORNING SMOOTHIE
INGREDIENTS

1 cucumber, peeled

3-4 carrots, scrubbed, ends cut, tops removed

1 lemon

1-inch chunk ginger root

3-4 green leaves (kale, collards, chard)

1 avocado, cut in quarters

2-3 tablespoons ground almonds, flaxseeds, or chia seeds to sprinkle on top (optional)

DIRECTIONS

Juice the cucumber, carrots, lemon, ginger, and greens. Pour the juice in a blender and add avocado. Blend well until smooth. Sprinkle ground almonds or seeds on top, as desired.
Serves 2.

Adapted from The Juice Lady's Turbo Diet *by Cherie Calbom*

CURB YOUR CRAVINGS SMOOTHIE
INGREDIENTS

½ apple, juiced

½ cup spinach

1 celery stalk

1 tablespoon tahini

1 banana, peeled, cut in chunks and frozen

6 ice cubes

DIRECTIONS

Put all ingredients in a blender and process until smooth.
Serves 1.

Recipe courtesy of The Ultimate Smoothie Book *by Cherie Calbom*

SAUCES/DRESSINGS

AMASAI SAUCE WITH LIME-CILANTRO
INGREDIENTS

2 cups plain Amasai

1 cup cucumber, peeled and diced

1 cup fresh cilantro, chopped

2 tablespoons fresh lime juice

sea salt and freshly ground pepper, to taste

add a bit of water to thin to desired consistency for a dressing

DIRECTIONS

Blend all ingredients in processor using on/off turns until cucumber is well blended. Add a bit of water, if needed, for desired consistency for salad dressing. Season with salt and pepper and transfer to small bowl.

This sauce can be prepared 1 hour ahead; cover and chill.

Yield: 4 cups (about 12 servings)

Adapted from The Coconut Diet *by Cherie Calbom*

RAW PESTO
INGREDIENTS

2-4 cloves garlic

2 bunches spinach

1 bunch fresh basil

juice of ½ medium lemon

1 cup pine nuts

½ teaspoon sea salt

½ cup olive oil

DIRECTIONS

Place garlic into a food processor. Process until the garlic is well minced. Add all remaining ingredients and process until completely smooth. Serve as a dip or over pasta. Makes 4 servings.

Recipe courtesy of Paul Nison, author of Raw Food: Formula for Health

RAW TAHINI DRESSING
INGREDIENTS

½ cup raw tahini

juice of ½ medium-size lemon

1 clove garlic

pinch of cayenne

Nama Shoyu

DIRECTIONS

Combine tahini, lemon juice, garlic, and cayenne in a blender and process until completely smooth. With blender running, add water, 1-2 teaspoons at a time, until dressing is the consistency you desire. Season with Nama Shoyu, a raw, unpasteurized Japanese soy sauce, to taste. This delicious, all-purpose salad dressing can be used year round. Store covered in the refrigerator.

Makes 5 servings.

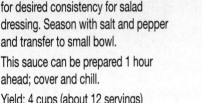

NEED RECIPES?

You'll find healthy and delicious recipes in the Appendix, "Beyond Organic Recipes." For additional recipes, please visit **LiveBeyondOrganic.com**

BEYOND ORGANIC FAN FAVORITES

Over the years, we have shared a lot of recipes with our fans. And we've also received a lot of feedback on what they like and what they don't like. The following section is a group of recipes that consistently "hit the mark" with our fans. Enjoy! And be sure to let us know what your favorite recipes are and even new recipes that you create.

Email us at recipes@livebeyondorganic.com.

SPAGHETTI WITH GREENFED MEAT SAUCE

INGREDIENTS

1 lb. GreenFed ground beef

2 14.5 ounces cans Italian-style diced tomatoes

1 8 ounces can tomato sauce

1 6 ounces can tomato paste

2 teaspoons extra virgin olive oil

1 teaspoon minced garlic

1 teaspoon dried oregano

1 teaspoon dried basil

½ teaspoon garlic powder

¼ teaspoon thyme

¼ teaspoon dried crushed red pepper

½ teaspoon salt or Herbamare or mixed spice blend to taste

½ large onion, chopped

1 cup button mushrooms, washed and quartered (optional)

1 tablespoon butter

1½ boxes of whole grain spelt spaghetti or angel hair pasta (whole wheat is a substitute for spelt)

parmesan cheese (optional)

DIRECTIONS

Combine the diced tomatoes, tomato sauce, tomato paste, olive oil, garlic, oregano, basil, garlic powder, thyme, dried red pepper, and salt in a medium- or large-sized pot and bring to a slight boil. Reduce to low heat.

In the meantime, sauté the onion and mushrooms in butter over medium heat until tender. Brown the beef in a large skillet, stirring until it crumbles. Drain the meat. Add the cooked meat, mushrooms, and onions to the sauce. Prepare 1 ½ boxes of spelt spaghetti or angel hair pasta according to the directions on the package. Adding a small amount of olive oil to the boiling water helps the pasta not to stick. Drain pasta. Top pasta with meat sauce and sprinkle with parmesan cheese.

Serves 6.

BEYOND ORGANIC FAN FAVORITES

JUICY ROSEMARY BAKED LAMB

INGREDIENTS

5-6 pounds boneless lamb leg, trimmed of excess fat

2 tablespoons dry rosemary leaves

1 tablespoon dry marjoram

2 tablespoons dry thyme leaves

4 large garlic cloves

½ cup Spanish onions, finely chopped

2 teaspoons ground cloves

1 teaspoon dry ground ginger

⅔ cup balsamic vinegar

⅓ cup organic cane sugar

1 teaspoon sea salt

1 cup mix nuts, finely chopped

DIRECTIONS

Make 1-inch cuts into meat, 3-4 inches apart; combine all diced and chopped herbs and spices. Stuff ½ teaspoon of seasoning mix into openings. Rub meat with remainder of seasoning mix. Marinate covered in refrigerator for 7 hours (preferably overnight).

Mirepoix (mixture of diced vegetables)

INGREDIENTS

1 large onion, rough chopped

4 stalks celery, rough chopped

3 large carrots, rough chopped

In shallow roasting pan, spread mirepoix. Place marinated lamb leg on mirepoix in preheated oven at 325 degrees. Bake for 2½ hrs., or until internal temperature is 155 degrees. During the last 15 minutes of cooking, apply chopped nuts over meat. Allow lamb to rest 15-20 minutes before slicing.

Yield is 12-15 servings.

Recipe courtesy of Sheila Barcelo of Eden's Wellness Lifestyle in Lakeland, Florida

CRANBERRY APPLE CRUNCH

INGREDIENTS

3 cooking apples (Granny Smith, etc.) peeled and cut into cubes

1 bag fresh or frozen cranberries

1 cup organic cane sugar

1 stick melted butter

extra-virgin coconut oil

⅓ cup honey

2¼ cups honey oats

1½ cups chopped walnuts

DIRECTIONS

Mix apples, cranberries, and organic sugar and place in casserole dish greased with extra-virgin coconut oil. Mix melted butter, honey oats, and chopped walnuts and pour over apples and cranberries. Bake in a covered dish for 1 hour at 350 degrees.

Serves 6-8.

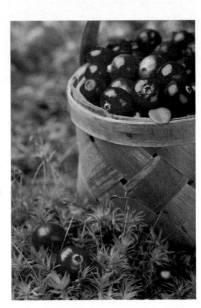

BEYOND ORGANIC FAN FAVORITES

TROPICAL CHICKEN AND VEGETABLE KABOBS

INGREDIENTS

2 pounds boneless skinless chicken breast, cut into bite-size pieces

2 cups red and green bell peppers, cut into 1-inch squares

1 cup cherry tomatoes

2 cups pineapples, bite-size chunks

MARINADE INGREDIENTS FOR FRUITS AND VEGGIES:

½ cup chicken stock

½ cup pineapple juice

2 tablespoons lemon juice

2 tablespoons extra virgin olive oil

1 tablespoon honey

GARNISH:

2 tablespoons lemon zest

SEASONING FOR CHICKEN:

2 tablespoons paprika

1 tablespoon minced garlic

$\frac{1}{8}$ teaspoon onion flakes or powder

1 teaspoon Herbamare or mixed spice blend

2 tablespoons apple cider vinegar

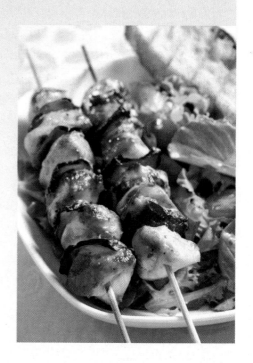

DIRECTIONS

Combine vinegar, herbs, and spices with chicken and marinate for minimum of 2 hours. Combine all juices, chicken stock, and honey, and marinate veggies and fruit. Stir-fry chicken for 20 minutes until almost done, then cool until comfortable to skewer.

Remove veggies and fruit from marinate, skewer with chicken, pineapple, red and green peppers together, with chicken and tomato at the end. Finish under broiler, lower rack, or on grill for 5 minutes, turning once.

Serves 2 people with 4-6 kabobs.

Recipe courtesy of Sheila Barcelo of
Eden's Wellness Lifestyle in Lakeland, Florida

BEYOND ORGANIC FAN FAVORITES

SWEET POTATO PIE

INGREDIENTS

4 cups mashed sweet potatoes
(4 medium sweet potatoes)

1 teaspoon vanilla

2 well-beaten eggs

½ stick melted butter

½ cup organic sugar

¼ cup honey

1 teaspoon extra virgin coconut
oil to grease pan

DIRECTIONS

Boil potatoes with skins on for 25-30 minutes, or until tender. Remove from pot, let cool and peel. Mix all ingredients with a fork, and pour into greased 9x13 baking dish.

TOPPING INGREDIENTS

1 cup chopped pecans

½ cup spelt or kamut flour

½ cup organic sugar

¼ cup honey

¾ stick butter, melted

DIRECTIONS

Combine ingredients and sprinkle over potato mixture. Bake 30 minutes at 350 degrees.

Yield: 8 servings.

RAW MUSHROOM PIZZA

INGREDIENTS

1 large Portobello mushroom

1 lemon

¼ cup raw tahini or almond butter

1 ripe tomato, thinly sliced

¼ ripe avocado, peeled, pitted and thinly sliced (optional)

DIRECTIONS

Remove and discard stem of the mushroom and clean the mushroom cap. Turn cap upside down and place on a serving plate. Squeeze the lemon juice over it, then pour on the tahini. Top with the tomato and optional avocado. Makes 1 serving.

Recipe courtesy of Paul Nison, author of Raw Food: Formula for Health

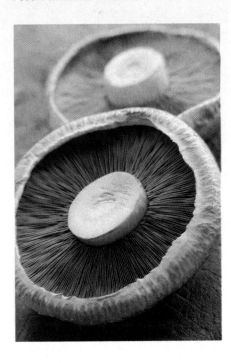

BEYOND ORGANIC FAN FAVORITES

RAW CAULIFLOWER "MASHED POTATOES" WITH MUSHROOM GRAVY

INGREDIENTS

cauliflower florets

½ cup pine nuts

½ cup fresh thyme leaves

¼ cup freshly squeezed lemon juice

2 cloves garlic

sea salt

olive oil

DIRECTIONS

Combine all ingredients in a food processor, adding salt and olive oil to taste. Process until mixture is consistency of mashed potatoes. Add a small amount of water, if necessary, to facilitate processing and achieve the desired consistency.

Makes 5 servings.

Recipe courtesy of Paul Nison, author of Raw Food: Formula for Health

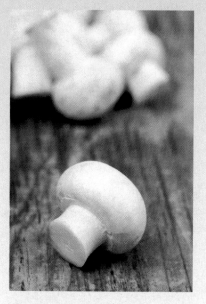

RAW MUSHROOM GRAVY

INGREDIENTS

4 Portobello mushrooms

1 jar (8 ounces) raw almond butter

1 cup water

2 ripe plum tomatoes, coarsely chopped

1 medium-size red onion, coarsely chopped

2 cloves garlic, coarsely chopped

sea salt

DIRECTIONS

Remove and discard the stems of the mushroom. Clean and coarsely chop the cups. Transfer to food processor along with all of the remaining ingredients, adding salt to taste. Process until completely smooth. Serve this over the Cauliflower "Mashed Potatoes."

Makes 8-12 servings.

Recipe courtesy of Paul Nison, author of Raw Food: Formula for Health

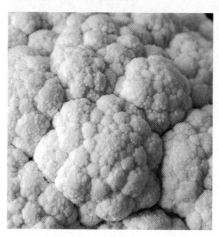

BEYOND ORGANIC FAN FAVORITES

SWISS ALMOND SMOOTHIE

INGREDIENTS

10 ounces Amasai (plain)

1-2 organic eggs

1 tablespoons extra virgin coconut oil

1 tablespoon flaxseed oil or hemp seed oil

1-2 tablespoons unheated honey

2 tablespoons cocoa or carob powder

2 tablespoons almond butter

1-2 fresh or frozen bananas

½ teaspoon vanilla extract

DIRECTIONS:

Combine the listed ingredients in
a high-speed blender.

Yield: 2 8-ounce servings.

TUNA MELT

INGREDIENTS

2 cans tuna—albacore is best; salmon
is another variation

4 Tablespoons mayonnaise

4 Tablespoons garlic-chili flaxseed oil

1 small red onion, finely chopped

1 celery stalk, finely chopped

½ red pepper, finely chopped

Herbamare® to taste

sprouted grain English muffins

2-4 ounces cheddar cheese

DIRECTIONS

Mix all ingredients in a medium-sized bowl. Toast English muffin halves. Spread tuna
mixture over English muffin halves. Top with cheddar cheese slices. Bake at 400 degrees
until cheese is melted.

Serves 4

Recipe courtesy of Jordan Rubin

ALL-DAY BEEF STEW

INGREDIENTS

3 pounds stew beef, cut into 1-inch pieces

1 cup red wine

3-4 cups beef stock

4 tomatoes, peeled, seeded, and chopped
or 1 can tomatoes

2 tablespoons tomato puree

½ teaspoon black peppercorns

several sprigs fresh thyme, tied together

2 cloves garlic, peeled and crushed

2-3 small pieces orange peel

8 small red potatoes

1 pound carrots, peeled and cut into sticks

Celtic sea salt and freshly ground pepper

DIRECTIONS

Marinate meat in red wine overnight.
(This step is optional.) Place all ingredients
except for potatoes and carrots in an
oven-proof casserole and cook at 250
degrees for 12 hours. Add carrots and
potatoes during the last hour. Season to
taste.

Serves 6-8

Sally Fallon, author of Nourishing Traditions

BEYOND ORGANIC FAN FAVORITES

PUMPKIN DELIGHT

INGREDIENTS

4 cups canned organic pumpkin

2 tablespoons ground cinnamon

¼ teaspoon allspice

¼ teaspoon nutmeg

1 teaspoon vanilla

2 well-beaten organically raised eggs

½ stick melted butter

½ cup rapadura sweetener

¼ cup honey

1 teaspoon coconut oil to grease pan

DIRECTIONS

Mix all ingredients with a fork and pour into greased 9x13 baking dish. Make topping.

TOPPING INGREDIENTS

1 cup chopped pecans

½ cup spelt or kamut flour

½ cup rapadura sweetener

¼ cup honey

¾ stick butter, melted

DIRECTIONS

Combine ingredients and sprinkle over pumpkin mixture. Bake 30 minutes at 350 degrees.

Serves 8

*Recipe courtesy of
Extraordinary Health Team*

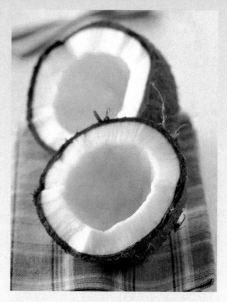

COCONUT BREAKFAST MIX

INGREDIENTS

2 cups of fresh coconut, cut into thin ribbons or flaked

2 cups of organic Granny Smith apples, diced

4 cups of organic dates, chopped

$\frac{1}{3}$ cup of chia seeds

½ cup of cacao nibs

¼ cup of pumpkin seeds

4 tablespoons cinnamon

DIRECTIONS

Place the $\frac{1}{3}$ cup of chia seeds in one cup of water and let stand for 10 minutes. In the meantime, mix all the other ingredients together in a mixing bowl. When chia seeds have set for 10 minutes, drain any remaining water and add to the mix. Stir mixture. Cover with whole organic milk or whole probiotic-rich yogurt and serve.

Serves 6

Recipe courtesy of Extraordinary Health Team

BEYOND ORGANIC FAN FAVORITES

CREAMY COCONUT PIE
CRUST INGREDIENTS

3 cups of fresh coconut, grated or flaked

¾ cup of dates, finely chopped

1 teaspoon organic vanilla extract

2 tablespoons extra virgin coconut oil

DIRECTIONS

Place all ingredients (except the dates) into a food processor with the S-blade on. Slowly add the dates until the crust begins to stick together. When done, press the crust into a coconut oil greased 9-inch glass pie pan.

FILLING INGREDIENTS

3 cups young coconut meat

1 cup young coconut water

½ cup of extra virgin coconut oil

1 teaspoon organic vanilla extract

¼ cup of raw honey

DIRECTIONS

Add all ingredients into a blender and blend until smooth. Pour mixture into the pie crust and let set in the refrigerator for about two hours. Serve.

Serves 8

Recipe courtesy of Extraordinary Health Team

DARK CHOCOLATE-COVERED STRAWBERRIES
INGREDIENTS

16 ounces of organic dark chocolate, squares or morsels (at least 60% cocoa preferred)

2 pounds of large, organic strawberries—washed and allowed to dry

DIRECTIONS

Lay out enough parchment paper to hold dipped strawberries. Fill a large saucepan with about an inch of water and simmer. Turn off the heat. Put the chocolate in a bowl and then place the bowl in the hot water until the chocolate is melted. Stir the chocolate until it is smooth. Remove from heat once it is melted and smooth.

Working quickly, hold each strawberry by its stem and dip it into the dark chocolate. Lift and slightly twist the strawberry over the bowl, allowing any excess chocolate to drip. Set dipped strawberries on the parchment paper and allow to set for about 45 minutes. Chill. Serve.

Makes 24-36

Recipe courtesy of Extraordinary Health Team

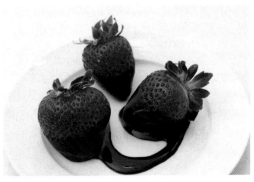

BEYOND ORGANIC FAN FAVORITES

CHOCOLATE CHEESECAKE

CRUST INGREDIENTS

6 dark chocolate squares, melted (at least 60% cocoa)

2 cups of organic pecans

1/3 cup of fresh dates

DIRECTIONS

Fill a small saucepan with about an inch of water and simmer. Turn off the heat. Put the chocolate in a bowl and then place the bowl in the hot water until the chocolate is melted. Stir the chocolate until it is smooth. Remove from heat once it is melted and smooth. Process the pecans and dates in a food processor—adding chocolate when blended. Press mixture into a coconut oil-greased pie plate or into a springform pan.

CHEESECAKE INGREDIENTS

4 cups of organic cashews, soaked

1 cup of rapadura

1 cup of cocoa butter (or coconut oil)

8 dark chocolate squares, melted (at least 60% cocoa)

½ cup of pure water

2 teaspoons of vanilla

DIRECTIONS

Fill a small saucepan with about an inch of water and simmer. Turn off the heat. Put the chocolate in a bowl and then place the bowl in the hot water until the chocolate is melted. Stir the chocolate until it is smooth. Remove from heat once melted and smooth. Process the remaining ingredients in a food processor—adding the water slowly and the chocolate when blended. Pour mixture onto the crust. Place in freezer to set up. Serve.

Serves 8

Recipe courtesy of Extraordinary Health Team

TANTALIZING TRUFFLES

Makes about 2 dozen

INGREDIENTS

3 cups of dates, processed into a paste

2 cups of tahini

2 cups of organic cocoa powder, reserving a small amount to roll mixture in

2/3 cup of raw honey

DIRECTIONS

In a large mixing bowl, mix together all the ingredients. Roll the mixture into about two dozen small, ball-shaped servings. Roll truffles into the reserved cocoa powder and place on parchment paper. Chill for about an hour. Serve.

Makes about 2 dozen

Recipe courtesy of Extraordinary Health Team

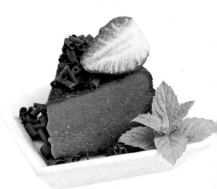

BEYOND ORGANIC FAN FAVORITES

FAMILY ROAST BEEF

INGREDIENTS

4 to 5 pound chuck roast (or pot roast), from grassfed beef

¼ pound butter

½ cup Worcestershire sauce

Celtic sea salt

black pepper, freshly ground

DIRECTIONS

Preheat oven to 325 degrees. Rub the roast with salt and pepper and place in a baking dish with 2-inch sides. In a saucepan, melt the butter and add an equal volume of Worcestershire sauce. Pour the sauce over the roast. Bake slowly at 325 degrees until a meat thermometer reads 150-155 degrees (for medium). Remove the roast from the oven and allow it to rest and redistribute the juices before carving. The temperature will climb to 180 degrees.

Note: Grassfed beef should be cooked more slowly at a lower temperature than commercial beef. Grassfed beef should also be allowed to "coast in" to the desired level of doneness by removing it from the oven several minutes before you think it is done. This preserves the juiciness and produces meat that is more tender.

Serves 4-6

Recipe courtesy of Keith Tindall from White Egret Farm

GRILLED MARINATED CHICKEN

INGREDIENTS

1¼ cups extra virgin olive oil

⅓ cup fresh parsley, chopped

3 tablespoons lime juice

3 tablespoons hot pepper sauce

1 small tomato, diced

1 teaspoon sea salt

1 teaspoon black pepper, ground

2 cloves of garlic, minced

1 tablespoon dried oregano

6 boneless chicken breasts (organic)

DIRECTIONS

Mix together all of the ingredients listed above—except for the chicken. Line chicken breasts in a long, shallow glass pan; pour marinade over the chicken and let marinate in the refrigerator for at least two hours. When ready to cook, preheat the grill on medium heat. Place chicken on the grill and cook for 20 minutes or until cooked all the way through. Serve.

Serves 6

Recipe courtesy of Extraordinary Health Team

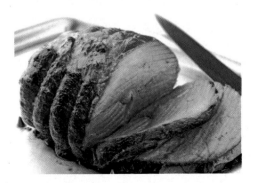

BEYOND ORGANIC FAN FAVORITES

SALMON PASTA SALAD

INGREDIENTS

1 large can of salmon, with bones

1 12-ounce package of whole-grain pasta

2 cups finely chopped red or green bell peppers

½ cup chopped onion

2 cups cooked whole-kernel corn

1 Tablespoon basil

sea salt and pepper to taste

1 cup mayonnaise

1 cup whole fat plain organic yogurt

1 large bag of spinach leaves (washed)

grated Swiss cheese

sliced almonds

DIRECTIONS

Cook pasta; drain, cool and set aside.
Drain canned salmon and break it into chunks.
Place in a large bowl. Add cooled pasta, cooked corn, peppers, onion, basil, sea salt and pepper. Mix gently, but well. Blend together mayonnaise and whole fat plain yogurt. Fold mixture into the other salad ingredients.

Line salad plates with washed spinach leaves and then spoon out the salmon pasta salad over the spinach leaves. Sprinkle with grated Swiss cheese and sliced almonds. Serve.

Serves 4-6

Recipe courtesy of Extraordinary Health Team

BLACK BEAN SALAD

INGREDIENTS

2 cups of freshly cooked black beans

½ cup of chopped green onions

2 avocados, peeled, seeded and chunked

¼ cup of fresh basil, chopped

2 fully ripened large tomatoes, chopped

2 cups frozen corn, thawed and drained

¼ cup fresh cilantro, chopped

1 lime, juiced

1 tablespoon extra virgin olive oil

sea salt, to taste

pepper, to taste

grated mozzarella cheese

DIRECTIONS

Drain the freshly cooked black beans; set aside and cool. After the beans have cooled, use a large bowl and combine the black beans, green onions, avocados, basil, tomatoes, corn, cilantro, juice of one lime, olive oil, sea salt, and pepper.

Chill. Top with grated mozzarella cheese. Serve.

Serves 4-6

*Recipe courtesy of
Extraordinary Health Team*

BEYOND ORGANIC FAN FAVORITES

GRILLED CHICKEN SALAD WITH SAVORY STRAWBERRY DRESSING

INGREDIENTS

One pound of organic, boneless, skinless chicken breasts; grilled and sliced

10 cups of arugula

10 ounces of snow peas, stemmed

8 ounces of goat cheese

½ cup of sliced pecans

1 quart of fresh strawberries, sliced

SAVORY STRAWBERRY DRESSING INGREDIENTS

1 cup of fresh strawberries

1 tablespoon of apple cider vinegar

1 teaspoon ground black pepper

¼ teaspoon sea salt

1 teaspoon raw honey

1 tablespoon almond oil

DIRECTIONS

Grill the chicken; let cool slightly and slice. Set aside. Combine arugula, snow peas, goat cheese, pecans and strawberries—adding the pecans and strawberries to top the salad. In a blender, blend together the ingredients for the dressing until at desired consistency. Pour dressing on salad and serve.

Serves 5

Recipe courtesy of Extraordinary Health Team

RASPBERRY-ALMOND SALAD

INGREDIENTS

10 cups organic spring salad mix

1 medium avocado, sliced

1 small red onion, thinly sliced

2 cups fresh raspberries

⅓ cup sliced raw almonds

healthy salad dressing of your choice—i.e. raspberry walnut or extra virgin olive oil & apple cider vinegar mixture

DIRECTIONS

In a large serving bowl, combine the spring salad mix, the sliced avocado, red onions slices, raspberries and almonds—with almonds going on last. Serve with your choice of healthy salad dressing.

Serves 5

Recipe courtesy of Extraordinary Health Team

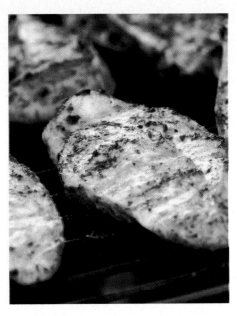

BEYOND ORGANIC FAN FAVORITES

ESPRESSO-CHOCOLATE DESSERT

INGREDIENTS

12 ounces of organic dark chocolate bar, ground up in a blender or broken into small pieces

¼ cup of fresh espresso, still warm

2 tablespoons organic vanilla

2 tablespoons organic ground cinnamon

¼ cup of unsweetened cocoa baking powder

¼ cup of raw honey

¼ cup of powdered stevia

2 sticks of organic butter (at room temperature)

6 free-range organic eggs, room temperature

DIRECTIONS

Preheat oven to 350 degrees and coat a springform pan with butter or extra virgin coconut oil. In a large mixing bowl, mix together all the ingredients, adding the espresso last. Place the mixture in the coated springform pan and place in the oven. Bake for 50 minutes or until the middle is done and an inserted toothpick comes out clean. Remove from the oven; cool. Serve.

Serves 4-6

Recipes courtesy of Extraordinary Health Team

BERRY TRIO DESSERT

INGREDIENTS

2 cups fresh blueberries

2 cups fresh blackberries

2 cups fresh raspberries

5 tablespoons stevia

3 cups steel-cut oats

2 cups whole grain flour

3 tablespoons ground cinnamon

1 teaspoon ground nutmeg

1 cup of organic butter

DIRECTIONS

Preheat oven to 350 degrees. In a large bowl, mix together the blueberries, blackberries, raspberries and 1 Tablespoon of the stevia. In a separate large bowl, combine the rest of the stevia, the steel-cut oats, whole grain flour, cinnamon and nutmeg—and then cut in the butter until the mixture is crumbly. Press half of the oats & flour mixture into the bottom of a buttered 9 x 13 inch pan. Pour the berry mixture on top and then sprinkle the remaining half of the oats & flour mixture over the berries. Bake at 350 degrees for 35-45 minutes or until the fruit bubbles and the topping is golden-brown. Serve warm—with or without organic ice cream.

Serves 10-15

Recipe courtesy of Extraordinary Health Team

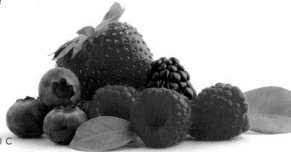

BEYOND ORGANIC FAN FAVORITES

CURRIED LENTILS & RICE BAKE
INGREDIENTS

2 tablespoons butter

6 cups filtered water

1½ cups brown basmati rice

1½ cups dry, brown lentils

3 garlic cloves, diced

1 teaspoon sea salt

1 teaspoon fresh, crushed ginger

2 tablespoons (gluten-free) curry powder or red curry paste

DIRECTIONS

Preheat oven to 350 degrees. In a large pot, melt 2 tablespoons butter. Add rice and curry powder or red curry paste and cook until lightly toasted—about one minute or so. Add water, lentils, garlic, salt and ginger. Bring to a boil. Cover, turn off heat and let stand for about 10 minutes. Use the other 1 tablespoon of butter to butter a large baking dish and set aside. After 10 minutes, place mixture into the large, buttered baking dish with lid. Bake at 350 degrees for about an hour or until rice and lentils are tender. Fluff and serve.

Serves 6

Recipe courtesy of Extraordinary Health Team

BEEF CEVAPCICI
INGREDIENTS

2 pounds GreenFed ground beef

1 egg, slightly beaten (free-range, organic)

4 tablespoons beef broth

1 teaspoon sea salt

¼ teaspoon freshly ground pepper

1 garlic clove, crushed

1 teaspoon paprika

1 tablespoon marjoram

½ teaspoon Tabasco sauce

DIRECTIONS

In a large mixing bowl, combine all ingredients and mix together thoroughly. Next, form the beef mixture into sausages about 1 inch thick and 4 inches long. Cook slowly until well-cooked on a grill or under a broiler, turning often to make sure they're cooked through. Serve.

Serves 6-8.

Recipe courtesy of Extraordinary Health Team

GREENFED MEATLOAF
INGREDIENTS

2 pounds of GreenFed ground beef

2 eggs, slightly beaten (free-range, organic)

4 tablespoons flaxseeds, ground

¼ cup raw walnuts, ground

⅓ cup of organic catsup or barbecue sauce

1 cup of flaxseed bread crumbs

¼ cup of organic whole milk

sea salt and pepper, to taste

pinch of garlic

DIRECTIONS

In a large mixing bowl, mix all the ingredients together. Pour into a loaf pan or a casserole dish. Bake at 350 degrees Fahrenheit for about an hour. Serve.

Serves 6-8

Recipe courtesy of Extraordinary Health Team

BEYOND ORGANIC FAN FAVORITES

CAJUN-STYLE SALMON

INGREDIENTS

4 6-ounce wild Alaskan salmon fillets

1/3 cup of cultured butter

2 garlic cloves, minced

2 tablespoons Cajun blackened seasoning

1 teaspoon Tabasco sauce

1 teaspoon oregano

2 teaspoons pepper

1 tablespoon chili powder

1/2 cup lemon juice

1/4 cup of Worcestershire sauce

2 lemons, sliced in half

DIRECTIONS

In a large skillet, melt butter over medium-high heat. Stir in the garlic and Cajun seasoning and cook for about 2 minutes, stirring constantly. Remove from heat and set aside on the stovetop. In a medium bowl, mix together the remaining ingredients, except for the lemon slices. When mixed, pour into the skillet with the Cajun and garlic mixture. Cook for 3 minutes, stirring continuously. Add salmon fillets and cook for 10 minutes per inch of fish thickness (measured at the thickest part) or until fish just flakes when tested with a fork. Squeeze lemon juice from sliced lemons over the salmon and serve immediately.

Serves 4

Recipe courtesy of
Extraordinary Health Team

MANGO-TUNA SALAD

INGREDIENTS

4 6-ounce wild tuna steaks

extra virgin coconut oil

1 large mango, pitted, peeled and cut into 1/4-inch strips

1/2 cup of red onion, thinly sliced

1 red bell pepper, thinly sliced

4 Tablespoons fresh cilantro, chopped

2 Tablespoons raw apple cider vinegar

2 Tablespoons extra virgin olive oil

1 Tablespoon flaxseed oil

sea salt and freshly ground pepper, to taste

DIRECTIONS

Mix the mango, red onion, red bell pepper, cilantro, vinegar, olive oil and flaxseed oil in a large bowl. Sprinkle with sea salt and pepper, to taste. Melt the coconut oil and brush the tuna with the coconut oil and broil until the fish is opaque in color or about 4 minutes per side. Divide the mango salad on 4 salad plates. Top with tuna when it's finished cooking. Serve.

Serves 4

Recipe courtesy of
Extraordinary Health Team

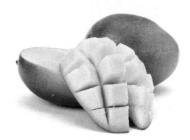

BEYOND ORGANIC FAN FAVORITES

STRAWBERRIES & FLAXSEED SHORTCAKE

INGREDIENTS

12 cups fresh organic strawberries, rinsed and sliced

²/₃ cup rapadura

4 cups flaxseed flour

¼ cup flaxseeds, ground

½ cup rapadura

1 tablespoon baking powder

1 teaspoon sea salt

2 cups organic, cultured butter

4 eggs, beaten (free-range, organic)

3 cups whole organic milk

DIRECTIONS

In a large mixing bowl, stir together the strawberries and rapadura and set in the refrigerator. Mix together the flaxseed flour, ground flaxseeds, rapadura, baking powder and sea salt. Cut in the butter until the mixture is coarse and crumbly. Combine the eggs and milk and slowly add to the dry ingredients until it is moist. Spread the shortbread mixture into a large baking pan (12 x 16) or two smaller baking pans and bake at 425 degrees Fahrenheit for about 30 minutes. Cool. Slice shortcake and top with strawberry mixture. Top with whipped cream, if desired.

Serves 10-12

Recipe courtesy of Extraordinary Health Team

ZUCCHINI, WALNUT & FLAX BREAD

INGREDIENTS

1½ cups of flaxseed flour

1 tablespoon flaxseeds, ground

1 teaspoon baking powder

¼ teaspoon sea salt

¼ teaspoon baking soda

1 teaspoon cinnamon, ground

¼ teaspoon nutmeg, ground

2 eggs (free-range, organic)

1 cup rapadura

½ cup unsweetened organic applesauce

3 tablespoons extra virgin coconut oil

1 cup grated zucchini

2 tablespoons chopped walnuts

DIRECTIONS

Preheat the oven to 350 degrees Fahrenheit. Coat 2 mini 6 x 3 inch loaf pans with 1 Tablespoon of coconut oil. Mix the flaxseed flour, flaxseeds, baking powder, baking soda, salt, cinnamon and nutmeg together in a large mixing bowl. Mix the eggs, rapadura, applesauce, and 2 Tablespoons coconut oil. Once mixed, then slowly add the grated zucchini. Add the entire zucchini mixture to the dry ingredients—slowly, so that it mixes well. Fold in the walnuts, then fold the batter in the prepared loaf pans. Bake at 350 degrees for about 45 minutes or until an inserted toothpick comes out clean. Cool and then serve.

Serves 12-14

Recipe courtesy of Extraordinary Health Team

BEYOND ORGANIC FAN FAVORITES

MEDITERRANEAN VEGGIE & CHEESE SALAD

INGREDIENTS

3 fresh cucumbers, diced

3 fresh red tomatoes, diced

1 container of kalamata olives

1 small onion, diced

½ cup raw feta cheese

3 ounces organic extra virgin olive oil

sea salt & pepper, to taste

raw apple cider vinegar, to taste

4 tablespoons probiotic-rich yogurt

DIRECTIONS

In a large salad bowl, toss all the ingredients together and serve.

Serves 2-4

Recipe courtesy of
Extraordinary Health Team

YOGURT & AVOCADO DIP

INGREDIENTS

4 ripe avocados, peeled and chopped

1 cup of organic, plain, whole fat probiotic-rich yogurt

4 Tablespoons fresh cilantro, chopped

2 Tablespoons ground cumin

½ teaspoon Celtic sea salt

1 garlic clove, minced

½ cup finely chopped onion

3 tablespoons fresh lime juice

DIRECTIONS

Place all the ingredients in a food processor or blender and process until smooth. Serve with sprouted tortillas, pita or chips.

Serves 8

Recipe courtesy of
Extraordinary Health Team

HEALTHY YOGURT HUMMUS

INGREDIENTS

2 pounds of garbanzo beans

2 cloves of garlic

1 cup of probiotic-rich plain yogurt or sour cream

½ cup raw tahini

1 teaspoon Celtic sea salt

2 teaspoons Tabasco sauce

1 teaspoon fresh ground pepper

¾ cup flat leaf parsley

DIRECTIONS

Place the garlic and parsley in a food processor and chop until finely diced; then add remaining ingredients and process until smooth. Serve with fresh vegetables or sprouted pita or tortillas.

Serves 8

Recipe courtesy of
Extraordinary Health Team

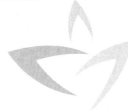

BEYOND ORGANIC FAN FAVORITES

PROBIOTIC FRUIT DIP

INGREDIENTS

2 cups of probiotic-rich plain yogurt

½ cup raw honey

¾ cup raw tahini

DIRECTIONS

Combine all ingredients, mixing until smooth. Serve with apples, strawberries or bananas.

Makes about 3 cups

Recipe courtesy of Extraordinary Health Team

ENZYME-RICH FRUIT TREATS

INGREDIENTS

1 cup dried figs

1 cup dates

1 cup raisins

raw walnuts, crushed

shredded coconut

DIRECTIONS

Mash together the figs, dates and raisins. Form mixture into 12 small bars. Coat with crushed raw walnuts and shredded coconut.

Makes about 12 bars

Recipe courtesy of Extraordinary Health Team

QUICK SPROUTED APPLE CRISP

INGREDIENTS

4 medium baking apples

1 ounce purified water

⅔ cup sprouted cereal (like Ezekiel 4:9 brand)

1 tablespoon butter

2 tablespoons raw honey, separated

DIRECTIONS

Preheat oven to 375 degrees. Peel, core, and chop the apples. Place apples in medium-sized pot with water and butter. Cover and cook on medium heat for 15 minutes or until apples can be mashed with a fork to the consistency of apple sauce. Stir in 1 Tablespoon of honey. Pour mixture into a medium-sized baking dish.

Pour cereal evenly over apple mixture and press down with a fork. Drizzle with remaining 1 Tablespoon of honey. Bake for 15 minutes. Remove from heat, let cool, and serve.

Serves 4

Recipe courtesy of Nicki Rubin

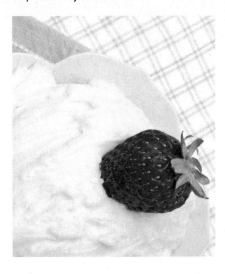

BEYOND ORGANIC FAN FAVORITES

SEASONAL PUMPKIN BREAD
INGREDIENTS

3 cups of freshly ground spelt flour

1½ cups of mashed pumpkin or sweet potatoes

1 cup of water

3 tablespoons of kefir, probiotic-rich yogurt, or raw apple cider vinegar

¾ cup of extra virgin coconut oil

3 omega-3 eggs

1 teaspoon of ground cinnamon

1 teaspoon ground cloves

¾ teaspoon of sea salt

1 teaspoon of baking soda

½ teaspoon of baking powder

1 cup of raisins

1 cup crispy nuts (chopped)

DIRECTIONS

Mix together the flour, mashed pumpkin or sweet potatoes, water and kefir in a large bowl. Cover the bowl and let the mixture sit at room temperature for at least 8 hours.

When you're ready to bake the pumpkin bread, preheat the oven to 350 degrees Fahrenheit. Grease two loaf pans with coconut oil. Uncover the pumpkin mixture and add the remaining ingredients—except for the raisins and nuts—and mix well. When mixed, then add the raisins and nuts.

Pour the batter into to the two loaf pans and then bake them for 45 minutes until golden brown. Cool for about 30 minutes. Serve warm.

Serves 10-12

Recipe courtesy of Extraordinary Health Team

SALMON WRAPPED IN GRAPE LEAVES
INGREDIENTS

1 pound of cooked wild salmon fillets; cooled and chunked

2 tablespoons whole milk plain yogurt

1 teaspoon lemon juice

½ teaspoon sea salt

¼ teaspoon cayenne pepper

chopped fresh chive and dill

10 grape leaves in brine

DIRECTIONS

In a large bowl, mix all ingredients (except the grape leaves), adding the cooked wild salmon chunks last. Pat dry the grape leaves with a paper towel. Wrap one-fifth of the salmon mixture in 2 overlapping grape leaves; repeat this procedure until all the salmon mixture is gone and all the grape leaves are filled.

You can serve them chilled or heated by baking them at 450 degrees for 10 minutes prior to serving. For variety, you can top with a sauce made of whole milk plain yogurt mixed with diced cucumbers with a dash of garlic powder.

Serves 5

Recipe courtesy of Extraordinary Health Team

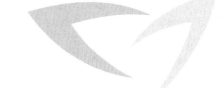

BEYOND ORGANIC FAN FAVORITES

FRESH TZATZIKI

INGREDIENTS

3 cups of fresh whole milk plain yogurt

2 fresh organic cucumbers; peeled, seeded and finely grated

1/3 cup of organic extra virgin olive oil

4 fresh, mashed garlic cloves

2 tablespoons lemon juice

Fresh basil, thyme, turmeric and dill to taste

Dash of sea salt

DIRECTIONS

Placed finely grated cucumbers in a strainer and let drip for about 10 minutes. Combine the rest of the ingredients in a mixing bowl and mix well, adding the fresh herbs and sea salt last. Add drained cucumbers. Mix well. Cover and refrigerate for at least 30 minutes prior to serving so that flavors are accentuated.

Serves 6

*Recipe courtesy of
Extraordinary Health Team*

CURRIED CARROT SOUP

INGREDIENTS

4 tablespoons coconut oil, melted

6 cups of chicken broth

5 cups of peeled carrots, thinly sliced into rounds

2 cups fresh chopped onions

2 teaspoons curry powder

1 tablespoon fresh ginger, minced

1 teaspoon coriander seeds, powdered

¾ teaspoon yellow mustard seeds, powdered

2 teaspoons lime peel, finely grated

3 teaspoons fresh lime juice

sea salt and fresh ground pepper to taste

plain whole milk yogurt (for garnish)

DIRECTIONS

Melt coconut oil over medium heat in a large soup pot. Add ground coriander and mustard seeds, curry and ginger. Stir one minute. Sprinkle with sea salt and ground pepper. Add onions and sauté them until they slightly soften. Add 6 cups chicken broth and sliced carrots and cook on medium-low heat for about 30 minutes or until carrots are tender. Cool. Working in batches, puree in blender until smooth and return the soup to the pot. Stir in lime juice and season with more sea salt and ground pepper to taste. Ladle soup into bowls and garnish with yogurt. Serve.

Serves 6-8

Recipe courtesy of Extraordinary Health Team

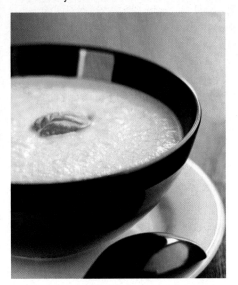

BEYOND ORGANIC FAN FAVORITES

ROASTED VEGGIE SOUP

INGREDIENTS

4 stalks of coarsely chopped celery

4 large carrots, coarsely chopped

2 medium onions, coarsely chopped

2 tablespoons extra virgin olive oil

8 garlic cloves, chopped

5 cups filtered water

½ cup porcini mushroom pieces

1 teaspoon turmeric

Sea salt and red pepper to taste

DIRECTIONS

Preheat oven to 500 degrees. Coat the carrots, celery and onion with the olive oil and then place on a small nonstick pan and bake for 10 minutes. Remove pan from the oven and add garlic; mix well and bake for another 10 minutes. Remove pan from the oven and add a little water to loosen the vegetables from the baking pan. Pour this mixture and the rest of the ingredients into a large soup pot and simmer for about 30 minutes. Serve.

Serves 4

Recipe courtesy of Extraordinary Health Team

ROASTED RED PEPPER AND SWEET POTATO SOUP

INGREDIENTS

4 red peppers, roughly chopped with seeds and stems removed

3 tablespoons olive oil

4 sweet potatoes, peeled and roughly chopped

1 onion, medium, diced

2 garlic cloves, chopped

3 thyme sprigs

6 cups veggie or chicken stock

½ cup heavy cream

DIRECTIONS

Preheat oven to 450 degrees. Drizzle 1 tablespoon of olive oil on peppers, rub to coat, and place skin side up on baking sheet, and place in oven. Roast until the skins turn black, 20 – 25 minutes. Remove from oven and using tongs or a fork, transfer the peppers to a plastic bag and seal. Let stand for 15 minutes, and then peel the black skins off the pepper.

In a large pot, heat 2 tablespoons of olive oil over medium-high heat. Add the onions and sweat for 5 minutes, then add the garlic and cook for 3 minutes more. Add the roasted peppers and thyme sprigs and cook for 5 minutes. Add potatoes and stock, and bring to a boil. Boil until sweet potatoes are tender, about 12 -14 minutes.

Remove from heat, remove thyme sprigs and puree using either a stick blender or an upright blender. Stir in cream and serve.

Serves 4-6

Recipe courtesy of Jason Longman of Atlanta

BEYOND ORGANIC FAN FAVORITES

BABY ARUGULA SALAD WITH PAN-SEARED SALMON

INGREDIENTS FOR THE SALMON:

2 6-ounce wild salmon fillets

2 tablespoons fresh lemon juice

2 tablespoons organic extra-virgin oil

sea salt and ground black pepper to taste

INGREDIENTS FOR THE SALAD:

3 cups of organic bagged baby arugula salad

$^2/_3$ cup cherry tomatoes, halved

¼ cup red onion, thinly sliced

1 tablespoon olive oil

1 tablespoon red wine vinegar

sea salt and pepper to taste

$^1/_8$ cup of slivered almonds (topping)

DIRECTIONS

In a shallow bowl, mix lemon juice, olive oil, salt and pepper and place the salmon fillets into this mixture. Let stand for 15 minutes, then cook the salmon fillets in a pan over medium-high heat for 2-3 minutes. Reduce the heat and cook the fillets through for about 3-4 minutes more or until done. Meanwhile, combine the salad ingredients in a large salad bowl. Top with cooked salmon and slivered almonds. Serve.

Serves 2

Recipe courtesy of Extraordinary Health Team

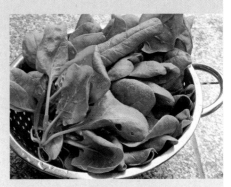

SPINACH AND GOAT CHEESE SALAD

INGREDIENTS

5 cups organic baby spinach leaves, coarsely chopped

2 large red bell peppers, diced

2 cups of celery, diced

½ cup red onion, chopped

1 tablespoon fresh oregano

2 tablespoons fresh lime juice

3 tablespoons organic extra-virgin olive oil

1 cup fresh goat cheese, crumbled

¼ cup slivered almonds

sea salt and fresh-ground pepper to taste

DIRECTIONS

Mix olive oil, lime juice and oregano together in a large mixing bowl. Season with salt & pepper (to taste). Add spinach, red bell peppers, celery and red onion to the oil mix. Top with goat cheese and slivered almonds. Divide on to five chilled salad plates and serve.

Serves 5

Recipe courtesy of Extraordinary Health Team

BEYOND ORGANIC FAN FAVORITES

AVOCADO & QUINOA SALAD
INGREDIENTS

2 organic avocados, cut into pieces

1 cup red quinoa

1 medium tomato, cut into pieces

¼ cup diced red onion

2 fresh basil leaves, crushed

DRESSING INGREDIENTS

⅓ cup organic extra-virgin olive oil

¼ teaspoon cayenne pepper

1 garlic clove, minced

juice of two limes

sea salt and pepper to taste

DIRECTIONS

In a small saucepan, bring two cups of water to a boil and add rinsed quinoa. Cover and simmer for 15-20 minutes or until water is absorbed. Cool and set aside.

Mix the dressing ingredients together in a small mixing bowl. Mix all the other ingredients together in a large mixing bowl and then add cooled quinoa. Toss with dressing. Chill and serve.

Serves 2

Recipe courtesy of Extraordinary Health Team

DELECTABLE SPINACH SALAD
INGREDIENTS

1 large bag of organic baby spinach, washed

2 medium-sized tomatoes, cut in small pieces

6 scallions, trimmed and thinly sliced

5 tablespoons whole milk plain yogurt

3 tablespoons organic extra-virgin olive oil

2 garlic cloves, minced

½ teaspoon fresh thyme, ground

sea salt and ground pepper to taste

DIRECTIONS

Tear the spinach into large pieces and place in a large salad bowl. Add cut tomatoes and scallions. In a separate bowl, combine the whole milk yogurt, olive oil, garlic, thyme and salt and pepper. Mix well. Pour the yogurt mixture onto the spinach, tomatoes and scallion mixture. Season to taste with salt & pepper. Serve.

Serves 4

Recipe courtesy of Extraordinary Health Team

NAVY BEAN AND SPINACH DIP
INGREDIENTS

1 can navy beans, drained

1 pound fresh spinach

5 cloves garlic

2 tablespoons olive oil

1 lemon

½ teaspoon cumin, freshly ground

½ teaspoon coriander, freshly ground

salt to taste

Serves 6-8

DIRECTIONS

Heat a large, heavy-bottom sauté pan over medium heat. Add olive oil and whole garlic cloves, and sauté for 4 minutes. Add spinach and cook until wilted, working in batches if the pan is not big enough.

Place beans, spinach, garlic, lemon and spices in food processor and blend to desired consistency (add water for a thinner dip.) Serve with fresh vegetables or whole wheat pita for dipping.

Recipe courtesy of Jason Longman of Atlanta

BEYOND ORGANIC FAN FAVORITES

AMAZING SWEET POTATO SALAD

INGREDIENTS

2 pounds of sweet potatoes

2 red bell peppers, thinly sliced and diced

4 tablespoons of raisins

3 tablespoons lemon juice

3 tablespoons chopped parsley

4 tablespoons organic extra-virgin olive oil

3 tablespoons chopped fresh rosemary leaves

$1/3$ cup sliced raw almonds

DIRECTIONS

Bake sweet potatoes in 400-degree oven for 45 minutes. Cool and cube. Place in large mixing bowl and set aside. Mix olive oil, red pepper, rosemary, parsley, lemon juice and raisins. Add to the cooled sweet potato cubes. Mix well. Chill. Top with sliced almonds and serve.

Serves 4

Recipe courtesy of Extraordinary Health Team

AVOCADO & BROCCOLI SALAD

INGREDIENTS

2 ripe avocados

1 pound of fresh broccoli

4 tablespoons extra virgin olive oil

2 tablespoons lime juice

1 teaspoon of fresh oregano

1 tablespoon of brown mustard

DIRECTIONS

Wash the broccoli and cut it into small, bite-sized pieces. Peel and pit the avocados and cut them into small cubed pieces. Place the broccoli and avocado bits in a bowl. Meanwhile, whisk the olive oil, lime juice, fresh oregano and brown mustard together. Pour the oil mixture on the broccoli and avocado bits; toss well and serve.

Serves 4

Recipe courtesy of Extraordinary Health Team

CHERRY CRUNCH

INGREDIENTS

1 pound of frozen pitted tart cherries

2 medium organic Granny Smith apples

$1/4$ cup raw honey

$1/2$ teaspoon almond extract

2 tablespoons arrowroot powder

$1/2$ cup unsweetened cherry juice

1 teaspoon stevia mixed with 3 Tablespoons cinnamon

$1/3$ cup old-fashioned rolled oats

$1/3$ cup walnuts

2 Tablespoons whole wheat flour

3 Tablespoons grape seed oil

DIRECTIONS:

Preheat the oven to 400 degrees. In a large bowl, mix together the cherries, apples, and cinnamon and the almond extract. Set aside. In a small cup, mix the arrowroot powder with the unsweetened cherry juice and add to the fruit mixture. Stir well. Pour this mixture into a non-stick 8-inch square baking dish. Mix together the remaining ingredients and crumble the mixture on top of the fruit. Bake for 30 minutes. Remove and serve warm.

Serves 6-8

Recipe courtesy of Extraordinary Health Team

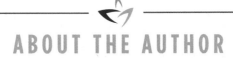

ABOUT THE AUTHOR

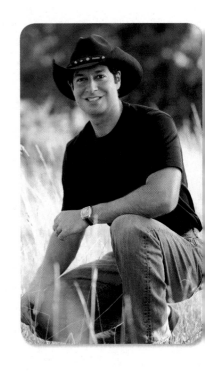

Jordan Rubin, one of the most respected and beloved natural health experts in the United States, has dedicated his life to transforming the health of others one life at a time. A successful entrepreneur, *New York Times* best-selling author, international motivational speaker, and television personality, Jordan's message of health and hope is a beacon to those looking for answers to help take control of their health.

Jordan is the founder and CEO of Beyond Organic, a new company on a mission to transforming people's health and lives through a commitment to sustainable agricultural practices and a goal to produce the world's healthiest foods and beverages. He is also the founder of Garden of Life, a health and wellness company that produces whole food nutritional supplements and health resources.

He and his wife, Nicki, are the parents of three children, Joshua, Samuel, and Alexis. They make their home in Palm Beach Gardens, Florida.

OTHER BOOKS BY JORDAN S. RUBIN

Jordan Rubin is the prolific author of more than twenty books with over five million copies in print. His most successful book is *The Maker's Diet*, which spent forty-seven weeks on the *New York Times* Best Seller list and remains popular today with 2.5 million copies in print.

Because of his successful books, Jordan has been featured on *Good Morning America*, *NBC Nightly News*, *Fox & Friends*, and *Inside Edition*, and in publications such as *Newsweek*, *Time*, *USA Today*, *Reader's Digest*, *Prevention*, and the *New York Times*.

HERE IS A COMPLETE LISITING OF THE BOOKS AUTHORED BY JORDAN RUBIN:

- *Patient Heal Thyself: A Remarkable Health Program Combining Ancient Wisdom with Groundbreaking Clinic Research* by Jordan Rubin (Freedom Publishing Company, 2002)

- *Restoring Your Digestive Health: How the Guts and Glory Program Can Transform Your Life* by Jordan Rubin and Joseph Brasco, M.D. (Kensington, 2003)

- *The Maker's Diet: The 40-Day Health Experience That Will Change Your Life Forever* by Jordan Rubin (Siloam, 2004)

- *The Great Physician's Prescription for Health and Wellness* by Jordan Rubin (Thomas Nelson, 2006)

- *The Great Physician's Prescription for Women's Health* by Jordan and Nicki Rubin (Thomas Nelson, 2007)

- *The Great Physician's Prescription for Children's Health* by Jordan Rubin (Thomas Nelson, 2008)

- *The Great Physician's Rx for Cancer* by Jordan Rubin (Thomas Nelson, 2006)

- *The Great Physician's Rx for Weight Loss* by Jordan Rubin (Thomas Nelson, 2006)

- *The Great Physician's Rx for Diabetes* by Jordan Rubin (Thomas Nelson, 2006)

- *The Great Physician's Rx for a Healthy Heart* by Jordan Rubin (Thomas Nelson, 2006)

- *The Great Physician's Rx for IBS* by Jordan Rubin (Thomas Nelson, 2006)

- *The Great Physician's Rx for Colds and Flu* by Jordan Rubin (Thomas Nelson, 2006)

- *The Great Physician's Rx for Arthritis* by Jordan Rubin (Thomas Nelson, 2007)

- *The Great Physician's Rx for Heartburn* by Jordan Rubin (Thomas Nelson, 2007)

- *The Great Physician's Rx for High Cholesterol* by Jordan Rubin (Thomas Nelson, 2007)

- *The Great Physician's Rx for Chronic Fatigue and Fibromyalgia* by Jordan Rubin (Thomas Nelson, 2007)

- *The Great Physician's Rx for Depression* by Jordan Rubin (Thomas Nelson, 2007)

- *The Great Physician's Rx for High Blood Pressure* by Jordan Rubin (Thomas Nelson, 2007)

- *Perfect Weight America* by Jordan Rubin (2008)

- *Perfect Weight Canada* by Jordan Rubin (2008)

- *Perfect Weight South Africa* by Jordan Rubin (2008)

- *The Maker's Diet for Weight Loss* by Jordan Rubin (a revision of Perfect Weight America, Strang, 2009)

- *Raw Truth* by Jordan Rubin (Garden of Life, 2010)

- *Live Beyond Organic* by Jordan Rubin (Beyond Organic, 2011)

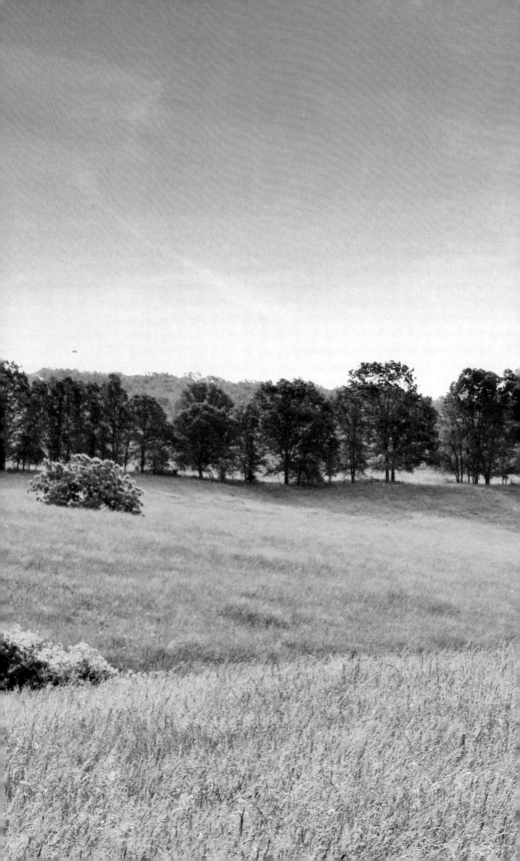

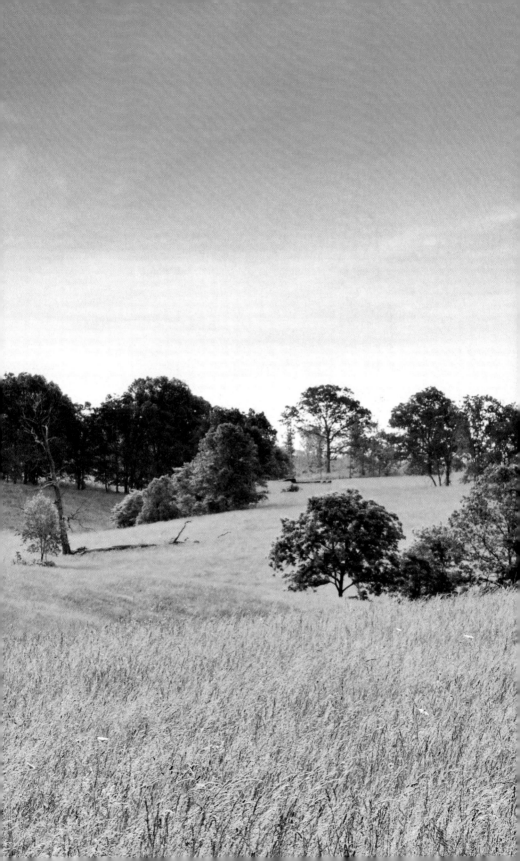

NOTES

NOTES

NOTES